Your *Clinics* subscription just got better!

You can now access the FUL[...] [...]n online at no additional co[...] subscription today[...]

- Full text of all issues from 2002 t[...]
- Photographs, tables, illustrations, and references
- Comprehensive search capabilities
- Links to MEDLINE and Elsevier journals

Activate Your Online Access Today!

Plus, you can also sign up for E-alerts of upcoming issues or articles that interest you, and take advantage of exclusive access to bonus features!

To activate your individual online subscription:

1. Visit our website at **www.TheClinics.com**.

2. Click on "Register" at the top of the page, and follow the instructions.

3. To activate your account, you will need your subscriber account number, which you can find on your mailing label (note: the number of digits in your subscriber account number varies from six to ten digits). See the sample below where the subscriber account number has been circled.

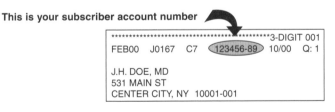

This is your subscriber account number

```
**************************************************3-DIGIT 001
FEB00   J0167   C7   (123456-89)  10/00   Q: 1

J.H. DOE, MD
531 MAIN ST
CENTER CITY, NY  10001-001
```

4. That's it! Your online access to the most trusted source for clinical reviews is now available.

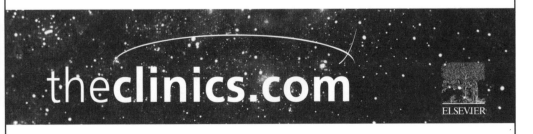

theclinics.com

ELSEVIER

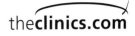

IMMUNOLOGY AND ALLERGY CLINICS OF NORTH AMERICA

Asthma Triggers

GUEST EDITOR
Leonard B. Bacharier, MD

February 2005 • Volume 25 • Number 1

SAUNDERS

An Imprint of Elsevier, Inc.
PHILADELPHIA   LONDON   TORONTO   MONTREAL   SYDNEY   TOKYO

W.B. SAUNDERS COMPANY
A Division of Elsevier Inc.

The Curtis Center • Independence Square West • Philadelphia, Pennsylvania 19106

http://www.theclinics.com

IMMUNOLOGY AND ALLERGY CLINICS OF NORTH AMERICA
February 2005
Editor: Sarah E. Barth

Volume 25, Number 1
ISSN 0889-8561
ISBN 1-4160-2674-6

The ideas and opinions expressed in *Immunology and Allergy Clinics of North America* do not necessarily reflect those of the Publisher. The Publisher does not assume any responsibility for any injury and/or damage to persons or property arising out of or related to any use of the material contained in this periodical. The reader is advised to check the appropriate medical literature and the product information currently provided by the manufacturer of each drug to be administered to verify the dosage, the method and duration of administration, or contraindications. It is the responsibility of the treating physician or other health care professional, relying on independent experience and knowledge of the patient, to determine drug dosages and the best treatment for the patient. Mention of any product in this issue should not be construed as endorsement by the contributors, editors, or the Publisher of the product or manufacturers' claims.

Immunology and Allergy Clinics of North America (ISSN 0889-8561) is published quarterly by W.B. Saunders Company. Corporate and editorial Offices: The Curtis Center, Independence Square West, Philadelphia, PA 19106-3399. Accounting and circulation offices: 6277 Sea Harbor Drive, Orlando, FL 32887-4800. Periodicals postage paid at Orlando, FL 32862, and additional mailing offices. Subscription prices are $165.00 per year for US individuals, $266.00 per year for US institutions, $83.00 per year for US students and residents, $205.00 per year for Canadian individuals, $320.00 per year for Canadian institutions, $220.00 per year for international individuals, $320.00 per year for international institutions, $110 per year for Canadian and international students. To receive student/resident rate, orders must be accompanied by name of affiliated institution, date of term, and the *signature* of program/residency coordinator on institution letterhead. Orders will be billed at individual rate until proof of status is received. Foreign air speed delivery is included in all *Clinics* subscription prices. All prices are subject to change without notice. POSTMASTER: Send address changes to *Immunology and Allergy Clinics of North America,* W.B. Saunders Company, Periodicals Fulfillment, Orlando, FL 32887-4800. **Customer Service: 1-800-654-2452 (US). From outside of the US, call 1-407-345-4000. E-mail: hhspcs@wbsaunders.com**

Reprints. For copies of 100 or more, of articles in this publication, please contact the Commercial Reprints Department, Elsevier Inc., 360 Park Avenue South, New York, New York 10010-1710. Tel. (212) 633-3813 Fax: (212) 633-3820 e-mail: reprints@elsevier.com

Immunology and Allergy Clinics of North America is covered in *Index Medicus, Current Contents/Life Sciences, Science Citation Index, ISI/BIOMED, Chemical Abstracts,* and *EMBASE/Excerpta Medica*

Printed in the United States of America.

GUEST EDITOR

LEONARD B. BACHARIER, MD, Assistant Professor of Pediatrics, Division of Pediatric Allergy and Pulmonary Medicine, Washington University School of Medicine and St. Louis Children's Hospital, St. Louis, Missouri

CONTRIBUTORS

LEONARD B. BACHARIER, MD, Assistant Professor of Pediatrics, Division of Pediatric Allergy and Pulmonary Medicine, Washington University School of Medicine and St. Louis Children's Hospital, St. Louis, Missouri

BRUCE G. BENDER, PhD, Head, Division of Pediatric Behavioral Health, National Jewish Medical and Research Center, Denver, Colorado; and Professor, Department of Psychiatry, Division of Psychology, University of Colorado School of Medicine, Denver, Colorado

SARAH E. BENDER, BS, Department of Psychology, Pennsylvania State University, State College, Pennsylvania

GORDON R. BLOOMBERG, MD, Associate Professor of Pediatrics, Division of Allergy and Pulmonary Medicine, Washington University Medical School, St. Louis, Missouri

EDITH CHEN, PhD, Canada Research Chair, Assistant Professor, Department of Psychology, University of British Columbia, Vancouver, British Columbia

RONINA A. COVAR, MD, Assistant Professor, Department of Pediatrics, National Jewish Medical and Research Center, Denver, Colorado

ELIZABETH A. ERWIN, MD, Instructor, Department of Medicine, Division of Allergy and Immunology, University of Virginia, Charlottesville, Virginia

JOEL FIEDLER, MD, Associate Clinical Professor, Department of Pediatrics, Division of Allergy and Immunology, The Children's Hospital of Philadelphia, University of Pennsylvania School of Medicine, Philadelphia, Pennsylvania

MITCHELL H. GRAYSON, MD, Assistant Professor, Department of Medicine, Division of Allergy and Immunology, Washington University School of Medicine, St. Louis, Missouri

SUSAN M. HARDING, MD, Associate Professor, Department of Medicine, Division of Pulmonary, Allergy & Critical Care Medicine, University of Alabama at Birmingham, Birmingham, Alabama

BETH A. MACOMBER, MD, Department of Pediatrics, Pediatric Allergy/Immunology Fellow, National Jewish Medical and Research Center, Denver, Colorado

ANA L. MacDOWELL, MD, Fellow in Allergy and Immunology, Washington University School of Medicine, St. Louis, Missouri

THOMAS A.E. PLATTS-MILLS, MD, PhD, Professor, Department of Medicine and Head, Division of Allergy and Immunology, University of Virginia, Charlottesville, Virginia

GAIL G. SHAPIRO, MD, Northwest Allergy and Asthma Center; Clinical Professor of Pediatrics, University of Washington School of Medicine, Seattle, Washington

RAYMOND G. SLAVIN, MD, Division of Allergy and Immunology, Saint Louis University School of Medicine, St. Louis, Missouri

BRIAN A. SMART, MD, Asthma and Allergy Center, DuPage Medical Group, Glen Ellyn, Illinois

JONATHAN M. SPERGEL, MD, PhD, Assistant Professor, Department of Pediatrics, Division of Allergy and Immunology, The Children's Hospital of Philadelphia, University of Pennsylvania School of Medicine, Philadelphia, Pennsylvania

WILLIAM W. STORMS, MD, Clinical Professor, University of Colorado Health Sciences Center, Denver; Asthma & Allergy Associates, P.C., Colorado Springs, Colorado

STANLEY J. SZEFLER, MD, Helen Wohlberg and Herman Lambert Chair in Pharmacokinetics; Professor, Department of Pediatrics, National Jewish Medical and Research Center, Denver, Colorado

ASHLEY JERATH TATUM, MD, Northwest Allergy and Asthma Center; Clinical Instructor of Medicine, University of Washington School of Medicine, Seattle, Washington

PAUL G. VIGO, MD, Senior Fellow, Department of Medicine, Division of Allergy and Immunology, Washington University School of Medicine, St. Louis, Missouri

CONTENTS

of suspicion. Treatment usually controls exercise-induced asthma but usually requires therapy tailored for each individual patient.

There is abundant evidence that asthma is frequently exacerbated by infectious agents. Several viruses have been implicated in the inception and exacerbation of asthma. Recent attention has been directed at the role of infections with the atypical bacteria *Mycoplasma pneumoniae* and *Chlamydia pneumoniae* as agents capable of triggering asthma exacerbations and potentially as inciting agents for asthma. This article examines the evidence for interaction between specific infectious agents and exacerbations of asthma, including the immunopathology of infection-triggered asthma, and the current therapeutic options for management.

Rhinosinusitis is a common disease in patients of all age groups. Rhinosinusitis arises from a variety of infectious and inflammatory mechanisms. There is ample evidence that rhinosinusitis can directly influence asthma. There is also growing evidence that rhinosinusitis may be associated with asthma as different manifestations of the same disorder. A great deal of future research is required to fully elucidate the different mechanisms whereby rhinosinusitis influences or associates with asthma, but it is clear that rhinosinusitis needs to be considered in patients with severe or refractory asthma.

The psychologic influence on childhood asthma has long been a subject of investigation and controversy. This article illustrates the evidence that psychologic stress is related to children with asthma. Individual experience, the impact of family and neighborhood, the effect of caregiver mental status, and the presence of negative psychologic events affect symptoms and management. The pathways through which these factors influence asthma are mediated through cognitive and biologic mechanisms, with evidence indicating changes in behavior and alteration in immune response as underlying mechanisms. Psychologic issues are important in the patient with severe asthma. The mind-body paradigm that links psychologic stress to disease is necessary when considering the global evaluation of childhood asthma.

on inhalation without ingestion. However, isolated asthma or rhinitis symptoms without concomitant cutaneous or gastrointestinal symptoms are rare events.

Certain medications can generate asthma symptoms, with the potential to cause considerable morbidity. This article focuses on the common drugs that have the potential to cause distinct respiratory reactions in asthmatics: aspirin and other nonsteroidal anti-inflammatory drugs, β-blockers, and angiotensin-converting enzyme inhibitors. The means by which these medications can trigger asthma vary in terms of acuity of onset, severity, and the mechanisms involved. The general and most practical approach is avoidance and cautious use of these drugs in asthmatics. However, these classes of medications can exert a major role in the management of common and serious diseases. Fortunately, controller therapy for asthma and alternative or more selective medications for the treatment of these conditions are now available.

The prevalence of occupational asthma is rising, possibly due to the introduction of different chemicals and substances in the workplace. Etiologic agents include organic and inorganic compounds that are encountered in a variety of industries. Early diagnosis, adequate management of inflammation, and prevention of further exposure are essential to occupational asthma management. Reducing complications and disability while providing work rehabilitation should be the ultimate goal of the health care provider. This article discusses these issues and gives guidance to the clinician treating patients with possible occupational asthma.

FORTHCOMING ISSUES

RECENT ISSUES

VISIT THESE RELATED WEB SITES

Access your subscription at:
www.theclinics.com

ELSEVIER
SAUNDERS

Immunol Allergy Clin N Am
25 (2005) xi–xii

IMMUNOLOGY
AND ALLERGY
CLINICS
OF NORTH AMERICA

Preface

Asthma Triggers

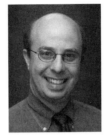

Leonard B. Bacharier, MD
Guest Editor

The continued rise in the prevalence and burden of asthma worldwide over the past decades has occurred in parallel with substantial advances in the understanding of the pathophysiology that underlies asthma. Furthermore, therapeutic options have expanded to include several new classes of medications, and substantial efforts have been devoted to the dissemination of guidelines to improve the management of patients with asthma. These advances have not eliminated asthma-related morbidity or mortality, and patients continue to experience symptoms and exacerbations of asthma.

A major element of national and international guidelines for asthma management is the identification and minimization of exposure to factors that commonly trigger asthma symptoms and episodes. Avoidance or elimination of a multitude of asthma triggers may lead to improved asthma control, along with reductions in asthma medication use and exacerbation-related morbidities. This issue of *Immunology and Allergy Clinics of North America* has been compiled with the goal of increasing the knowledge and recognition of such triggers, ideally leading to further investigation and interventions aimed at decreasing exposures.

In this issue, attention is focused upon several factors that are consistently recognized as triggers of asthma, such as exercise, allergens, pollutants, environmental tobacco smoke, occupational exposures, and infections. In addition, articles examining the roles of psychologic stress, medication nonadherence, gas-

doi:10.1016/j.iac.2004.09.010

troesophageal reflux, foods and food additives, and medications are presented to complete the discussion of other less obvious factors that contribute to asthma severity. Through increased recognition of the multitude of conditions and agents that influence asthma activity, physicians may provide more comprehensive and effective advice for their patients, ideally leading to improved asthma control and reduction in asthma exacerbations and their related morbidities.

Although the identification of asthma triggers has been derived from complete patient histories and often confirmed by clinical studies, the exact relationships between many asthma triggers and asthma exacerbations remain incompletely understood. Furthermore, although the identification of a trigger is often straightforward, interventions aimed at avoidance of the trigger are often difficult and are frequently insufficiently studied to fully appreciate their true efficacies. Even with our broad understanding of the many factors that contribute to asthma severity and symptoms, more investigation is needed to elucidate the mechanisms by which these factors influence asthma, along with the most effective avoidance approaches.

This volume is the combined work of many fine physicians and researchers who have provided insight and clarity into the role of asthma triggers, and I thank them for their scholarly contributions. I also want to acknowledge the strong support and guidance from Sarah Barth (Senior Editor, Elsevier). Finally, thanks to my wonderful family for their endless support and encouragement.

Leonard B. Bacharier, MD
Division of Pediatric Allergy and Pulmonary Medicine
Washington University School of Medicine and St. Louis Children's Hospital
One Children's Place
St. Louis, MO 63110, USA
E-mail address: Bacharier_L@kids.wustl.edu

ELSEVIER
SAUNDERS

Immunol Allergy Clin N Am
25 (2005) 1–14

IMMUNOLOGY
AND ALLERGY
CLINICS
OF NORTH AMERICA

Allergens

Elizabeth A. Erwin, MD,
Thomas A.E. Platts-Mills, MD, PhD*

*Department of Medicine, Division of Allergy and Immunology, University of Virginia, PO Box 801355,
Charlottesville, VA 22908, USA*

An increase in the prevalence and severity of asthma has been observed in developed countries throughout the world. Concurrently, societal changes have been complex, inter-related, and far reaching. The shift toward single-parent families and families in which both parents work has led to an increased number of children in daycare. At the same time, childhood vaccinations have changed the incidence of common childhood diseases. With parents spending less time at home or perhaps questioning their children's safety outside and with the pervasiveness of television in our culture, children spend far more time indoors. Home environments have changed, resulting in differences in allergen exposure. Furthermore, exposure to some pollutants, diesel particulates, and ozone has increased. Given the complexity of the interactions, it is likely that a combination of factors has resulted in the overall increase in disease prevalence and severity that has been observed.

Sensitization to allergens found indoors, such as dust mite, cat, and cockroach, is a risk factor for asthma. As molecular knowledge of allergens becomes greater and our understanding of the immune system increases, differences in allergens and in responses to them have become apparent. In the past, attempts to evaluate the role of allergens in asthma looked to knowledge of dust mite as the model. It may not be that simple; we do not believe that the tendency to develop IgE ab is the same regardless of the allergen. It also may be that allergens affect the respiratory or immune systems directly to cause wheezing. In this article, current information is presented on the immune response to dust mite, pets, cockroach, and Alternaria, and thus their role as asthma triggers.

This work was supported by Asthma Center grant AI-20565.

* Corresponding author.

E-mail address: tap2z@virginia.edu (T.A.E. Platts-Mills).

Dust mite

As the major allergen associated with atopic asthma, dust mites have been the center of much research. Dust mites are arthropods, but being in the order *acari* they are not closely related to insects [1]. They acquire water from water vapor in the environment. Thus, dust mite growth varies throughout the world depending on the climate. There is virtually no measurable dust mite allergen present in the frigid (and consequently dry) areas of northern Sweden, whereas some of the highest levels are found in New Zealand. Between those extremes, a wide range of levels is found in the United States, United Kingdom, and South America. In temperate areas, the prominent species are *Dermatophagoides pteronyssinus* and *D farinae*. A study of eight regions within the United States determined that most homes have both species, with the dominant species varying within homes in each region [2]. *Euroglyphus maynei* was found in the most humid, southern regions. In tropical and subtropical regions, *Blomia tropicalis* is clinically important. Many different dust mite allergens have been characterized. Recently Der f 18, a 60-kD protein with chitinase homology, was purified and cloned [3]. Those most extensively studied are the group 1 and 2 allergens, a 25-kD cysteine protease and 14-kD epididymal protein, respectively (Table 1) [4,6–8]. Several other mite allergens are enzyme proteases secreted in mite feces. Group 10 allergens (Der p 10 and Der f 10) are of interest because they are tropomyosins that may lead to IgE ab cross-reactivity between mites and other invertebrates, such as shrimp and cockroaches [9].

Table 1
Properties of allergens associated with asthma

Allergen	Molecular weight (kD)	Function (homology)	Mode of exposure
Mite			
Der p 1	25	Cysteine protease	Fecal particles
Der p 2	14	(epididymal protein)	
Der p 9	24	Serine protease	
Der p 10	36	Tropomyosin	
Cat			
Fel d 1	36	Uteroglobin	Sebaceous glands
Fel d 2		Albumin	
Dog			
Can f 1	25	Lipocalin	
Cockroach			
Bla g 1		(Mosquito protein)	Saliva
Bla g 2	36	Aspartic protease	Fecal particles
Bla g 4	21	Lipocalin	
Bla g 5	22	Glutathione transferase	
Per a 7	37	Tropomyosin	
Alternaria			
Alt a 1	28	Unknown	Spores
Rye grass			
Lol p 1	27	Unknown	Pollen

Data from Refs. [4,52] and www.allergen.org.

Longitudinal studies have confirmed the relevance of the relationship between allergy to house dust mite and asthma. Recently published results of a large population-based birth cohort in New Zealand revealed that sensitivity to dust mite (by skin test results) was associated with persistent symptoms and relapse of asthma in adulthood [10]. The 21.2% who reported wheezing at only one assessment had a markedly increased prevalence of sensitivity to dust mite. Nonetheless, atopy seems to be a major determinant of continued wheeze.

It remains confusing that many children are exposed and exhibit evidence of sensitivity to dust mite but do not report symptoms. Several groups have examined the relationship between dust mite exposure and incident asthma. In a group of children at risk due to family history, Sporik et al [11], with a geometric mean exposure level of 18.4 μg/g mattress dust in 1979 and 10.6 μg/g in 1989, showed a strong correlation between wheezing and sensitization to dust mite (relative risk of asthma of 19.7 in a child sensitized to dust mite). Furthermore, there was a correlation between early high exposure to dust mite and wheezing. By contrast, in Germany, with mean exposure to dust mite up to 5.6 μg/g, wheezing was strongly associated with sensitivity to mite (30% of wheezing children), but a dose-response relationship between mite exposure and wheezing was not evident [12]. In a recent study in the United States in which the geometric mean concentration of mite allergen was 2.8 μg/g and only 19% of children were exposed to > 10 μg/g of dust, there was no evidence that high levels of exposure were associated with increased risk of asthma [13].

In addition to a high prevalence of IgE ab to mite, there is evidence that the titer of IgE ab to mite can be markedly elevated. From the standpoint of the general ability of the dust mite allergen to induce the production of IgE ab, the highest IgE ab responses in patients with atopic dermatitis (AD) were observed to dust mite [14]. We have also observed high titers of IgE ab to mite among children living in New Zealand. In children with and without wheezing, the geometric mean titer of IgE ab to mite was 22.1 IU/mL. This IgE ab response to mite comprised up to 20% of the total IgE measurement in > 15% of the children with wheezing. These observations may be consistent with in vitro evidence that Der p 1 has the ability to cleave CD23 [15]. One isoform of the CD23 molecule is found on activated B cells and can function as an Fc receptor, binding IgE and interacting with CD21. Through these roles, it may have an immune regulatory function over IgE ab production. At high levels, IgE ab binds CD23, causing feedback inhibition of further IgE synthesis. Thus, a decrease in surface expression of CD23 by dust mite allergen could be viewed as "proallergic." The ability of Der p 1 to effect cleavage of CD23 would be expected to be inhibited by normal function of respiratory antiproteases, but patients with asthma may have reduced defenses due to inflammation.

Immunologically, asthma is viewed as a complex disease that results from a combination of IgE-mediated and cell-mediated mechanisms. Dust mite particles (and allergen) have been shown to have non-IgE–mediated direct inflammatory action. Specifically, nitric oxide (NO), which is elevated in the airways of patients with asthma, has been shown to increase in rat alveolar macrophages exposed to dust mite fecal particles or Der p 1 and Der p 2 [16]. The concentration of NO produced was dose dependent and time dependent, with maximal production at 48 hours, which is consistent with persistent inflammation in response to exposure that is observed clinically. The mechanism was believed to be through induction of iNOS.

Respiratory epithelial cells have been shown to release inflammatory mediators. The allergens Der p 1 and Der p 9 (cysteine and serine proteases, respectively) were shown to directly stimulate release of granulocyte/macrophage colony-stimulating factor, interleukin (IL)-6, and IL-8 from human bronchial epithelial cells (in transformed and freshly cultured cells) [17]. The action of the proteases was dose dependent, with significant cytokine release at 8 hours. Only 30 minutes of exposure was necessary, and the response was inhibited by antiproteases.

Pet paradox

Reviewing the evidence for a relationship between pet ownership and prevalence and symptoms of asthma presents a contrast with the evidence in relation to dust mites. Specifically, the immune response to cat exposure is markedly different from the dose-dependent development of sensitization observed to dust mite. The underlying concept is that high exposure to cat allergen results in a lower prevalence of sensitization to cat. This observation was initially presented by a group of investigators in Sweden [18]. It was confirmed in several areas throughout the world, including the United States, the United Kingdom, northern Sweden, and New Zealand (Table 2) [19–21]. In the initial report of Hesselmar et al [18], pet exposure during the first year of life was associated with decreased allergic diagnoses, including allergic rhinitis, asthma, and cat sensitization.

Table 2
Studies that show reduced risk of sensitization and asthma among children living with a pet

		Allergen		Sensitization		
Study	Region	Cat	Dog	Specific	Nonspecific	Asthma
Hesselmar et al [18]	Sweden	√	√	√		√
Roost et al [72]	Europe/ New Zealand/Australia	√		√		
Platts-Mills et al [19]	Los Alamos, NM/ Charlottesville, VA	√		√		√
Remes et al [73]	Tucson, AZ		√			√
Custovic et al [20]	United Kingdom	√		√		
Litonjua et al [29]	Boston, MA	√	√			√
Perzanowski et al [21]	Northern Sweden	√			√	√
Ownby et al [22]	Detroit, MI		√		√	
Svanes et al [74]	Europe/New Zealand/Australia		√		√	
Ronmark et al [66]	Northern Sweden	√	√		√	
Gern et al [23]	Madison, WI		√		√	

Eczema and sensitization to other allergens tested were not decreased with early pet exposure. The lower prevalence of asthma (odds ratio [OR] 0.34 in those who lived with a cat) was not explained by selection bias due to family history of allergy. A careful review of their results reveals several related issues that have emerged, including the importance of timing of pet exposure and the possibility of selection bias of patients, with a family history of allergy, against keeping pets. In this study, the relationship between pet ownership and asthma remained significant even when families who chose not to own a pet because of family history of allergy were excluded [18]. In addition, family history did not influence the results seen in Detroit or the United Kingdom [20,22].

The next question is whether exposure to dogs has the same effect on the immune system and the development of allergic sensitization and asthma. In Detroit, a decreased prevalence of allergic sensitization to any allergen was observed among children who were living with two or more dogs or cats [22]. Similarly, in Wisconsin it was observed that children living with dogs were significantly less likely to have a positive RAST test result at 1 year of age [23]. In these studies, cat exposure did not decrease sensitization in general. Almqvist [24] found that dog exposure early in life was associated with a decrease in sensitization to other allergens and a decrease in asthma.

The contrast in responses to cat and dog introduces a further question about the mechanism underlying the relationship between pet ownership and allergic response: Is it a shared response or allergen specific? One theory has focused on the role of endotoxin, a component of bacterial cell walls. The idea came from observations of decreased atopy and, in some studies, wheezing among children growing up on farms [25–27]. Bräun-Fahrlander et al [28] measured endotoxin levels in rural Germany and found that exposure to increased amounts of endotoxin was associated with decreased atopic sensitization. The relationship between endotoxin exposure and wheezing was dependent upon the type of wheezing. Only atopic wheezing was reduced in association with high endotoxin levels. Others have shown that exposure to endotoxin was associated with increased risk of wheezing in early life [29]. Alternatively, it has been proposed that cats induce an immune-specific response characterized by the production of IgG ab without IgE ab. Because this IgG was largely of the IgG_4 subclass (which is IL-4 dependent), this has been termed the modified Th2 response [19]. Investigation of T-cell responses further supported the concept of specific immune control because allergic and "tolerant" individuals exhibited increased levels of IL-10 in cultures stimulated with peptides of Fel d 1 [30].

The major allergen in cat dander, Fel d 1, was isolated in 1974 [31]. It is found in saliva and sebaceous secretions. Purification and measurement became possible with the development of monoclonal antibodies in 1994 [32,33]. It was found to predominate over cat albumin in terms of prevalence of IgE ab in the sera of allergic individuals [34]. The crystal structure of the molecule, formed by two heterodimers, was recently characterized [35]. In so doing, the similarity of the tertiary structure of the molecule to that of the secretogogue uteroglobin was confirmed. This similarity suggests that Fel d 1 may share some of the abilities of uteroglobin to influence the immune response [36]. By contrast, the major dog allergen, Can f 1, is a lipocalin similar to those of other animals, including mouse (Mus m 1) and rat (Rat n 1).

In conclusion, pets present a paradox immunologically because cat allergen is a significant risk factor for asthma in the sensitized individual, but exposure does not result in dose-dependent sensitization. There is strong evidence to the contrary; high exposure to cat and dog allergen results in decreased sensitization. However, the underlying process seems to be different. Although high exposure to cat is specifically associated with decreased allergy to cat, the effect of high exposure to dog seems to be nonspecific. Although it is premature to say that all children should have pets, this knowledge must influence the recommendation allergists have made for many years that allergic children should not have pets.

Other animals

In the United States, attention has recently turned toward an assessment of the significance of other, sometimes unwanted, animals found in homes, including mice and rats. In the laboratory, a dose-response association has been observed to the allergens of these animals. Atopic workers were more likely to develop animal allergy with increased exposure [37]. In a subsample from the National Cooperative Inner-City Asthma Study (NCICAS), almost all of the homes studied (95%) had measurable mouse allergen in at least one room [38]. Examination of the children living in those homes revealed that 18% were sensitized to mouse, with high levels of exposure in the kitchen and other allergy as risk factors [39]. In that study, sensitization to mouse was not significantly related to asthma morbidity. Another study of the Baltimore area that included children with asthma living in city or suburban homes found a dose-response relationship between exposure and sensitization but did not directly relate exposure and symptoms [40]. In a recent analysis of NCICAS data for rat exposure, fewer homes (33%) had measurable rat allergen in any room by comparison to mouse allergen [41]. However, the prevalence of sensitization to rat (21%) was slightly higher than that to mouse. Although sensitization to rat was not significantly related to exposure, children who were sensitized and exposed to rat allergen were more likely to be hospitalized for asthma.

Cockroach

One area known for a high prevalence of severe asthma is inner-city areas of the United States. This argues against improved hygiene as a cause for increases in the disease. Thus, allergen exposure provides an appealing explanation in these areas. A correlation between cockroach sensitization and asthma has also been reported in Europe and Brazil and in suburbs in the United States [42–45]. Studies of emergency departments have shown an association between cockroach allergy and severe asthma [46,47]. Rosenstreich's analysis of inner-city children strengthened evidence for the cockroach allergen effect by showing that the combination of exposure and allergic sensitization increased the risk of hospitalization [48]. They found a high prevalence of sensitization to cockroach (37%), dust mite (35%), and cat (23%); however, high levels of exposure were found primarily to cockroach (50% of houses). Furthermore, cockroach-allergic children with exposure had increased rates of hospitalization, wheezing, and missed school. Litonjua et al [49] reported a dose-response relationship between cockroach exposure and asthma in children living in Boston. Exposure to 2 U Bla g 1 or Bla g 2/g dust was associated with a high risk (OR >10) for developing asthma.

Appreciation of the significance of cockroach allergy is not new. Bernton and Brown [50] reported sensitization to cockroach and noted an increased prevalence (58%) in urban areas. Kang [51] showed a relationship between sensitization and asthma when she performed bronchial provocation testing with cockroach antigen. A significant decrease in pulmonary function occurred in 88% of sensitized patients, whereas none of the asthmatics who were not sensitized to cockroach reacted.

The major species infesting United States homes is German cockroach (*Blattella germanica*), whereas the American cockroach (*Periplaneta americana*) is more common in tropical areas such as Taiwan and Brazil. Initial studies to characterize the major allergens revealed two molecules, Cr-I and Cr-II (25.5 and 69 kD, respectively), to which 70% of sensitive patients exhibited positive skin tests [52]. In that early study, results were similar for American and German species. More recently, additional allergens have been described primarily from German cockroach. The function of Bla g 1 is unknown; it has an unusual structure containing tandem repeats [5]. Typically, the cockroach allergens do not seem to be cross-reactive between the two species, but Bla g 1 and Per a 1 are exceptions. Unlike some dust mite allergens, the allergens of cockroach are not active enzymes. Bla g 2 is an inactive aspartic protease resembling mammalian pregnancy-associated glycoproteins believed to function as binding proteins [53]. Bla g 4 is a lipocalin, as are many of the animal allergens, and Bla g 5 is a glutathione transferase [52]. Per a 7 was recently identified and has homology with tropomyosins, especially those in other invertebrates, such as shrimp and dust mite [54]. Bla g 1 and Bla g 2 are most frequently measured for exposure data.

In spite of the difficulty in isolating and identifying enzymatically active cockroach allergens, cockroach extract has been shown to have in vitro proteolytic effects [55]. Cockroach extract increased IL-8 production through a G-protein receptor. In addition to regulation of cytokines like IL-8, activation of this specific G-protein may influence airway function as evidenced through action on guinea pig smooth muscle.

Alternaria

Alternaria is unique among the important allergens associated with asthma in that it is primarily considered to be an outdoor exposure. Initial search for a major allergen in Alternaria extracts showed a carbohydrate-rich fraction with RAST binding in >80% of sensitized individuals, ALT-I [56]. These results were observed by several other investigators who isolated a 29- to 31-kD fraction termed Alt a 1 [57]. Studies of Alternaria revealed that allergen measurements were extremely sensitive to culture conditions and extraction techniques [58]. Little is known about dose response to mold allergen. It has been shown that Alt a 1 is increased in germinated spores [59]. Outdoors, a warm, dry climate has been associated with increased levels of Alternaria. Recently, standards for indoor measurement have been proposed; however, studies to confirm their effectiveness are lacking. Thus, measurements of indoor exposure are limited.

In stark contrast to the paucity of biochemical data, evidence that Alternaria is clinically significant in relation to asthma is abundant. O'Hollaren et al [60] at the Mayo Clinic reported that patients with positive skin test to Alternaria had an increased risk of severe or fatal attacks. Subsequently, it became clear from cross-sectional studies that sensitization to Alternaria was a major risk factor for wheezing in Arizona and New Mexico [61,62].

Alternaria has been shown to induce increased quantities of specific IgE ab among subjects with atopic dermatitis and asthma. Using Pharmacia CAP to measure IgE ab, the mean quantity of IgE ab to Alternaria in those with AD and asthma was 4.1 IU/mL and 3.7 IU/mL, respectively; both were significantly higher than the control group [13].

Some of the inflammatory effects of fungi may be antibody independent. The cell walls of fungi, which contain β-glucans and polysaccharide (glucomannan), must have an effect on the immune system. However, most of the research has examined the influence of Aspergillus and has not focused on the inflammatory effects seen in asthma. In addition to observation of inhibition of the mucociliary system by Aspergillus, Wang et al [63] suggested that Aspergillus hyphae may activate monocytes through toll-like receptor-4 (TLR-4) and CD14.

Grass

Similar to molds, exposure to grasses occurs primarily outdoors and in most population-based or cohort studies has not been found to be an independent risk factor for asthma. Nonetheless, ragweed pollen or grass pollen exposure has been shown to be a dramatic trigger for asthma symptoms in areas where pollen counts are very high. In 1986, during a 1-week period in May when rye grass pollen counts reached >2000 counts per cm^2, 205 patients were treated for acute asthma at Travis Air Force Base in northern California [64]. This was 40% of the total number of patients seen for asthma during the period from July 1985 to June 1986. The patients with asthma were significantly more likely to be sensitized to grass pollen than control subjects. The specific IgE ab levels were markedly elevated. In this study, grass pollen levels were measured inside the homes of a subset of patients. All of the homes measured had >2 μg Lol p 1/g dust, and most

(13/15) had > 10 μg Lol p 1/g dust, providing evidence that sufficient quantities could be found indoors during the pollen season.

Summary

Given that children and adults spend little time outdoors, it is not surprising that sensitization to allergens found indoors is common. It may well be the fact that exposure to these allergens persists year round that explains their importance in relation to bronchial hyper-reactivity and asthma symptoms. Understanding the increase in asthma is more complex because this may reflect increased concentrations of allergens indoors, increased time spent indoors, and changes in immune response. However, the risk for asthma is consistently related to sensitization to one or more of the perennial allergens. In general, this risk relates to the presence of high concentrations of the allergens in the community [4,65]. Thus, for dust mites, cockroach, or rodent urinary allergens, there are good studies showing that sensitization is rare in communities where the allergens are not present [61,62,66]. The recent evidence that sensitization is not increased by the presence of a cat or a dog has added considerable confusion primarily because the results from different studies are not the same (Table 2). It is not resolved whether the effect of animals (1) requires exposure early in life, (2) is nonspecific (ie, reduces sensitization to other allergens), or (3) can be explained by family choice (this is unlikely). The most recent evidence argues that exposure to cats in childhood can produce an allergen-specific form of tolerance that controls the prevalence of sensitization and the titer of IgE ab among sensitized children [30,67].

The evidence about cat argues strongly that all allergens are not created equal. This implies that there is a biologic or immunologic difference between the response to dust mite and cat allergens (Table 3). Whether other allergens can be classified is not clear, but the preliminary evidence suggests that cockroach and pollen allergens may be comparable to dust mite (ie, Class I), whereas dog and rodent allergens may induce tolerance (ie, Class II). There is another consequence of the results that may be equally relevant to understanding the role of allergens

Table 3
Biologic and immunologic differences between dust mite and cat allergens

	Class I	Class II
Source	Dust mite (cockroach, grass)	Cat (dog)
Particles	10–30 μm (fecal)	2.5–20 μm
Airborne	Airborne only with disturbance	Remain airborne
Nature of protein	Enzymatic potential: known to cleave CD23, CD25, and open tight junctions	Not enzymes: homology with uteroglobin (known immunomodulator) by sequence and structure
Immune response	No evidence for tolerance, includes high titer of IgE ab	Induces tolerance at high exposure, lower titers of IgE ab

in asthma. The presence of IgE ab to cat (or dog) is strongly associated with asthma regardless of the exposure levels [68]. Thus, it seems clear that it is the IgE ab, not IgG ab, IgG$_4$ ab, or T cells, that creates the risk of asthma [69]. It is important to recognize that all the evidence about the association between allergens and asthma relates to immediate skin tests or serum IgE ab. At a simple level it could be argued that this implies an immediate relationship between allergen exposure and asthma that is comparable to an immediate challenge response. However, there is plenty of evidence that the response is delayed in time course and that the effect of prolonged exposure persists for weeks or months even in an allergen-free environment. Also, there is evidence that T cells are involved. Thus, the correct conclusion is that IgE ab plays a critical role in the initial development of symptoms or in establishing inflammation of the lungs. A possible scenario would be that sensitization of the lungs with IgE ab would allow the local recruitment of specific T cells, which contribute to prolonged inflammation in the lungs.

Attempts to establish that allergen exposure correlated directly with acute episodes of asthma have not been convincing. Many attacks occur during a period when the patient has had continuing high exposure, but only a minority can be ascribed to a recent increase in exposure. Thus, the primary triggers of symptoms are nonspecific factors, such as cold air, exercise, passive smoke, etc. In most cases these triggers are acting on lungs that have been inflamed by chronic, perennial, low-grade allergen exposure. Similarly, a major cause of moderate or severe episodes of wheezing is a rhinovirus infection in a patient with underlying allergen-induced inflammation [70]. The situation with rhinovirus infection is striking because multiple studies have shown that rhinovirus challenge has an effect only on the lungs of allergic individuals. Among children and adults presenting to hospital with asthma, it is the combination of allergy and positive polymerase chain reaction for rhinovirus that is associated with the strongest risk [71].

Summary

The association between allergen sensitization and asthma is so strong that it is inevitable that allergens play a role in the disease. This conclusion is strongly supported by a wide range of experiments where patients are removed from their houses. Further, it is the allergens found in homes of the community that are relevant to asthma. On the other hand, the detailed triggers of attacks come from many different nonspecific factors acting on an inflamed lung.

References

[1] Arlian LG, Platts-Mills TA. The biology of dust mites and the remediation of mite allergens in allergic disease. J Allergy Clin Immunol 2001;107:S406–13.

[2] Arlian LG, Bernstein D, Bernstein IL, et al. Prevalence of dust mites in the homes of people with asthma living in eight different geographic areas of the United States. J Allergy Clin Immunol 1992;90:292–300.

[3] Weber E, Hunter S, Stedman K, et al. Identification, characterization, and cloning of a complementary DNA encoding a 60-kD house dust mite allergen (Der f 18) for human beings and dogs. J Allergy Clin Immunol 2003;112:79–86.

[4] Platts-Mills TAE, Vervloet D, Thomas WR, et al. Indoor allergens and asthma: report of the Third International Workshop. J Allergy Clin Immunol 1997;100:S1–24.

[5] Arruda LK, Vailes LD, Ferriani VPL, et al. Cockroach allergens and asthma. J Allergy Clin Immunol 2001;107:419–28.

[6] Chapman MD, Platts-Mills TAE. Purification and characterization of the major allergen from Dermatophagoides pteronyssinus-antigen P1. J Immunol 1980;125:587–92.

[7] Chua KY, Stewart GA, Thomas WR, et al. Sequence analysis of cDNA coding for a major house dust mite allergen, Der p 1, homology with cysteine proteases. J Exp Med 1988;167:175–82.

[8] Thomas W, Chua K. The major mite allergen Der p 2: a secretion of the male mite reproductive tract? Clin Exp Allergy 1995;25:667–9.

[9] Witteman AM, Akkerdass JH, van Leeuwen J, et al. Identification of a cross-reactive allergen (presumably tropomyosin) in shrimp, mite and insects. Int Arch Allergy Immunol 1994;105: 56–61.

[10] Sears MR, Greene JM, Willan AR, et al. A longitudinal, population-based, cohort study of childhood asthma followed to adulthood. N Engl J Med 2003;349:1414–22.

[11] Sporik R, Holgate ST, Platts-Mills TAE, Cogswell JJ. Exposure to house-dust mite allergen (Der p 1) and the development of asthma in childhood: a prospective study. N Engl J Med 1990; 323:502–7.

[12] Lau S, Illi S, Sommerfeld C, et al. Early exposure to house-dust mite and cat allergens and development of childhood asthma: a cohort study. Multicentre Allergy Study Group. Lancet 2000;356:1392–7.

[13] Cole Johnson C, Ownby DR, Havstad SL, et al. Family history, dust mite exposure in early childhood, and risk for pediatric atopy and asthma. J Allergy Clin Immunol 2004;114:105–10.

[14] Scalabrin DM, Bavbek S, Perzanowski MS, et al. Use of specific IgE in assessing the relevance of fungal and dust mite allergens to atopic dermatitis: a comparison with asthmatic and non-asthmatic control subjects. J Allergy Clin Immunol 1999;104:1273–9.

[15] Hewitt CR, Brown AP, Hart BJ, et al. A major house dust mite allergen disrupts the immunoglobulin E network by selectively cleaving CD23: innate protection by antiproteases. J Exp Med 1995;182:1537–44.

[16] Peake HL, Currie AJ, Stewart GA, et al. Nitric oxide production by alveolar macrophages in response to house dust mite fecal pellets and the mite allergens, Der p 1 and Der p 2. J Allergy Clin Immunol 2003;112:531–7.

[17] King C, Brennan S, Thompson PJ, et al. Dust mite proteolytic allergens induce cytokine release from cultured airway epithelium. J Immunol 1998;161:3645–51.

[18] Hesselmar B, Åberg N, Åberg B, et al. Does early exposure to cat or dog protect against later allergy development? Clin Exp Allergy 1999;29:611–7.

[19] Platts-Mills TAE, Vaughan J, Squillace S, et al. Sensitization, asthma, and a modified Th2 response in children exposed to cat allergen: a population-based cross-sectional study. Lancet 2001;357:752–6.

[20] Custovic A, Hallam CL, Simpson BM, et al. Decreased prevalence of sensitization to cats with high exposure to cat allergen. J Allergy Clin Immunol 2001;108:537–9.

[21] Perzanowski MS, Ronmark E, Platts-Mills TAE, et al. Effect of cat and dog ownership on sensitization and development of asthma among preteenage children. Am J Respir Crit Care Med 2002;166:696–702.

[22] Ownby DR, Johnson CC, Peterson EL. Exposure to dogs and cats in the first year of life and risk of allergic sensitization at 6 to 7 years of age. JAMA 2002;288:963–72.

[23] Gern JE, Reardon CL, Hoffjan S, et al. Effects of dog ownership and genotype on immune development and atopy in infancy. J Allergy Clin Immunol 2004;113:307–14.

[24] Almqvist C, Egmar AC, Hedlin G, et al. Direct and indirect exposure to pets- risk of sensitization and asthma at 4 years in a birth cohort. Clin Exp Allergy 2003;33:1190–7.

[25] Braun-Fahrländer D, Gassner M, Grize L, et al. Prevalence of hay fever and allergic sensitization in farmer's children and their peers living in the same rural community. SCARPOL team. Clin Exp Allergy 1999;29:28–34.

[26] Riedler J, Eder W, Oberfeld G, et al. Austrian children living on a farm have less hay fever, asthma and allergic sensitization. Clin Exp Allergy 2000;30:194–200.

[27] von Ehrenstein OS, von Mutius E, Illi S, et al. Reduced risk of hay fever and asthma among children of farmers. Clin Exp Allergy 2000;30:187–93.

[28] Braun-Fährlander C, Riedler J, Herz U, et al. Environmental exposure to endotoxin and its relation to asthma in school-age children. N Engl J Med 2002;347:869–77.

[29] Litonjua AA, Milton DK, Celedon JC, et al. A longitudinal analysis of wheezing in young children: the independent effects of early life exposure to house dust endotoxin, allergens, and pets. J Allergy Clin Immunol 2002;110:736–42.

[30] Reefer AJ, Carneiro RM, Custis NJ, et al. A role for IL-10-mediated HLA-DR7-restricted T-cell dependent events in development of the modified Th2 response to cat allergen. J Immunol 2004; 172:2763–72.

[31] Ohman JL, Lowell FC, Bloch KJ. Allergens of mammalian origin. III: properties of a major feline allergen. J Immunol 1974;113:1668–77.

[32] Chapman MD, Aalberse RC, Brown MJ, et al. Monoclonal antibodies to the major feline allergen Fel d 1. II: single step affinity purification of Fel d 1, N-terminal sequence analysis, and development of a sensitive two-site immunoassay to assess Fel d 1 exposure. J Immunol 1988; 140:812–8.

[33] Luczynska CM, Li Y, Chapman MD, et al. Airborne concentrations and particle size distribution of allergen derived from domestic cats (Felis domesticus): measurements using cascade impactor, liquid impinger, and a two-site monoclonal antibody assay for Fel d 1. Am Rev Respir Dis 1990;141:361–7.

[34] van Ree R, Van Leeuwen WA, Bulder I, et al. Purified natural and recombinant Fel d 1 and cat albumin in in vitro diagnostics for cat allergy. J Allergy Clin Immunol 1999;104:1223–30.

[35] Kaiser L, Gronlund H, Sandalova T, et al. The crystal structure of the major cat allergen Fel d 1, a member of the secretoglobin family. J Biol Chem 2003;278:37730–5.

[36] Mandal AK, Zhang Z, Ray R, et al. Uteroglobin represses allergen-induced inflammatory response by blocking PGD2 receptor-mediated functions. J Exp Med 2004;199:1317–30.

[37] Bush RK, Wood RA, Eggleston PA. Laboratory animal allergy. J Allergy Clin Immunol 1998; 102:99–112.

[38] Phipatanakul W, Eggleston PA, Wright EC, et al. Mouse allergen. I: the prevalence of mouse allergen in inner-city homes. J Allergy Clin Immunol 2000;106:1070–4.

[39] Phipatanakul W, Eggleston PA, Wright EC, et al. Mouse allergen. II: the relationship of mouse allergen exposure to mouse sensitization and asthma morbidity in inner-city children with asthma. J Allergy Clin Immunol 2000;106:1075–80.

[40] Matsui EC, Wood RA, Rand C, et al. Mouse allergen exposure and mouse skin test sensitivity in suburban, middle-class children with asthma. J Allergy Clin Immunol 2004;113:910–5.

[41] Perry T, Matsui E, Merriman B, et al. The prevalence of rat allergen in inner-city homes and its relationship to sensitization and asthma morbidity. J Allergy Clin Immunol 2003;112:346–52.

[42] Stelmach I, Jerzynska J, Stelmach W, et al. Cockroach allergy and exposure to cockroach allergen in Polish children with asthma. Allergy 2002;57:701–5.

[43] Santos AB, Chapman MD, Aalberse RC, et al. Cockroach allergens and asthma in Brazil: identification of tropomyosins as a major allergen with potential cross-reactivity with mite and shrimp allergens. J Allergy Clin Immunol 1999;104:329–37.

[44] Matsui EC, Wood RA, Rand C, et al. Cockroach allergen exposure and sensitization in suburban middle-class children with asthma. J Allergy Clin Immunol 2003;112:87–92.

[45] Sporik R, Squillace SP, Ingram JM, et al. Mite, cat, and cockroach exposure, allergen sensitization, and asthma in children: a case-control study of three schools. Thorax 1999;54:675–80.

[46] Gelber LE, Seltzer LH, Bouzoukis JK, et al. Sensitization and exposure to indoor allergens as risk factors for asthma among patients presenting to hospital. Am Rev Respir Dis 1993;147: 573–8.

[47] Call RS, Smith TF, Morris E, et al. Risk factors for asthma in inner city children. J Pediatr 1992;121:862–6.

[48] Rosenstreich DL, Eggleston P, Kattan M, et al. The role of cockroach allergy and exposure to cockroach allergen in causing morbidity among inner-city children with asthma. N Engl J Med 1997;336:1356–63.

[49] Litonjua AA, Carey VJ, Burge HA, et al. Exposure to cockroach allergen in the home is associated with incident doctor-diagnosed asthma and recurrent wheezing. J Allergy Clin Immunol 2001;107:41–7.

[50] Bernton HS, Brown H. Insect allergy-preliminary studies of the cockroach. J Allergy Clin Immunol 1964;35:506–13.

[51] Kang B. Study on cockroach antigen as a probable causative agent in bronchial asthma. J Allergy Clin Immunol 1976;58:357–65.

[52] Twarog FJ, Picone FJ, Strank RS, et al. Immediate hypersensitivity to cockroach: isolation and purification of the major antigens. J Allergy Clin Immunol 1977;59:154–60.

[53] Pómes A, Chapman MD, Vailes LD, et al. Cockroach allergen Bla g 2: structure, function, and implication for allergic sensitization. Am J Respir Crit Care Med 2002;165:391–7.

[54] Santos AR, Chapman MD, Aalberse RC, et al. Cockroach allergen and asthma in Brazil: identification of tropomyosin as a major allergen with potential cross-reactivity with mite and shrimp allergens. J Allergy Clin Immunol 1999;104:329–37.

[55] Page K, Strunk VS, Hershenson MB. Cockroach proteases increase IL-8 expression in human bronchial epithelial cells via activation of protease-activated receptor (PAR)-2 and extracellular-signal-regulated kinase. J Allergy Clin Immunol 2003;112:1112–8.

[56] Yunginger JW, Jones RT, Nesheim ME, et al. Studies on Alternaria allergens. III: isolation of a major allergenic fraction (ALT-I). J Allergy Clin Immunol 1980;66:138–47.

[57] Paris S, Debeaupuis JP, Prevost MC, et al. The 31 kD major allergen, Alt a I1563 of *Alternaria alternata*. J Allergy Clin Immunol 1991;88:902–8.

[58] Portnoy J, Pacheco F, Ballam Y, et al. The effect of time and extraction buffers on residual protein and allergen content of extracts derived from four strains of Alternaria. J Allergy Clin Immunol 1993;91:930–8.

[59] Zinovia-Mitakakis T, Barnes C, Tovey ER. Spore germination increases allergen release from Alternaria. J Allergy Clin Immunol 2001;107:388–90.

[60] O'Hollaren MT, Yunginger JW, Offord KP, et al. Exposure to an aeroallergen as a possible precipitating factor in respiratory arrest in young patients with asthma. N Engl J Med 1991; 324:359–63.

[61] Halonen M, Stern DA, Wright AL, et al. Alternaria as a major allergen for asthma in children raised in a desert environment. Am J Respir Crit Care Med 1997;155:1356–61.

[62] Perzanowski MS, Sporik R, Squillace SP, et al. Association of sensitization to Alternaria allergens with asthma among school age children. J Allergy Clin Immunol 1998;101:626–32.

[63] Wang JE, Warris A, Ellingsen EA, et al. Involvement of CD14 and toll-like receptors in activation of human monocytes by *Aspergillus fumigatus* hyphae. Infect Immunol 2001;69:2402–6.

[64] Pollart SM, Reid MJ, Fling JA, et al. Epidemiology of emergency room asthma in northern California: association with IgE antibody to ryegrass pollen. J Allergy Clin Immunol 1988; 82:224–30.

[65] Asher MI, Stewart A, Crane J. Worldwide variations in the prevalence of asthma symptoms: the International Study of Asthma and Allergies in Childhood (ISAAC). Eur Respir J 1998;12: 315–35.

[66] Ronmark E, Perzanowski M, Platts-Mills TAE, et al. Four-year incidence of allergic sensitization among schoolchildren in a community where allergy to cat and dog dominates sensitization: report from the Obstructive Lung Disease in Northern Sweden Study Group. J Allergy Clin Immunol 2003;112:747–54.

[67] Erwin EA, Wickens K, Custis NJ, et al. Cat and dust mite sensitivity and tolerance in relation to wheezing among children raised with high exposure to both allergens. J Allergy Clin Immunol, in press.

[68] Sporik R, Squillace SP, Ingram JM, et al. Mite, cat and cockroach exposure, allergen sensitization, and asthma in children: a case-control study of three schools. Thorax 1999;54:675–80.

[69] Platts-Mills TAE, Erwin EA, Allison AB, et al. The relevance of maternal immune responses to inhalant allergens to maternal symptoms, passive transfer to the infant, and development of antibodies in the first 2 years of life. J Allergy Clin Immunol 2003;111:123–30.

[70] Zambrano JC, Carper HT, Rakes GP, et al. Experimental rhinovirus challenges in adults with mild asthma: response to infection in relation to IgE. J Allergy Clin Immunol 2003;111:1008–16.

[71] Heymann PW, Carper HT, Murphy DD, et al. Viral infections in relation to age, atopy, and the season of admission among children hospitalized for wheezing. J Allergy Clin Immunol 2004; 114:239–47.

[72] Roost HP, Kunzli N, Schindler C, et al. Role of current and childhood exposure to cat and atopic sensitization. European Community Respiratory Health Survey. J Allergy Clin Immunol 1999; 104:941–7.

[73] Remes ST, Castro-Rodriguez JA, Holberg CJ, et al. Dog exposure in infancy decreases the subsequent risk of frequent wheeze but not of atopy. J Allergy Clin Immunol 2001;108:509–15.

[74] Svanes C, Heinrich J, Jarvis D, et al. Pet-keeping in childhood and adult asthma and hay fever: European community respiratory health survey. J Allergy Clin Immunol 2003;112:289–300.

ELSEVIER
SAUNDERS

Immunol Allergy Clin N Am
25 (2005) 15–30

IMMUNOLOGY
AND ALLERGY
CLINICS
OF NORTH AMERICA

The effects of outdoor air pollution and tobacco smoke on asthma

Ashley Jerath Tatum, MD*, Gail G. Shapiro, MD

Northwest Asthma and Allergy Center, 4540 Sand Point Way NE, #200, Seattle, WA 98105, USA

Asthma is characterized by increased bronchial hyper-reactivity to a number of stimuli. Persons with asthma are especially sensitive to the impact of air contaminants. Increased levels of ozone, particulate matter (PM), and environmental tobacco smoke (ETS) have been associated with increased asthma symptoms, reduced lung function, and increased admissions to the emergency department (ED). Ozone, diesel exhaust (an important contributor to PM), and ETS are known to have proinflammatory actions. These air contaminants may affect allergen-induced inflammation by initiating TH_2 responses to antigens or by exacerbating such inflammation in persons already sensitized [1–3]. This article examines the influence of outdoor air pollutants and ETS on asthma, with an emphasis on ozone, PM, and ETS on asthma exacerbations.

Outdoor air pollutants include oxides of nitrogen, ozone, PM, carbon monoxide, and sulfur dioxide. These pollutants derive from a number of sources. In the United States, it is estimated that nonmobile sources of pollution (eg, power and chemical plants and steel mills) emit approximately 93% of the sulfur dioxide, 51% of the nitrogen oxide, 9% of the carbon monoxide, and 52% of the volatile organic compound emissions found outdoors. Mobile sources, such as automobiles, aircraft, water vessels, and lawn mowers, are thought to generate 2% of the sulfur dioxide, 45% of the nitrogen oxide, 81% of the carbon monoxide, and 37% of the volatile organic compound emissions. Mobile and nonmobile sources contribute to respirable particulate matter with an aerodynamic diameter of $\leq 10\ \mu m$ (PM_{10}) and particulate matter with an aerodynamic diameter of $\leq 2.5\ \mu m$ ($PM_{2.5}$) [1,2].

---

* Corresponding author.
E-mail address: atatum@nwasthma.com (A.J. Tatum).

0889-8561/05/$ – see front matter © 2005 Elsevier Inc. All rights reserved.
doi:10.1016/j.iac.2004.09.003

Table 1
United States Environmental Protection Agency standards for ozone and PM_{10}

Pollutant	NAAQS[a]
Ozone (ppm, 1-h mean)	0.12
Ozone (ppm, 8-h mean)	0.08
PM_{10} ($\mu g/m^3$, 24-h mean)	150
$PM_{2.5}$ ($\mu g/m^3$, 24-h mean)	65

Abbreviation: NAAQS, National Ambient Air Quality Standards.

[a] Air quality index: 0.20 ppm, alert; 0.40 ppm, warning; 0.50 ppm, emergency; 0.60 ppm, significant harm.

Data from Peden DB. Air pollution: indoor and outdoor. In: Adkinson NF, Yunginger JW, Busse WW, Bochner BS, Holgate ST, Simons FE, editors. Middleton's allergy: principles and practice. 6th edition. Philadelphia: Mosby; 2003. p. 515–28.

Ozone is a by-product of atmospheric reactions that require nitrogen oxide, hydrocarbons (volatile organic compounds), and ultraviolet light. Thus, ozone is elevated in areas with substantial amounts of sunlight and nitrogen oxide, which is sometimes studied as a proxy for ozone. Automobile exhaust is the most significant source for outdoor nitrogen dioxide [2]. The United States Environmental Protection Agency (EPA) proposed National Ambient Air Quality Standards for ozone, PM_{10}, and $PM_{2.5}$ are listed in Table 1. The EPA is considering revising the standards for PM in response to the emerging importance of $PM_{2.5}$.

The Clean Air Act of 1970, amended in 1990, mandates that standards protect the health of persons (eg, children, elderly persons, and persons with asthma) who are thought to be the most sensitive to the impact of pollutants [2]. The effect of air pollutants can depend on (1) the concentration of pollutant, (2) the duration of pollutant exposure, (3) the level of exercise of the subject studied (exercise increases minute ventilation), and (4) the population studied (eg, asthmatic or nonasthmatic subjects). Data from the National Cooperative Inner-City Asthma Study conducted in children in eight urban areas in the United States revealed that at levels below current United States air quality standards, summer air pollution is significantly related to symptoms and decreased pulmonary function (morning peak expiratory flow [PEF] rate) among children with asthma (using a 4–5 day moving average) [4]. In children with mild to moderate asthma, ozone within international air quality standards was associated with an increase in the occurrence of asthma attacks, respiratory infections, and changes in lung function, measured by a decrease in PEF and an increase in PEF variability [5].

Ozone

Numerous studies have documented an increase in morbidity, mortality, and prevalence of asthma in different populations. The causes of this trend remain controversial. Compared with emissions from nonvehicular sources, the relative amounts of nitrogen oxide, carbon monoxide, and PM emitted from vehicles has increased disproportionately due to the dramatic increase in worldwide automobile use in the past 30 years. Many studies have found positive associations between traffic density on the street of residence and asthma events or asthma prevalence. During the Olympic games in Atlanta (19 July through 4 August 1996), local government acted to decrease ozone generation from vehicle exhaust via implementation of an integrated 24-hour-a-day public transportation system and alternative work hours. Ozone concentration decreased to 58.6 parts per billion (ppb), a 13% reduction compared with the baseline period of 4 weeks before and 4 weeks after the Olympic games. Weekday 1-hour morning peak traffic counts decreased 22.5% during the Olympic games, and total 24-hour traffic counts decreased 2.8%. One-hour morning peak traffic counts correlated with peak ozone concentration. Information from Medicaid, health maintenance organization, pediatric emergency department, and Georgia Hospital Discharge databases revealed a reduction in acute asthma events in children of 41.6%, 44.1%, 11.1%, and 19.1%, respectively [6]. An increase in daily acute asthma events was associated with levels of 1-hour ozone concentration of > 60 to 89 ppb [6,7].

Summer asthma camp studies are designed to allow for daily lung function measurements and daily air monitoring values from a central site at the camp that is representative for all children. These studies have found linear decrements in PEF and forced expiratory volume in 1 second (FEV_1) associated with 1-hour ozone concentrations. Mortimer et al [4] reported that a 0.5% decline in PEF accompanied a 15-ppb increase in ozone. Thurston et al [8] reported that asthma exacerbations and chest symptoms increased approximately 40% on the highest pollution day.

Some persons may be more susceptible to the effects of ozone. Among children with asthma, those with low birth weight or premature birth demonstrated a greater decline in morning PEF and a higher incidence of morning symptoms upon ozone exposure [9]. Children with asthma requiring maintenance medication, a marker for persistent disease, are particularly vulnerable to ozone. In Mexico City, an 8% increase in cough in children with asthma was calculated for a 50-ppm increase in ozone on the same day or on the previous day [7]. In adults with asthma, heavy personal tobacco use may be an effect modifier for ozone-associated morbidity. Cassino et al [10] reported that heavy smokers (≥13 pack-year tobacco history) displayed an increased relative risk of ED visits for asthma compared with nonsmokers with similar asthma severity in response to increases in 2-day lagged ozone levels. There can be a time lag between increased ozone levels and ED admissions. A lag from 24 hours to up to 5 days has been reported. The lag time between symptom onset and ED visit may lie in the time course for the development of airway inflammation in response to ozone exposure [10]. Because ozone effects can be delayed, they may not be captured by short-term laboratory studies exposing individuals to ozone [7].

Ozone exposure leads to a neutrophilic inflammatory response in the airway. Studies using airway sampling with bronchial alveolar lavage (BAL) or mucosal biopsy have revealed inflammatory responses from subjects exposed to 0.08 to 0.40 ppm ozone [1]. The influx of neutrophils occurs 1 to 6 hours after exposure, peaks 6 to 18 hours later, and continues beyond 24 hours [1,11]. Inflammatory mediators, such as interleukin (IL)-6, IL-8, granulocyte/macrophage colony-stimulating factor (GM-CSF), myeloperoxidase, prostaglandin E_2 (PGE_2), leukotriene B_4, thromboxane B_2, fibronectin, plasminogen activator, and elastase, are increased by ozone [2,12]. With the exception of PGE_2, an increase in inflammatory mediators and cells does not correlate with immediate changes in lung function in normal subjects [2]. In subjects with allergic rhinitis or allergic asthma, ozone inhalation increased neutrophil influx as seen in nonallergic subjects and eosinophil numbers in the nasal samples [2]. Two studies have demonstrated that an increased number of neutrophils occur in BAL fluid from persons with asthma exposed to ozone compared with healthy volunteers, with no effect on eosinophils [12,13]. Others have observed that persons with asthma experience an increase in neutrophils and eosinophils in the lower airway after exposure to 0.16-ppm ozone when compared with clean air exposure [1,14]. Evidence of eosinophil activation after ozone exposure has been reported [15]. In children, ozone exposure was significantly linked with increased levels of eosinophilic cationic protein (ECP) in urine samples [2]. Ozone-induced upregulation of TH_2-related cytokines and neutrophil chemoattractants in subjects with asthma differs from the inflammatory response seen in healthy control subjects. This may contribute to subsequent worsening of airway inflammation and may help explain the differential sensitivity to ozone in persons with asthma [16]. Therefore, it seems likely that chronic lower airway inflammation seen in asthma has an impact on the inflammatory response to ozone [1].

Epithelial cells play a central role in mediating ozone-induced inflammation in the airway. Bronchial epithelial cell release of GM-CSF and sICAM-1 after ozone is significantly greater in atopic asthmatics compared with nonatopic non-asthmatics [17,18]. It has been demonstrated with cultures of primary epithelial cells that ozone induces IL-1, IL-6, IL-8, and GM-CSF generation and activates NF-κB. It is likely that NF-κB activation is important to ozone-induced airway inflammation. The toll-like receptor 4 (TLR4) was identified as a key component in the signal transduction pathway for endotoxin. Genetic linkage studies in rodents have found a strong association between ozone-induced effects in the airway and the TLR4 locus [1]. Ozone stimulates epithelial cells to generate lipid peroxides and aldehydes, which can mediate inflammation [2]. Airway monocytes and macrophages are less responsive after ozone exposure, with blunting of the oxidative burst and phagocytosis [2,19]. Mucociliary clearance is reduced secondary to ozone exposure [20].

Airway responses in humans to ozone studied via challenge studies indicate that ozone exposure results in a relatively rapid decrease in forced vital capacity (FVC) and FEV_1, with an increase in nonspecific bronchial hyper-responsiveness [2]. Silverman et al [21] demonstrated that challenge with 0.25-ppm ozone for 2 hours decreased pulmonary function in some subjects with asthma within 30 to 60 minutes. Ozone seems to worsen airflow in subjects with asthma to a greater extent than in healthy volunteers. Exposure to 0.40-ppm ozone for 2 hours with rigorous exercise resulted in a significantly greater percent decrease in FEV_1

within 60 to 90 minutes in patients with asthma compared with nonasthmatic subjects [22].

Air pollution and allergen exposure can have a synergistic effect on the exacerbation of asthma. Significant statistical interactions are demonstrated between ozone and temperature and ozone and pollen count for asthma exacerbations [5]. The profile of the airway inflammatory response induced by ozone exposure can change when acute pre-existing airway inflammation is present. Ozone exposure after a late airway response elicited by allergen challenge can potentiate the eosinophilic inflammatory response induced by the allergen challenge in subjects with mild atopic asthma. Ozone exposure of 0.27 ppm for 2 hours occurring 24 hours after an allergen challenge increased airway eosinophils induced by allergen in subjects with mild asthma; however, the number of neutrophils remained the same. There was also a greater reduction in FEV_1 and FVC. Inhalation of ozone can lead to airway epithelial damage and increased airway permeability. ECP released by eosinophils can lead to epithelial damage. Thus, an increase in eosinophils with the addition of ozone after allergen challenge can create a greater pathologic and clinical response [11].

Also of interest is the effect of pre-exposure to ozone on the acute response to allergen challenge. Ozone pre-exposure increases allergen-induced bronchoconstriction in subjects with asthma and primes eosinophils for activity by allergens in the nose [11]. It is reported that exposure to 0.12-ppm ozone for 1 hour increases sensitivity to inhaled allergen as measured by a provocation dose of allergen that induces a 20% fall in FEV_1 as an endpoint; however, these results have not been consistent. Exposure to 0.16-ppm ozone has also been demonstrated to increase the response to inhaled allergens [2]. A resting exposure for 1 hour to 0.12-ppm ozone did not potentiate an immediate bronchoconstrictive response to grass allergen in subjects with mild atopic asthma [23]. Short-term exposure to 250-ppb ozone during 3 hours of intermittent exercise was shown to increase bronchial allergen responsiveness in subjects with mild allergic asthma or rhinitis when these individuals were first exposed to ozone and then challenged with allergen [24].

Repeated exposure to ozone, at a peak ambient air level, can enhance functional and inflammatory responses to inhaled allergen in subjects with pre-existing allergic airway disease [25]. There was no correlation between the change in sputum neutrophils and lung function [26]. Ozone can potentiate the effect of aeroallergens in subjects with bronchial hyper-responsiveness under natural exposure conditions. Exposure of subjects with mild atopic asthma to ozone levels sufficient to cause modest decrements in lung function increased the reactivity to allergen (house dust mites) [27]. A statistically significant interaction was demonstrated between total spore count and ozone. Mean PEF fell in association with increased spore count, but the change was greater with higher prior ozone levels [28].

The response to ozone varies between individuals and may be due to genetic susceptibility. Ozone oxidizes biomolecules in the lung, thereby generating reactive oxygen species, and activates inflammatory cells, which release reactive oxygen species. Antioxidants and antioxidant enzymes are present in the lung and provide protection against oxidative stress. Levels of the antioxidants alpha-tocopherol (vitamin E) and ascorbic acid (vitamin C) are reduced in the lung lining of patients with asthma. Therefore, polymorphisms in genes involved in the response to oxidative stress may play a role in asthma susceptibility in humans. Nicotinamide adenine dinucleotide phosphate–reduced quinone oxido-reductase (NQ01) and glutathione S-transferase M1 (GSTM1) are phase II enzymes important in the response to oxidative stress. Reactive oxygen species generated during NQ01-mediated activation of quinones and polyaromatic hydrocarbons present in diesel exhaust and ETS may interact with ozone in increasing oxidative stress in the lung. Quinones can be conjugated by GSTM and excreted and are thus unavailable for activation by NQ01. Functionally significant polymorphisms in NQ01 and GSTM-1 affect asthma risk in children of nonsmoking parents in Mexico City, an area with high ozone levels. A protective effect has been observed for the inactive NQ01 Ser allele among GSTM1-null children [29].

Particulate matter

Identifying the specific causative agents in PM is difficult because of its multiple constituents. Active agents include carbon black; a variety of metals including iron, nickel, and copper; organic residues; and biologic contaminants such as endotoxin. Organic residues include diesel exhaust particles, which consist of immunologically important polyaromatic hydrocarbons [1,2].

The Utah Valley studies have linked an increase in asthma morbidity to PM concentrations in subjects with asthma aged 8 to 72 years. In the 1980s, a strike occurred in the industrial plant thought to be the major source of particulate pollution in the Utah Valley. During the strike year, levels of $PM_{2.5}$ and admissions to the hospital for respiratory illnesses, including asthma exacerbations, decreased. Examination of particles recovered during the years before and after the strike and during the strike were analyzed for oxidant activity. Per milligram of PM, the oxidant activity and metal content of samples collected during the strike year were significantly lower than the previous and following years. Aqueous extracts from these samples were found to have proinflammatory activity on epithelial cells in vitro. This activity was inhibited by chelators and antioxidants, suggesting that the metal content of these particles is an important irritant. These same extracts were used in segmental challenge studies of normal volunteers. Reflecting the in vitro results, it was observed that extracts from samples collected during the strike year induced a significantly smaller amount of neutrophil influx than samples from the years before and after the strike [1,30,31].

The APHEA2 (Air Pollution and Health: a European Approach) Project initiated in 1998 investigated short-term health effects of particles in eight European cities. PM_{10} concentrations were positively associated with increased numbers of hospital admissions for respiratory diseases. The percent change in mean number of asthma admissions per 10 $\mu g/m^3$ increase in PM_{10} was 1.2% in persons 14 years of age and younger and 1.1% in persons 15 to 64 years of age [32].

In Seattle, Schwartz et al [33] demonstrated a 3.7% increase in ED admissions for asthma in persons 64 years of age and younger with an increase in PM_{10} of 10 $\mu g/m^3$. There was a significant decrement in FEV_1 and FVC associated with fine particles in children with asthma in Seattle compared with healthy subjects, with an average decline in lung function of 1.8 mL/$\mu g/m^3$ PM ≤ 2.5 μm [34]. A change of 11 $\mu g/m^3$ in $PM_{2.5}$ was associated with a 15% increase in asthma ED visits in Seattle [35]. Data from 133 children with asthma residing in the greater Seattle area participating in the Childhood Asthma Management Program study demonstrated an 11% increase in the odds of experiencing asthma symptoms for a 10 $\mu g/m^3$ increase in the previous day's PM_{10} [36]. Subsequent analysis revealed that an increase in asthma severity and medication use were associated with increases in $PM_{2.5}$ and PM_{10} in this study population [37]. Hospital admissions for asthma in patients younger than 65 years of age in Seattle showed a 5% increase associated with an interquartile range change in PM_{10} and a 4% increase with $PM_{2.5}$ [38].

Human challenge studies using chamber exposure to diluted diesel exhaust have revealed the following: (1) Exposure for 1 hour resulted in increased numbers of neutrophils, B lymphocytes, histamine, and fibronectin in BAL fluid; (2) bronchial biopsy specimens recovered 6 hours after challenge demonstrated mast cells, neutrophils, CD4+ and CD8+ T lymphocytes, increased IL-8, and ICAM-1 and VCAM-1 expression; (3) 4 hours after diesel exhaust particle exposure, increased airway neutrophils and myeloperoxidase were noted [2,39–41].

Animal and in vitro studies demonstrate that diesel exhaust particles (DEPs) shift primary immune responses to neoantigens toward a TH_2 phenotype, characterized by production of antigen-specific IgE, and enhance allergen-induced immune responses, including increased production of IgE, IL-4, IL-5, and GM-CSF. Diesel exhaust particles are reported to induce B lymphocyte immunoglobulin isotype switching to IgE [2]. It has been suggested that industrial air pollutants including DEPs are responsible for the increase in allergic disease seen in west Germans versus east Germans [42]. Challenge of the nasal mucosa with DEPs coupled with ragweed allergen in ragweed-sensitized atopic subjects was found to yield an enhanced ragweed-specific IgE response compared with ragweed challenge alone. This effect included increased expression of IL-4, IL-5, IL-6, IL-10, and IL-13 and decreased expression of IFN-γ and IL-2. A fourfold increase in ragweed-specific IgE in subjects challenged with DEPs coupled with ragweed was measured 1 day postchallenge, and a 16-fold difference was noted 4 days postchallenge [43]. Extracts from DEPs containing the polyaromatic hydrocarbon (PAH) fraction from these particles and the specific PAH compounds phenanthrene and 2,3,7,8-tetrachloro-dibenzo-p-dioxin are thought to mediate many of the effects of diesel exhaust particles on immune response [2]. Polyaromatic hydrocarbons can diffuse into cells, bind to cytosolic receptors, and alter ongoing transcriptional programs.

Diesel exhaust particles can activate the RANTES gene promoter via interactions with AP-1 and NF-κB, enhancing the production of allergen-specific IgE and other cytokines [2,44]. DEPs increase eosinophil adhesion to nasal epithelial cells and eosinophil degranulation [44]. It has been reported that DEPs can promote expression of CD80 in macrophages and enhance LPS-induced IL-1 responses [45]. The effects on macrophages and other antigen-presenting cells could account for the ability of DEPs to present antigen in such a way as to promote Th$_2$ responses [2]. It has been reported that increased PM$_{10}$ counts are synergistic with pollen counts as a predictor of asthma visits. A synergistic effect might be secondary to binding of pollens to DEPs, which increases the delivery of pollens to the lower respiratory tract [44].

Environmental tobacco smoke

ETS (sidestream smoke from the burning end of a cigarette and exhaled mainstream smoke from a smoker) is a complex mixture of more than 3800 compounds, including known respiratory irritants such as formaldehyde, ammonia, sulfur dioxide, and polyaromatic hydrocarbons [46]. Numerous case reports and studies suggest ETS is an important factor in asthma exacerbations. Individual differences in response to tobacco smoke may determine the impact of ETS in patients with asthma. Exposure to ETS can be assessed by the measurement of urinary, serum, or salivary cotinine, a metabolite of nicotine. Children living in homes where smoking occurs have increased levels of cotinine compared with children living in smoke-free homes, demonstrating a clear exposure to ETS. Increased ETS as assessed by urine cotinine levels was associated with acute exacerbations of asthma and reduction in FEV$_1$ and the ratio of FEV$_1$ to FVC [47]. ETS exposure has been associated with otitis media, upper and lower respiratory tract infections, wheezing, decreased lung function, and increased bronchial hyper-reactivity [2,48].

Increased asthma mortality and morbidity among minority inner-city children is closely linked to socioeconomic status, poverty, and environmental exposures. Up to one third of low-income children who do not live with a smoker spend time in a place with smokers [49]. In the Third National Health and Nutrition Examination Survey (1988–1991), 87.9% of nontobacco users in the United States had detectable levels of serum cotinine [50]. Nearly 40% of children aged 2 months to 2 years live with at least one smoker and might have their condition made worse by ETS exposure [51]. Exposure to higher levels of ETS ($\geq$10 cigarettes per day) was associated with a nearly threefold increase in nocturnal asthma symptoms in inner-city children. There was no association between ETS exposure and severity of nocturnal symptoms, limitation in physical activity, or missed school days [48].

An association between long-term ETS exposure and exacerbation of asthma in children is not limited to inner-city samples. Parental smoking is associated with an increased prevalence of asthma and respiratory symptoms. Among children who have already developed asthma, parental smoking is associated with more severe disease, with an increase in the incidence of ED visits, life-threatening attacks, and asthma symptoms [52]. Children with asthma who have high levels of tobacco smoke exposure, compared with those with low levels of exposure as measured by serum cotinine levels, were more likely to have moderate or severe asthma (odds ratio [OR] 2.7), decreased lung function (with a mean FEV_1 decrement of 8.1%, or 213 mL), and increased school absences [53].

Self-reported ETS exposure among nonsmoking adults with asthma is associated with greater asthma severity via asthma-QOL questionnaire, worse health status, and increased health care use (ie, greater odds of ED visits, urgent physician visits, and hospitalizations). Nearly one third of subjects reported some regular ETS exposure during an 18-month study interval. Subjects reporting the heaviest levels of newly initiated ETS exposure over the follow-up period had worsening of asthma severity and asthma-specific QOL. Subjects reporting ETS cessation showed improvement in asthma symptom severity and health status and decreased ED visits and hospitalizations [54].

A recent survey of adults presenting to the ED with acute asthma revealed that 35% were current smokers, and 22% to 43% were ex-smokers. Current smokers with asthma, compared with never-smokers, have more severe asthma, an accelerated decline in lung function, an increase in hospitalizations for asthma, and increased mortality after near-fatal asthma attacks [55]. The California EPA reported that the workplace accounts for the largest proportion of ETS exposure in adults. A significant decrement (~20%) in FEV_1 occurred after exposure of ETS for 1 hour in persons with asthma. Pretreatment with a bronchodilator prevented an acute decline in FEV_1 in previously reactive subjects [54,56]. Involuntary tobacco smoke exposure in the workplace, independent of exposure to other airborne contaminants, increased the risk of respiratory symptoms among German adults within the European Community Respiratory Health Survey, with an adjusted OR for asthma of 1.51. The OR for asthma was significantly increased (2.06) for subjects with >8 hours of self-reported exposure to passive tobacco smoke per day [57].

In addition to the eosinophilic airway inflammation observed in patients with asthma, smoking induces neutrophilic airway inflammation. A relationship is apparent between smoking history, airway inflammation, and lung function in smokers with asthma. Sputum IL-8 (neutrophil chemoattractant and activator) is increased in all smokers. In smokers with asthma, lung function (FEV_1) was negatively correlated with sputum IL-8 and neutrophil percentage. Sputum IL-8 correlated positively with smoking pack-years and neutrophil percentage [58]. Cigarette smoke can damage the bronchi via direct toxicity to bronchial epithelium, oxidative damage, inflammatory cell recruitment, and increased epithelial permeability. ETS exposure can result in airflow limitation and increased bronchial hyper-responsiveness. Cigarette smoke induces release of IL-8 from cultured human bronchial epithelial cells. In smokers, an increase in neutrophils, macrophages, IL-1β, IL-6, IL-8, and monocyte chemoattractant protein-1 compared with nonsmokers is demonstrated, with evidence of a cigarette dose-related relationship for some of these factors [58]. ETS may prime the airways of persons with asthma for inflammatory reactions to other airborne triggers. Alveolar macrophages of smokers are known to release greater amounts of reactive oxygen intermediates than those of nonsmokers. Increased levels of inflammatory mediators, including IL-6 and IL-8 in smokers, may translate into a more intense inflammatory response to ambient ozone [10].

The EGEA (Epidemiological Study of the Genetics and Environment of Asthma, Bronchial Hyperresponsiveness, and Atopy) data revealed that current smokers have significantly higher IgE than never smokers and that first-degree female relatives of asthmatics had increased IgE in relation to passive smoking. IgE plays a central role in the pathophysiology of asthma. Smoking has a direct effect on IgE regulation at the cellular level and an indirect action that may lead to increased permeability of airways to allergen. IgE production is controlled by TH_2 cytokines. Smoking, via an increase in IL-4 but no change in IFN-γ, leads to an increased IL-4/IFN-γ ratio and thus affects TH_2/TH_1 balance. These changes may be intensified in patients with asthma. With an increased permeability of bronchial epithelium, an already increased sensitization to allergens in allergic asthmatic patients can be enhanced [59].

A strong causal association between ETS exposure and induction of asthma in children has been reported. A meta-analysis of 37 studies conducted by the California EPA indicated an increased risk for asthma and wheezing disease in children exposed to ETS [60]. Risk factors for asthma and wheeze in school-aged children in Cape Town included maternal smoking in pregnancy (OR 1.87) and each additional household smoker (OR 1.15) as independent contributors [61]. ETS may enhance atopy development in susceptible individuals by a number of mechanisms, including increased airway mucosal permeability and direct effects on immune function. Maternal tobacco smoking is linked to increased rates of wheezing and asthma, increased bronchial reactivity, and increased total and antigen-specific IgE in exposed children [2,52]. Childhood exposure to ETS is associated with an increased prevalence of asthma among adult never-smokers without a family history of asthma. Physician-diagnosed asthma was reported in 6.8% of exposed subjects and in 3.8% of non-exposed subjects [46]. However, this study did not question respondents regarding the age of asthma onset and did not calculate asthma incidence. The relative risk of asthma in children with smoking mothers has been reported to be 1.2 to 2.6. The pooled OR for asthma prevalence was 1.37 if either parent smoked. The association between parental smoking and asthma seemed to be stronger in nonatopic children [46]. Childhood exposure to tobacco smoke has been associated with many asthma-related phenotypes. Other studies have suggested that an interaction between family history of asthma and atopy and exposure to tobacco smoke in early childhood influences the risk for asthma [62].

The inclusion of ETS as a potential risk factor for asthma was incorporated into asthma gene linkage analysis. Linkage results from regions on chromosomes 1, 5q, and 17p demonstrated significant changes in lod score in the exposed groups when ETS was taken into account. Therefore, it seems that a gene–

environment interaction may exist between ETS and unobserved susceptibility genes in these regions. Genes in three chromosomal regions (1p, 5q, and 7p) might interact with ETS to confer risk, whereas genes in two other regions (1q and 9q) might confer susceptibility through a pathway independent of ETS exposure. Region 5q contains genes for the β-adrenergic receptor, IL-4, and IL-13 [62].

The adverse effects of in utero exposure to maternal smoking on a broad range of asthma and wheezing outcomes were largely restricted to children with the GSTM1 null genotype. Among GSTM1-null children, in utero exposure to tobacco smoke was associated with increased prevalence of early-onset asthma (OR 1.6), asthma with current symptoms (OR 1.7), persistent asthma (OR 1.6), lifetime history of wheezing (OR 1.8), wheezing with exercise (OR 2.1), wheezing requiring medications (OR 2.2), and ED visits in the past year (OR 3.7). Among children with a GSTM1-positive genotype, in utero exposure was not associated with asthma or wheezing [63].

In utero exposure to maternal smoking in the USC Children's Health Study was independently associated with persistent deficits in lung function that were larger for children with asthma. School-aged children with asthma show large deficits in lung function, especially airway flows, that are associated with in utero exposure to maternal smoking that seem to be independent of ETS exposure. Boys and girls with a history of in utero exposure to maternal smoking showed deficits in maximum mid-expiratory flow (MMEF) and a decrease in FEV_1/FVC ratio. As compared with children without asthma, boys with asthma and in utero exposure had larger deficits in FVC, MMEF, and FEV_1/FVC, and girls had larger decreases in FEV_1/FVC. Perinatal deficits persist into childhood and adolescence. Newborns with a family history of asthma had a greater deficit in lung function from in utero exposure than did newborns without a family history of asthma. Small airway deficits from in utero exposure reflect damage during critical periods of development that permanently alters the structure or function of the lung, such as its elastic recoil properties and immune function [64].

Treatment

Treatment with oral or inhaled corticosteroids in smokers has been disappointing. Active smoking impairs the efficacy of short-term oral corticosteroid treatment, as measured by FEV_1, morning PEF, and asthma control score, in chronic asthma independent of asthma severity. Similarly, smoking was demonstrated to impair the efficacy of short-term inhaled corticosteroids in steroid-naive asthma, with no improvement in lung function, bronchial hyper-responsiveness, or sputum eosinophils [55]. The effect of smoking on asthma may be partially reversible because the ex-smokers had a significant improvement in morning and night-time PEF values after corticosteroids. The effect of corticosteroid insensitivity may be secondary to increased neutrophils in airways of smokers with asthma and to increased levels of TNF-α in smokers, leading to increased numbers of glucocorticoid β-receptors. ETS contains bacterial LPS that activates NF-κB. Smokers have decreased histone deacetylase expression and activity, from oxidative stress, which glucocorticosteroids require for maximal suppression of cytokine induction [55]. Inhaled budesonide did not inhibit the functional response to ozone exposure as detected by a reduction in FEV_1 and an increase in total symptom score, but it significantly blunted the increase in the percentage of sputum neutrophils and IL-8 concentrations in the supernatant. Thus, 4 weeks of inhaled budesonide blunted the airway neutrophilic inflammatory response but did not prevent the functional impairment of airways after ozone exposure in patients with mild persistent asthma. Ozone-induced inflammation is not closely related to a decrease in lung function in occurrence or in severity, suggesting that different pathophysiologic mechanisms underlie the two features. FVC and FEV_1 decrements seem to be neurally mediated, involving stimulation of airway C fibers. On the other hand, airway inflammation induced by ozone exposure results from increased vascular and epithelial permeability and an enhanced release of proinflammatory mediators by different cells. Thus, although corticosteroids can exert their anti-inflammatory effect, reducing the vascular and epithelial permeability of the airway and reducing the release of inflammatory cytokines, they cannot inhibit the neurogenic mechanism underlying early FEV_1 and FVC reduction [65].

In a nurse-led, behavior-changing strategy that incorporated basic asthma education with feedback on a child's urinary cotinine level, intervention significantly reduced asthma health care use in ETS-exposed, low-income, minority children. The proportion of children with more than one acute asthma-related visit decreased from 50% in the baseline year to 29.6% in the follow-up year, as contrasted with a slight increase (from 37.2% to 46.5%) in the control group [52].

Supplementation with antioxidants (50 mg/d of vitamin E and 250 mg/d of vitamin C) might modulate the impact of ozone exposure on the small airways of children with moderate to severe asthma [66]. Flavonoids and selenium may have a protective effect on asthma [67]. Children with asthma who have a genetic deficiency of GSTM1 might be more susceptible to the deleterious effects of ozone on the small airways and might derive a greater benefit from antioxidant supplementation [68].

Summary

Epidemiologic and human challenge studies demonstrate that exposure to outdoor air pollution and ETS can adversely affect health. Patients with asthma are particularly susceptible. Outdoor air pollution and ETS have proinflammatory actions that can exacerbate existing lower airway inflammation in persons with asthma. Exposure to these air contaminants can increase the risk of developing asthma in susceptible persons. Outdoor air pollution and ETS can influence allergen-induced inflammation by exacerbating such inflammation or by initiating TH_2 responses. Thus, efforts to reduce levels of outdoor air contaminants may reduce asthma morbidity and prevalence.

References

[1] Peden DB. Air pollution in asthma: effect of pollutants on airway inflammation. Ann Allergy Asthma Immunol 2001;87:12–7.

[2] Peden DB. Air pollution: indoor and outdoor. In: Adkinson NF, Yunginger JW, Busse WW, Bochner BS, Holgate ST, Simons FE, editors. Middleton's allergy: principles and practice. 6th edition. Philadelphia: Mosby; 2003. p. 515–28.

[3] Forster J, Kuehr J. The role of ozone. Pediatr Allergy Immunol 2000;11:23–5.

[4] Mortimer KM, Neas LM, Dockery DW, Redline S, Tager IB. The effect of air pollution on inner-city children with asthma. Eur Respir J 2002;19:699–705.

[5] Just J, Segala C, Sahraoui F, Priol G, Grimfeld A, Neukirch F. Short-term health effects of particulate and photochemical air pollution in asthmatic children. Eur Respir J 2002;20:899–906.

[6] Friedman MS, Powell KE, Hutwagner L, Graham LM, Teague WG. Impact of changes in transportation and commuting behaviors during the 1996 summer Olympic games in Atlanta on air quality and childhood asthma. JAMA 2001;285:897–905.

[7] Ghent JF, Triche EW, Holford TR, Belanger K, Bracken MB, Beckett WS, et al. Association of low-level ozone and fine particles with respiratory symptoms in children with asthma. JAMA 2003;290:1859–67.

[8] Thurston GD, Lippmann M, Scott MB, Fine JM. Summertime haze air pollution and children with asthma. Am J Respir Crit Care Med 1997;155:654–60.

[9] Mortimer KM, Tager IB, Dockery DW, Neas LM, Redline S. The effect of ozone on inner-city children with asthma. Am J Respir Crit Care Med 2000;162:1838–45.

[10] Cassino C, Ito K, Bader I, Ciotoli C, Thurston G, Reibman J. Cigarette smoking and ozone-associated emergency department use for asthma by adults in New York City. Am J Respir Crit Care Med 1999;159:1773–9.

[11] Vagaggini B, Taccola M, Cianchetti S, Carnevali S, Bartoli ML, Bacci E, et al. Ozone exposure increases eosinophilic airway response induced by previous allergen challenge. Am J Respir Crit Care Med 2002;166:1073–7.

[12] Scannell C, Chen L, Aris RM, Tager I, Christian D, Ferrando R, et al. Greater ozone-induced inflammatory responses in subjects with asthma. Am J Respir Crit Care Med 1996;154:24–9.

[13] Basha MA, Gross KB, Gwizdala CJ, Haidar AH, Popovich J. Bronchoalveolar lavage neutrophilia in asthmatic and healthy volunteers after controlled exposure to ozone and filtered purified air. Chest 1994;106:1757–65.

[14] Peden DB, Boehlecke B, Horstman D, Devlin R. Prolonged acute exposure to 0.16 ppm ozone induces eosinophilic airway inflammation in asthmatic subjects with allergies. J Allergy Clin Immunol 1997;100:802–8.

[15] Newson EJ, Krishna MT, Lau LC, Howarth PH, Holgate ST, Frew AJ. Effects of short-term exposure to 0.2 ppm ozone on biomarkers of inflammation in sputum, exhaled nitric oxide, and lung function in subjects with mild atopic asthma. J Occup Environ Med 2000;42:270–7.

[16] Bosson J, Stenfors N, Bucht A, Helleday R, Pourazar J, Holgate ST, et al. Ozone-induced bronchial epithelial cytokine expression differs between healthy and asthmatic subjects. Clin Exp Allergy 2003;33:777–82.

[17] Bayram H, Rusznak C, Khair OA, Sapsford RJ, Abdelaziz MM. Effect of ozone and nitrogen dioxide on the permeability of bronchial epithelial cell cultures of non-asthmatic and asthmatic subjects. Clin Exp Allergy 2002;32:1285–92.

[18] Bayram H, Sapsford RJ, Abdelaziz MM, Khair OA. Effect of ozone and nitrogen dioxide on the release of proinflammatory mediators from bronchial epithelial cells of nonatopic nonasthmatic subjects and atopic asthmatic patients in vitro. J Allergy Clin Immunol 2001;107:287–94.

[19] Devlin RB, McKinnon KP, Noah T, Becker S, Koren HS. Ozone-induced release of cytokines and fibronectin by alveolar macrophages and airway epithelial cells. Am J Physiol 1994;266: 612–9.

[20] Tarlo SM, Broder I, Corey P, Chan-Yeung M, Ferguson A, Becker A, et al. The role of symptomatic colds in asthma exacerbations: influence of outdoor allergens and air pollutants. J Allergy Clin Immunol 2001;108:52–8.

[21] Silverman F. Asthma and respiratory irritants (ozone). Environ Health Perspect 1979;29:131–6.

[22] Kreit JW, Gross KB, Moore TB, Lorenzen TJ, D'Arcy J, Eschenbacher WL. Ozone-induced changes in pulmonary function and bronchial responsiveness in asthmatics. J Appl Physiol 1989; 66:217–22.

[23] Ball BA, Folinsbee LJ, Peden DB, Kehrl HR. Allergen bronchoprovocation of patients with mild allergic asthma after ozone exposure. J Allergy Clin Immunol 1996;98:563–72.

[24] Jorres R, Nowak D, Magnussen H. The effect of ozone exposure on allergen responsiveness in subjects with asthma or rhinitis. Am J Respir Crit Care Med 1996;153:56–64.

[25] Holz O, Mucke M, Paasch K, Bohme S, Timm P, Richter K, et al. Repeated ozone exposures enhance bronchial allergen responses in subjects with rhinitis or asthma. Clin Exp Allergy 2002; 32:681–9.

[26] Holz O, Jorres RA, Timm P, Mucke M, Richter K, Koschyk S, et al. Ozone-induced airway inflammatory changes differ between individuals and are reproducible. Am J Respir Crit Care Med 1999;159:776–84.

[27] Kehrl HR, Peden DB, Ball B, Folinsbee LJ, Horstman D. Increased specific airway reactivity of persons with mild allergic asthma after 7.6 hours of exposure to 0.16 ppm ozone. J Allergy Clin Immunol 1999;104:1198–204.

[28] Higgins BG, Francis HC, Yates C, Warburton CJ, Fletcher AM, Pickering CAC, et al. Environmental exposure to air pollution and allergens and peak flow changes. Eur Respir J 2000; 16:61–6.

[29] David GL, Romieu I, Sienra-Monge JJ, Collins WJ, Ramirez-Aguilar M, del Rio-Navarro BE, et al. Nicotinamide adenine dinucleotide (phosphate) reduced quinine oxidoreductase and glutathione s-transferase M1 polymorphisms and childhood asthma. Am J Respir Crit Care Med 2003;168:1199–204.

[30] Pope III CA. Respiratory disease associated with community air pollution and a steel mill, Utah Valley. Am J Public Health 1989;79:623–8.

[31] Ghio AJ, Devlin RB. Inflammatory lung injury after bronchial instillation of air pollution particles. Am J Respir Crit Care Med 2001;164:704–8.

[32] Atkinson RW, Anderson HR, Sunyer J, Ayres J, Baccini M, Vonk JM, et al. Acute effects of particulate air pollution on respiratory admissions: results from the APHEA 2 project. Am J Respir Crit Care Med 2001;164:1860–6.

[33] Schwartz J, Slater D, Larson TV, Pierson WE, Koenig JQ. Particulate air pollution and hospital emergency room visits for asthma in Seattle. Am Rev Respir Dis 1993;147:826–31.

[34] Koenig JQ, Larson TV, Hanley QS, Rebolledo V, Dumler K, Checkoway H, et al. Pulmonary function changes in children associated with fine particulate matter. Environ Res 1993;63: 26–38.

[35] Norris G, YoungPong SN, Koenig JQ, Larson TV, Sheppard L, Stout JW. An association between fine particles and asthma emergency department visit for children in Seattle. Environ Health Perspect 1997;107:489–93.

[36] Yu O, Sheppard L, Lumley T, Koenig JQ, Shapiro GG. Effects of ambient air pollution on symptoms of asthma in Seattle-area children enrolled in the CAMP study. Environ Health Perspect 2000;108:1209–14.

[37] Slaughter JC, Lumley T, Sheppard L, Koenig JQ, Shapiro GG. Effects of ambient air pollution on symptom severity and medication use in children with asthma. Ann Allergy Asthma Immunol 2003;91:346–53.

[38] Sheppard L, Levy D, Norris G, Larson TV, Koenig JQ. Effects of ambient air pollution on non-elderly asthma hospital admissions in Seattle, 1987–1994. Epidemiology 1999;10:23–30.

[39] Salvi SS, Nordenhall C, Blomberg A, Rudell B, Pourazar J, Kelly FJ, et al. Acute exposure to diesel exhaust increases IL-8 and GRO-alpha production in healthy human airways. Am J Respir Crit Care Med 2000;161:550–7.

[40] Salvi S, Blomberg A, Rudell B, Kelly F, Sandstrom T, Holgate ST, et al. Acute inflammatory responses in the airways and peripheral blood after short-term exposure to diesel exhaust in healthy human volunteers. Am J Respir Crit Care Med 1999;159:702–9.

[41] Nightingale JA, Maggs R, Cullinan P, Donnelly LE, Rogers DF, Kinnersley R, et al. Airway inflammation after controlled exposure to diesel exhaust particulates. Am J Respir Crit Care Med 2000;162:161–6.

[42] Kramer U, Behrendt H, Dolgner R, Ranft U, Ring J, Willer H. Airway diseases and allergies in East and West German children during the first 5 years after reunification: time trends and the impact of sulphur dioxide and total suspended particles. Int J Epidemiol 1999;28:865–73.

[43] Diaz-Sanchez D, Tsien A, Fleming J. Combined diesel exhaust particulate and ragweed allergen challenge markedly enhances human in vivo nasal ragweed-specific IgE and skews cytokine production to a T helper cell 2-type pattern. J Immunol 1997;158:2406–13.

[44] Lierl MB, Hornung RW. Relationship of outdoor air quality to pediatric asthma exacerbations. Ann Allergy Asthma Immunol 2003;90:28–33.

[45] Nel AE, Diaz-Sanchez D, Li N. The role of particulate pollutants in pulmonary inflammation and asthma: evidence for the involvement of organic chemicals and oxidative stress. Curr Opin Pulm Med 2001;7:20–6.

[46] Larsson ML, Frisk M, Hallstrom J, Kiviloog J, Lundback B. Environmental tobacco smoke exposure during childhood is associated with increased prevalence of asthma in adults. Chest 2001;120:711–7.

[47] Chilmonczyk BA, Salmun LM, Megathlin KN, Neveux LM, Palomaki GE, Knight GJ, et al. Association between exposure to environmental tobacco smoke and exacerbations of asthma in children. New Engl J Med 1993;328:1665–9.

[48] Morkjaroenpong V, Rand CS, Butz AM, Huss K, Eggleston P, Malveaux FJ, et al. Environmental tobacco smoke exposure and nocturnal symptoms among inner-city children with asthma. J Allergy Clin Immunol 2002;110:147–53.

[49] Hopper JA, Craig KA. Environmental tobacco smoke exposure among urban children. Pediatrics 2000;106:E47.

[50] Pirkle JL, Flegal KM, Bernert JT, Brody DJ, Etzel RA, Maurer KR. Exposure of the US population to environmental tobacco smoke: the Third National Health and Nutrition Examination Survey, 1988 to 1991. JAMA 1996;275:1233–40.

[51] Gergen PJ, Fowler JA, Maurer KR, Davis WW, Overpeck MD. The burden of environmental tobacco smoke exposure on the respiratory health of children 2 months through 5 years of age in the United States: Third National Health and Nutrition Examination Survey, 1988 to 1994. Pediatrics 1998;101:E8.

[52] Wilson SR, Yamada EG, Sudhakar R, Roberto L, Mannino D, Mejia C, et al. A controlled trial of an environmental tobacco smoke reduction intervention in low-income children with asthma. Chest 2001;120:1709–22.

[53] Mannino DM, Homa DM, Redd SC. Involuntary smoking and asthma severity in children: data from the third national health and nutrition examination survey. Chest 2002;122:409–15.

[54] Eisner MD, Yelin EH, Henke J, Shiboski SC, Blanc PD. Environmental tobacco smoke and adult asthma: the impact of changing exposure status on health outcomes. Am J Respir Crit Care Med 1998;158:170–5.

[55] Chaudhuri R, Livingston E, McMahon AD, Thomson L, Borland W, Thomson NC. Cigarette smoking impairs the therapeutic response to oral corticosteroids in chronic asthma. Am J Respir Crit Care Med 2003;168:1308–11.

[56] Dahms TE, Bolin JF, Slavin RG. Passive smoking: effects on bronchial asthma. Chest 1981; 80:530–4.

[57] Radon K, Busching K, Heinrich J, Wichmann HE, Jorres RA, Magnussen H, et al. Passive smoking exposure: a risk factor for chronic bronchitis and asthma in adults? Chest 2002;122: 1086–90.

[58] Chalmers GW, MacLeod KJ, Thomson L, Little SA, McSharry C, Thomson NC. Smoking and airway inflammation in patients with mild asthma. Chest 2001;120:1917–22.

[59] Oryszczyn MP, Annesi-Maesano I, Charpin D, Paty E, Maccario J, Kauffmann F. Relationships of active and passive smoking to total IgE in adults of the epidemiological study of the genetics and environment of asthma, bronchial hyperresponsiveness, and atopy (EGEA). Am J Respir Crit Care Med 2000;161:1241–6.

[60] Schwartz J, Timonen KL, Pekkanen J. Respiratory effects of environmental tobacco smoke in a panel study of asthmatic and symptomatic children. Am J Respir Crit Care Med 2000;161: 802–6.

[61] Ehrlich RI, Du Toit D, Jordaan E, Zwarenstein M, Potter P, Volmink JA. Risk factors for childhood asthma and wheezing. Importance of maternal and household smoking. Am J Respir Crit Care Med 1996;154:681–8.

[62] Colilla S, Nicolae D, Pluzhnikov A, Blumenthal MN, Beaty TH, Bleecker ER, et al. Evidence for gene-environment interactions in a linkage study of asthma and smoking exposure. J Allergy Clin Immunol 2003;111:840–6.

[63] Gilliland FD, Li YF, Dubeau L, Berhane K, Avol E, McConnell R, et al. Effects of glutathione S transferase M1, maternal smoking during pregnancy, and environmental tobacco smoke on asthma and wheezing in children. Am J Respir Crit Care Med 2002;166:457–63.

[64] Li YF, Gilliland FD, Berhane K, McConnell R, Gauderman WJ, Rappaport EB, et al. Effects of in utero and environmental tobacco smoke exposure on lung function in boys and girls with and without asthma. Am J Respir Crit Care Med 2000;162:2097–104.

[65] Vagaggini B, Taccola M, Conti I, Carnevali S, Cianchetti S, Bartoli ML, et al. Budesonide reduces neutrophilic but not functional airway response to ozone in mild asthmatics. Am J Respir Crit Care Med 2001;164:2172–6.

[66] Romieu I, Sienra-Monge JJ, Ramirez-Aguilar M, Tellez-Rojo MM, Moreno-Macias H, Reyes-Ruiz NI, et al. Antioxidant supplementation and lung functions among children with asthma exposed to high levels of air pollutants. Am J Respir Crit Care Med 2002;166:703–9.

[67] Shaheen SO, Sterne JAC, Thompson RL, Songhurst CE, Margetts BM, Burney PGJ. Dietary antioxidants and asthma in adults: population-based case-control study. Am J Respir Crit Care Med 2001;164:1823–8.

[68] Romieu I, Sienra-Monge JJ, Ramirez-Aguilar M, Moreno-Macias H, Reyes-Ruiz NI, del Rio-Navarro BE, et al. Genetic polymorphism of GSTM1 and antioxidant supplementation influence lung function in relation to ozone exposure in asthmatic children in Mexico City. Thorax 2004; 59:8–10.

ELSEVIER
SAUNDERS

Immunol Allergy Clin N Am
25 (2005) 31–43

IMMUNOLOGY
AND ALLERGY
CLINICS
OF NORTH AMERICA

Asthma associated with exercise

William W. Storms, MD

Asthma & Allergy Associates, P.C., 2709 North Tejon Street, Colorado Springs, CO 80907, USA

One of the most common triggers for a patient with asthma is physical exertion. This may be anything from carrying groceries up the stairs to running a 10-km foot race, depending upon the patient's conditioning. Some patients with chronic asthma are able to perform only limited exercise, whereas others may become elite athletes and compete in the Olympics. Because exercise is a routine trigger for all patients with asthma, it is important to understand the best methods of diagnosing and treating this condition.

There is a subset of asthma patients who have only exercise-induced asthma (EIA) and do not have chronic daily asthma. These are usually recreational athletes (eg, high school students, college students, or adults who like to jog, bike, swim, etc.) who have asthma symptoms only with exercise. They should be worked up and treated because the treatment available can allow almost any patient to exercise at whatever level they desire.

Epidemiology

The epidemiology of EIA has not been well described. We have a large amount of information about the epidemiology of asthma in the United States and worldwide, but most studies focus on asthma in general and do not deal specifically with EIA. To get an idea of the incidence of exercise asthma, we need to look at small studies of specific populations. Studies have been done in normal school children and in athletes. Studies in school children who were not competitive athletes have shown that significant percentages of school children have EIA as determined by pulmonary testing before and after exercise; Hall-

E-mail address: sneezedoc@aacos.com

0889-8561/05/$ – see front matter © 2005 Elsevier Inc. All rights reserved.
doi:10.1016/j.iac.2004.09.007

strand [1] found that 9% of school children have EIA, and Rupp [2] found that 12% of school children have EIA. These findings showed that EIA occurred in many children who would otherwise not have been recognized as asthmatic. Other studies have been performed in athletes. A survey of athletes for the 1996 Atlanta Olympics [3] showed that 16% of the athletes had a history or medication use, which was compatible with EIA. In a study of collegiate cross-country runners, Thole [4] found incidence of 14% of EIA in these athletes. In winter sports, the incidence of EIA is higher: In competitive athletes it was found that 35% of figure skaters [5] and 35% of ice hockey players [6] had EIA. In the 1998 winter Olympics Games in Nagano [7], the overall incidence of EIA was 17%. In the winter Olympics in Salt Lake City in 2002, 14% of the cross-country skiers used inhaled beta-agonists for treatment of EIA [8]. Many of these studies on athletes were based on questionnaires, medical history, and medication usage. Some investigators have been more detailed in their evaluation of athletes by performing spirometric testing before and after a sport-specific challenge. The reason a sport-specific challenge was chosen rather than a standard treadmill exercise test or cycle ergometer test was the fact that well-trained athletes may not show evidence of EIA when subjected to the standard exercise challenge but may show some abnormalities after sport-specific challenge. Wilber [9] used sport-specific exercise challenge for athletes in winter sports. He found the overall incidence of EIA in winter sports was 23%, but some sports, such as cross-country skiing, had an incidence as high as 50%.

Pathophysiology: mechanisms of exercise-induced asthma

There are two theories regarding the pathogenesis of EIA [10,11]. The underlying mechanisms of EIA are not thought to be the same as chronic persistent asthma, in which inflammation of the airways is the primary underlying pathologic event. In EIA, the two theories that have been proposed are the hyperosmolarity theory [12] and the airway rewarming theory [13,14].

The hyperosmolarity theory states that water loss occurs during the hyperventilation of exercise and that this water comes from the airway surface liquid of the bronchi. Because of this water loss, there is hypertonicity and hyperosmolarity within the airway cells. This is felt to lead to the release of mediators that cause bronchoconstriction. These include histamine, prostaglandins, and leukotrienes. If this water loss occurs in a patient who has chronic persistent asthma and who has underlying airway inflammation, this inflammation may aggravate the postexercise bronchospasm caused by the exercise-related hyperosmolarity.

The airway rewarming theory states that the hyperventilation of exercise leads to cooling of the airway. After the exercise is finished, there is rewarming of the airway because of dilatation of the small bronchiolar vessels that wrap around the bronchial tree. This influx of warm blood into these vessels leads to congested vessels, fluid exudation from the blood vessels into the submucosa of the airway wall, and mediator release with subsequent bronchoconstriction.

Neither of these theories considers inflammation as the underlying pathophysiology of EIA. However, there is some evidence that inflammation may be involved in some patients with EIA. Sue-Chu [15] showed elevations in some inflammatory cells in the airway of athletes with EIA; however, not all the usual inflammatory cells associated with chronic asthma were elevated. Karjalainen [16] studied 40 elite cross-country skiers and looked for evidence of airway inflammation in bronchial biopsies. The skiers had elevated T lymphocytes, macrophages, and eosinophils in their airways as compared with the control group. They also had increased subepithelial basement membrane tenascin expression, which is a marker of airway remodeling. The authors concluded that cross-country skiers not only had symptoms and signs of exercise-induced asthma after exercise, but they also had evidence of chronic airway inflammation, which the authors proposed was caused by constant exercise and hyperventilation in cold air. Rundell et al [17] evaluated elite woman ice hockey players to identify whether continuous long-term exercise in cold air in ice rink athletes could lead to abnormalities in baseline lung function and chronic airway inflammation. They evaluated ice hockey players who had symptoms of EIA and those who did not have symptoms and performed spirometry at baseline and after an exercise challenge. They found that athletes who had EIA had lower baseline lung function, suggesting that prolonged exercise in the cold air of an ice rink may lead to chronic airway changes similar to those seen in chronic persistent asthma. Other studies have found evidence of inflammation using these and other markers of inflammation, but not all investigators have agreed. Gauvreau [18] studied subjects with mild asthma and found no change in the inflammatory cells in the sputum or the blood after exercise challenge. Nitric oxide (NO) is a surrogate marker of asthmatic inflammation and can be measured in exhaled air. Some authors have found changes in exhaled NO after exercise that correlated with the drop in FEV_1 and suggested the presence of inflammation in these patients with EIA [19–22]. Another surrogate marker for inflammation in asthma is plasma level of adenosine. Vizi [23] identified increased levels of plasma adenosine after exercise in patients with asthma. These data on inflammation suggest that subjects who exercise frequently, especially in cold air, may develop chronic inflammatory changes in the airways that are similar to the type of inflammation seen in chronic persistent asthma. This may not apply for the patient who has EIA only and no evidence of persistent asthma. The prevalence of the inflammatory changes in EIA is not known. One study tried to answer this question by looking for a late asthmatic response after exercise as is seen after allergen challenge; 50% of patients with EIA had a late response [24]. If this late response reflects airway inflammation in these patients, then we may find up to 50% of EIA patients having airway inflammation. Further studies are needed to give us a better understanding of the role of inflammation in EIA. Helenius [25] evaluated elite swimmers during and 5 years after their competitive careers. Some of the athletes continued to compete, albeit at a lower level, and some of them swam recreationally. Those swimmers who continued to compete continued to have asthma symptoms and bronchial hyper-responsiveness (by histamine inhalation challenge). The swimmers who stopped high-level training had reduced asthma symptoms and reduced bronchial responsiveness. This suggests that prolonged intense exercise may initiate changes in the airways, which we recognize as EIA, and that these changes may resolve when the intensity of the exercise is reduced.

Diagnosing exercise-induced asthma

The diagnosis of EIA requires an approach that is specific to the type of patient who presents with symptoms. For instance, the average school child or adult recreational athlete may have a different presentation than the competitive athlete. Most of our patients are school children who are doing exercise during physical education class or are recreational athletes. These patients present with common asthma symptoms, such as coughing, wheezing, shortness of breath, or chest tightness. The symptoms begin after about 6 to 8 minutes of strenuous exercise, but if the patient exercises for a longer period of time the symptoms may not be present until after exercise. In some cases the patient has symptoms during exercise, but then the exercise intensity is reduced for a short while and then the intensity is increased. This has been described by some as "running through" their asthma. Even if they "run through" their asthma, they may have asthma symptoms after stopping the exercise.

The diagnosis may be difficult to make in school children because the parents do not observe their child during gym or physical education class. The child may have asthma symptoms but may not recognize them as such and may just feel that they are unable to do the exercise that is required. In this setting it is important for the health care provider to question the child directly and ask about the type of exercise they do in school and whether or not they have any difficulty breathing during the exercise.

Some of the more subtle symptoms that may be associated with EIA are abdominal pain, muscle cramping, dizziness, fatigue, or "being out of shape." Another common symptom is a dry cough after exercise that may last for a few hours to a day. In most cases, the patient has symptoms that correlate with exercise intensity, and they are able to correlate and perceive their respiratory symptoms well. Some studies [26,27] have shown that self-reported symptoms from the patient are not good predictors for EIA and that there may be false-positive and false-negative findings when the symptoms are the only criteria used to the diagnosis. For that reason, anytime a diagnosis of EIA is raised, further evaluation (eg, exercise testing) should be performed. Other factors in history taking that support the diagnosis of EIA are increased symptoms upon exposure to cold dry air and with higher-intensity exercise (eg, running or cross-country skiing) as compared with intermittent sports (eg, racquetball, doubles tennis).

After a thorough history is taken, a physical examination should be performed including an ENT examination looking for nasal allergies, sinusitis, or otitis; a cardiac examination to evaluate for possible murmurs or arrhythmias; and a chest examination to check for wheezes, rhonchi, or rales. The physical examination is normal in most patients with EIA. Abnormal findings should be pursued and treated accordingly. Conditions such as allergic rhinitis or chronic sinusitis may aggravate EIA and require treatment to improve the EIA.

After the physical examination, spirometry needs to be performed. If the patient has EIA but not persistent asthma, the spirometry would be normal at rest, and the only changes would be after exercise. In most school-age children or recreational adult athletes, it is not necessary to perform an exercise challenge: As long as their resting FEV_1 is normal and they respond well to treatment, this is good evidence of EIA. $FEV_1 < 90\%$ normal suggests chronic daily asthma with an exercise-related exacerbation. In this situation, daily anti-inflammatory asthma therapy should be initiated, along with a beta-agonist before exercise, because this patient may have mild persistent asthma that has been previously unrecognized, and the EIA may be just an exercise-related worsening of the underlying asthma. Follow-up visits are important in EIA. A treatment trial may be enough to make the diagnosis, but if the treatment does not work, then further diagnostic evaluation may be necessary.

If the patient is an elite competitive athlete, the presenting symptoms may be different. EIA is more common in outdoor winter sports than it is in summer sports, so the winter athletes are at the highest risk. One common presenting symptom is a prolonged cough after exercise; less commonly there is wheezing, chest tightness, or shortness of breath. In elite athletes it is important to do spirometry before and after exercise (preferably in their sport); this may be the only way to identify EIA. Because of their high level of training, they may not realize that they have a significant drop in FEV_1 after exercise, and they may not seek medical attention. These athletes may be identified only by sport-specific exercise challenge.

Challenge testing

Challenge testing may be necessary in some patients because it can help confirm the diagnosis in a patient in whom the usual therapy has failed to give an effective result. Challenge testing is important in the screening of certain elite sport teams in whom it is known there is a high incidence of EIA (eg, cross-country skiers, ice skaters, etc.). The International Olympic Committee Medical Commission requires challenge testing for proof of the diagnosis of EIA so that athletes may take anti-asthmatic medications during competition. There are a number of challenge tests that can be performed to confirm the diagnosis of EIA, the standard treadmill or cycle ergometer exercise challenge being the most common. During the exercise challenge, the patient should inhale dry air from a large Douglas bag. An alternative to the treadmill test is the step test [28]. Free running (outdoors) is also an option, but the temperature and humidity cannot be controlled in this situation, and this test may not be as accurate. The best test is felt to be the sports-specific challenge [29], in which the athlete performs spirometry before and after intense exercise in his own sport (eg, interval sprints for track athletes, 1000-m sprint for speed skaters, etc.). This type of sports-specific exercise can be revealing because some athletes may have a drop in their FEV_1 when they are measured out in the field but may not have it when they are put on a treadmill. The drawback of the sports-specific exercise challenge is that the temperature and humidity cannot be controlled; high temperature or humidity may result in a negative test (this is not an issue for winter sports). Another type of challenge test that has been shown to be specific for EIA is the eucapnic voluntary hyperventilation (EVH) challenge with dry air [30,31]. The EVH challenge requires equipment that most physicians and hospital pulmonary function labs do not have and therefore is used primarily in exercise physiology labs. Methacholine challenge has also been used in the evaluation for asthma and EIA for many years. This does not predict EIA as well as some of the other challenges but may be more readily available in some physician's offices and some hospital pulmonary function labs. A recently developed test, the inhaled mannitol test, has been proposed as an excellent way to evaluate for EIA with minimal equipment. Holtzer [32] evaluated 27 summer elite athletes with the diagnosis of EIA and showed that the inhaled mannitol test was at least as accurate or more accurate than the EVH test in these athletes. The inhaled mannitol test is simple to perform because it requires only that the patient inhale dry powder mannitol; spirometry is done before and after the inhalation. There are no significant adverse events related to this challenge. Mannitol is not available in the United States for diagnostic testing, and until it is available for general use in the United States, and, until further data are generated on the specificity and sensitivity of this test, it will have to remain as a research tool.

A review of the athletes with EIA from the 2002 Winter Olympic Games was published by Rundell [33]. Before the games, the eucapnic voluntary hyper-ventilation (EVH) test was performed as a laboratory challenge to identify airway hyper-responsiveness that would be considered consistent with exercise asthma. All of the athletes were winter sports athletes, and the EVH test was performed in the laboratory at 19°C. The subjects also had exercise challenges performed outdoors in the cold (cross-country skiing, ice skating, or running) at 2°C and 45% relative humidity. The authors found that the EVH test for 6 minutes with cold dry air challenge had a greater chance of identifying airway hyper-responsiveness as compared with 6 to 8 minutes of field exercise in the cold. They suggested that the EVH test should be used as a challenge test for patients who are being evaluated for EIA.

Koskela et al [34] compared the sensitivity and validity of three different challenges (inhaled mannitol, inhaled histamine, and inhaled cold air) in patients with asthma to see which challenge was more predictive of airway hyper-responsiveness. This study was done in patients with chronic asthma, not specifically EIA. The tests were done before and after daily treatment with inhaled budesonide 800 µg/d. The authors concluded that the inhaled mannitol challenge is a sensitive and valid method for demonstrating airway hyper-responsiveness. They found that the histamine inhalation challenge was equally sensitive but not as valid as the mannitol challenge; cold air was less sensitive.

Treatment of exercised-induced asthma

The treatment of EIA invoves (1) education of the patient, including types of exercise to choose and warm-up before exercise; (2) treatment with pharmacologic agents; (3) treatment assessment at a follow-up visit; and (4) follow-up evaluations to monitor changes in the EIA. The first phase of treatment involves advising the patient regarding types of exercise that are less likely to cause asthma (Box 1). For instance, children who desire to participate in sports may choose swimming instead of ice skating because swimming is much less asthmagenic. This can be helpful in dealing with noncompetitive athletes, but competitive athletes have already picked their sport and are not likely to change the sport in which they are competing. Some athletes avoid exercising on days when the air is very cold because cold air worsens EIA. They might also be able to avoid high-pollen days [35,36]. The second educational part of treatment involves warm-up routines before exercise so that the EIA may be partially mitigated. Certain warm-up routines may reduce EIA if done before exercise; athletes should try to warm up at 80% to 90% of their maximum workload before they exercise or compete. This type of warm-up before the exercise reduces the severity of EIA [37]. This phenomenon has been referred to as a "refractory period" of protection against EIA by an intense warm-up; it has been shown to last as long as 2 hours. This effect may be different between individuals and in the same individual on different days, so it should not be the sole form of therapy. Albuterol and other medications noted below are important forms of therapy. Pharmacotherapy is the next step after patient education (Box 2). The drug most commonly chosen for EIA is inhaled albuterol (or another quick-acting beta-agonist) two to four puffs 15 minutes before exercise [11,38]. Other beta-agonists

---

Box 1. Exercise-induced asthma symptoms (during or after exercise)

Typical symptoms
- Wheezing
- Coughing
- Chest congestion
- Chest tightness
- Shortness of breath

Atypical symptoms
- Side ache
- Headache
- Fatigue
- Cramps

Box 2. Stepwise treatment of exercise-induced asthma

If the history, physical examination, and spirometry are consistent with EIA:

Empiric trial of albuterol MDI two puffs 15 minutes before exercise

If albuterol is not preventing symptoms:

Add four puffs Intal 15 minutes before exercise.

If symptoms are still present:

Consider exercise challenge, methacholine challenge, rhinolaryngoscopy, etc.
Add daily ICS, LTRA, LABA, Theo.
Trial of ipratropium three puffs before exercise

If additional medications have not improved the EIA:

Refer to an exercise asthma specialty center.

---

include metaproterenol (Alupent), pirbuterol (MaxAir), and formoterol (Foradil). If the beta-agonist does not prevent the EIA, then the patient should be evaluated again, and other diagnoses might be considered. If EIA is still the primary diagnosis, then four to eight puffs of cromolyn (Intal) or nedocromil (Tilade) should be added before exercise along with the beta-agonist. If this does not prevent the problem, then daily anti-asthmatic therapy should be initiated in combination with pretreatment. Another option that may be tried before daily therapy is the use of anticholinergic inhalers before exercise. There are no well-documented data on these, but an empiric trial of ipratropium (Atrovent) or tiotropium (Spiriva) may be considered. When daily anti-asthmatic therapy is necessary, consider the usual controller therapy used for persistent asthma. Daily controller medication can be used alone or in combination: (1) inhaled corticosteroids: budesonide (Pulmicort), triamcinolone (Azmacort), fluticasone (Flovent), flunisolide (AeroBid); (2) leukotriene receptor antagonist: zafirlukast (Accolate) or montelukast (Singulair); (3) long-acting beta-agonists: formoterol (Foradil) and salmeterol (Serevent); (4) or oral theophyllines (Uniphyl, Theo-24) [39–45]. The best stepwise approach to treatment is to add the inhaled steroids first and make sure the patient keeps taking the usual pre-exercise treatment. At this step, the patient is being put on long-term controller therapy on a daily basis to help prevent EIA; this is similar to treatment chronic asthma in the sense that the medications are increased if the asthma is not controlled, but here we are looking for control and prevention of EIA rather than control of spontaneous asthma symptoms. If inhaled steroids are not adequate as the daily add-on therapy, then add leukotriene receptor antagonists or long-acting beta-agonists. The only potential drawback to daily long-acting beta-agonists is the possibility of tachyphylaxis, with lower effectiveness after chronic usage [46]. Because Advair is a combination of salmeterol and fluticasone, it has the potential for tachyphylaxis when used daily, the same potential as salmeterol alone when used as monotherapy.

If daily controller therapy plus exercise pretreatment does not prevent EIA, then the physician needs to question the diagnosis and whether the patient is taking the medications properly. Proper medication use includes compliance with the dosing schedule and proper inhaler technique. It is important to have the patient demonstrate their inhaler technique in person. When metered-dose inhalers are used, it may be beneficial to use a spacer device along with the inhaler to improve coordination and drug deposition.

If the patient is not responding to the above-mentioned medications, then other diagnoses need to be investigated, including vocal cord dysfunction (VCD), cardiac arrhythmias, right to left shunts (pulmonary or cardiac), idiopathic arterial hypoxemia of exercise, cystic fibrosis, etc.

VCD is one of the more common conditions mimicking EIA (Box 3) [47]. This occurs when the vocal cords paradoxically adduct during inspiration rather than opening wide as they should. This produces an extrathoracic airway obstruction and therefore would not necessarily show any abnormalities on standard spirometric values. The diagnosis should be considered if multiple-flow volume curves with expiratory and inspiratory loops show truncated inspiratory segments of the flow volume curve. This is evidence of extrathoracic obstruction and may represent VCD. It is preferable to try to obtain these when the patient is having symptoms. If this is not diagnostic, then rhinolaryngoscopy before and

---

Box 3. Possible signs and symptoms of exercise-induced vocal cord dysfunction

- Tightness, wheezing, and a choking sensation localized to the larynx/neck area
- Symptoms usually beginning within minutes of exercise
- Stridor after exercise; stridorous sounds noted by auscultation over larynx
- Flattened expiratory and inspiratory loop of the flow volume curve when symptomatic
- Poor response to pre-exercise albuterol or other medications for EIA

after exercise should be done to obtain direct visualization of the vocal cords to see if they paradoxically adduct on inspiration. Rundell [29] reported that VCD may be identified in athletes if they have symptoms of inspiratory stridor during exercise and physical examination findings that note inspiratory stridor by auscultation over the larynx. If VCD is not the diagnosis, then further evaluation should be performed, such as a CT of the chest and a full metabolic exercise challenge with methacholine testing before and after exercise, rhinolaryngoscopy before and after exercise, bubble echocardiogram after exercise, and monitoring of arterial oxygenation, heart rate, and exhaled CO_2 during and after exercise. These studies help identify right to left shunts (pulmonary or cardiac), cardiac arrhythmias, and other diseases.

Future and emerging therapies

Symbicort, an inhaled controller medication, is a combination of budesonide (an inhaled steroid) and formoterol (a quick-onset, long-acting beta-agonist). This product is similar to Advair except for the fact that it is quick acting as compared with the slow onset of effects of the salmeterol in Advair. Phosphodiesterase-4 inhibitors roflumilast (Daxas) and cilomulast (Aeroflo) have potential efficacy in EIA, but studies have not been performed. Inhaled low-molecular-weight heparin may be available in the future [47]. Studies done with this chemical partially block EIA. The research was done with enoxaparin, a low-molecular-weight fraction of heparin. Further studies are required before this product is used.

A number of studies have looked at food supplements and dietary changes to try to improve symptoms of EIA. Mickleborough [48] evaluated 10 elite athletes with EIA and 10 control elite athletes without EIA. They performed a randomized, double blind, crossover study with dietary changes. The test material was fish oil capsules, and the placebo capsule was olive oil. The subjects took this dietary supplement daily for 3 weeks. The authors found that the fish oil supplement did not change the pre-exercise pulmonary function values, but, in subjects with EIA, it improved the postexercise pulmonary function compared with placebo. FEV_1 decreased 14% on the placebo diet and 3% on the diet supplemented with fish oil. The authors suggest that dietary fish oil sup-plementation has a protective effect in suppressing EIA in elite athletes.

Doping

Doping in athletics is defined as the use of any substance, product, or device that improves the performance of the athlete and potentially gives an unfair advantage. In the case of athletes with asthma, this includes certain oral and inhaled medications. Although physicians may not consider some of these pro-ducts to be performance enhancing, the International Olympic Committee (IOC) Medical Commission has identified certain medications that are prohibited and others that require special exemptions. A new organization, the World Anti-Doping Agency (WADA), has been formed to deal with these issues (www.wada-ama.org). The United States has its own anti-doping agency that works in conjunction with the WADA—the US Anti-Doping Agency (www.usantidoping.org). Some of the sports national governing bodies have separate rules and separate forms that athletes have to complete for participation that may be different from the IOC and USOC lists and forms. Examples of this are the National Collegiate Athletic Association and the International Skating Union. The physician has the responsibility of making sure that the athlete is not prescribed any prohibited substances and is responsible for completing the appropriate medical forms required for participation. These forms need to be filed long before the competition begins.

For asthma, oral beta-agonists and systemic steroids are banned, and only certain beta-agonists are allowed (see the WADA web site for details), but they are approved only with filing of a therapeutic use exemption form. Nasal steroids and inhaled steroids are allowed, but only with an exemption. The prescribing physician should review the prohibited substances and complete the appropriate forms for the athlete. The forms should be given to the athlete and faxed to the anti-doping agency. The WADA web site lists the various products that are prohibited.

Summary

EIA is a relatively common condition that frequently is unrecognized, especially in school children and competitive athletes. The symptoms are easily confused with "being out of shape." The health care provider can be helpful to his patients by having an inquiring mind and taking a good history regarding respiratory symptoms associated with exercise. The treatment of EIA is usually simple—two puffs of albuterol before exercise. When this does not work, multiple medications may be required to prevent the EIA. It is not unusual for competitive elite athletes to require multiple daily medications because of their frequent exercise. If EIA is not easily treated, then other conditions should be investigated, such as vocal cord dysfunction, cardiac arrhythmias, and right to left shunts.

References

[1] Hallstrand TS, Curtis JR, Koepsell TD, et al. Effectiveness of screening examinations to detect unrecognized exercise-induced bronchoconstriction. J Pediatr 2002;141:343–9.
[2] Rupp NT, Brudno DS, Guill MF. The value of screening for risk of exercise-induced asthma in high school athletes. Ann Allergy 1993;70:339–42.
[3] Weiler JM. Asthma in United States Olympic athletes who participated in the 1996 Summer Games. J Allergy Clin Immunol 1998;102:722–6.

[4] Thole RT, Sallis RE, Rubin AL, et al. Exercise-induced bronchospasm prevalence in collegiate cross-country runners. Med Sci Sports Exerc 2001;33:1641–6.

[5] Mannix ET, Farber MO, Palange P, et al. Exercise-induced asthma in figure skaters. Chest 1996;109:312–5.

[6] Leuppi JD, Kuhn M, Comminot C, et al. High prevalence of bronchial hyperresponsiveness and asthma in ice hockey players. Eur Respir J 1998;12:13–6.

[7] Weiler JM, Ryan EJ. Asthma in United States Olympic athletes who participated in the 1998 Olympic Winter Games. J Allergy Clin Immunol 2000;106:267–71.

[8] Anderson SD, Fitch K, Perry C, et al. Responses to bronchial challenge submitted for approval to use inhaled beta agonists before an event at the 2002 Winter Olympics. J Allergy Clin Immunol 2003;11:45–50.

[9] Wilber RL, Rundell KW, Szmedra L, et al. Incidence of exercise-induced bronchospasm in Olympic winter sport athletes. Med Sci Sports Exerc 2000;32:732–7.

[10] Anderson SD. The mechanism of exercise-induced asthma. J Allergy Clin Immunol 2000; 106:453–9.

[11] Storms W. Review of exercise-induced asthma. Med Sci Sports Exerc 2003;35:1464–70.

[12] Anderson SD, Argyros J, Magnussen H, et al. Provocation by eucapnic voluntary hyperpnoea to identify exercise-induced bronchoconstriction. Br J Sports Med 2001;35:344–7.

[13] McFadden ER, Gilbert IA. Vascular responses and thermally induced asthma. In: Holgate ST, Austen KF, Lichtenstein AM, Kay AB, editors. Asthma: physiology, immunopharmacology and treatment. San Diego: Academic Press; 1993. p. 337–55.

[14] McFadden ER, Gilbert IA. Vascular responses and thermally induced asthma. In: Holgate ST, Austen KF, Lichtenstein AM, Kay AB, editors. Asthma: physiology, immunopharmacology and treatment. San Diego: Academic Press; 1993. p. 337–55.

[15] Sue-Chu M, Karjalainen E-M, Laitinen A, et al. Placebo-controlled study of inhaled Budesonide on indices of airway inflammation in bronchoalveolar lavage fluid and bronchial biopsies in cross-country skiers. Respiration (Herrlisheim) 2000;67:417–25.

[16] Karjalainen E, Laitnen A, Sue-Chu M, et al. Evidence of airway inflammation and remodeling in ski athletes with and without bronchial hyperresponsiveness to methacholine. Am J Respir Crit Care Med 2000;161:2086–91.

[17] Rundell K, Anderson S, Spiering B, et al. Field exercise vs. laboratory eucapnic voluntary hyperventilation to identify airway hyperresponsiveness in elite cold weather athletes. Chest 2004;125:909–15.

[18] Gauvreau GM, Ronnen GM, Watson RM, et al. Exercise-induced bronchoconstriction does not cause eosinophilic airway inflammation or airway hyperresponsiveness in subjects with asthma. Am J Respir Crit Care Med 2000;162:1302–7.

[19] Kanazawa H, Asai K, Hirata K, et al. Vascular involvement in exercise-induced airway narrowing in patients with bronchial asthma. Chest 2002;122:166–70.

[20] Kotaru C, Coreno A, Skowronski M, et al. Exhaled nitric oxide and thermally induced asthma. Am J Respir Crit Care Med 2000;161:383–8.

[21] Scollo M, Zanconato S, Ongaro R, et al. Exhaled nitric oxide and exercised-induced bronchoconstriction in asthmatic children. Am J Respir Crit Care Med 1999;160:1047–50.

[22] Terada A, Fujisawa T, Togashi K, et al. Exhaled nitric oxide decreases during exercise-induced bronchoconstriction in children with asthma. Am J Respir Crit Care Med 2001;164:1879–84.

[23] Vizi É, Husár E, Csoma Z, et al. Plasma adenosine concentration increases during exercise: a possible contributing factor in exercise-induced bronchoconstriction in asthma. J Allergy Clin Immunol 2002;109:446–8.

[24] Chhabra SK, Ojha UC. Late asthmatic response in exercise-induced asthma. Ann Allergy Asthma Immunol 1998;80:323–7.

[25] Helenius I, Rytila P, Sarna S, et al. Effect of continuing or finishing high-level sports on airway inflammation, bronchial hyperresponsiveness, and asthma: a 5-year prospective follow-up study of 42 highly trained swimmers. J Allergy Clin Immunol 2002;109:962–8.

[26] Thole RT, Sallis RE, Rubin AL, et al. Exercise-induced bronchospasm prevalence in collegiate cross-country runners. Med Sci Sports Exerc 2001;33:1641–6.

[27] Rundell KW, Im J, Mayers B, et al. Self-reported symptoms and exercise-induced asthma in the elite athlete. Med Sci Sports Exerc 2001;33:208–13.

[28] Feinstein RA, Hains CS, Hemstreet MP, et al. A simple "step-test" protocol for identifying suspected unrecognized exercise-induced asthma (EIA) in children. Allergy Asthma Proc 1999;20:181–8.

[29] Rundell KW, Wilber RL, Szmedra L, et al. Exercise-induced asthma screening of elite athletes; field versus laboratory exercise challenge. Med Sci Sports Exerc 1999;32:309–16.

[30] Anderson SD, Lambert S, Brannan JD, et al. Laboratory protocol for exercise asthma to evaluate salbutamol given by two devices. Med Sci Sports Exerc 2001;33:893–900.

[31] Eliasson AH, Phillips YY, Rajogopal KR, et al. Sensitivity and specificity of bronchial provocation testing: an evaluation of four techniques in exercise-induced bronchospasm. Chest 1992;102:347–55.

[32] Holtzer K, Anderson SD, Chan H-K, et al. Mannitol as a challenge test to identify exercise-induced bronchoconstriction in elite athletes. Am J Respir Crit Care Med 2003;167:534–7.

[33] Rundell K, Spiering B, Evans T, et al. Baseline lung function, exercise-induced bronchoconstriction, and asthma-like symptoms in elite women ice hockey players. Med Sci Sports Exerc 2004;36:405–10.

[34] Koskela H, Hyvarinen L, Brannan J, et al. Sensitivity and validity of three bronchial provocation tests to demonstrate the effect of inhaled corticosteroids in asthma. Chest 2003;124:1341–9.

[35] Holzer K, Anderson SD, Douglass J. Exercise in summer athletes: challenges for diagnosis. J Allergy Clin Immunol 2002;110:374–80.

[36] Katelaris H, Carrozzi FM, Burke TV, et al. A springtime Olympics demands special consideration for allergic athletes. J Allergy Clin Immunol 2000;106:260–6.

[37] McKenzie DC, McLuckie SL, Stirling DR. The protective effects of continuous and interval exercise in athletes with exercise-induced asthma. Med Sci Sports Exerc 1994;26:951–6.

[38] Ferrari M, Balestreri F, Baratieri S, et al. Evidence of the rapid protective effect of formoterol dry-powder inhalation against exercise-induced bronchospasm in athletes with asthma. Respiration (Herrlisheim) 2000;67:510–3.

[39] Jonasson G, Carlsen K-H, Hultquist C. Low-dose budesonide improves exercise-induced bronchospasm in school children. Pediatr Allergy Immunol 2000;11:120–5.

[40] Vidal C, Fernández-Ovide E, Piñeiro J, et al. Comparison of montelukast versus budesonide in the treatment of exercise-induced bronchoconstriction. Ann Allergy Asthma Immunol 2001;86:655–8.

[41] Coreno A, Skowronski M, Kotaru C, et al. Comparative effects of long-acting B_2-agonists, leukotriene receptor antagonists, and a 5-lipoxygenase inhibitor on exercise-induced asthma. J Allergy Clin Immunol 2000;106:500–6.

[42] Edelman JM, Turpin JA, Bronsky EA, et al. Oral montelukast compared with inhaled salmeterol to prevent exercise-induced bronchoconstriction. Ann Intern Med 2000;132:97–104.

[43] Bronsky EA, Pearlman DS, Pobiner BF, et al. Prevention of exercise-induced bronchospasm in pediatric asthma patients: a comparison of two salmeterol powder delivery devices. Pediatrics 1999;104:501–5.

[44] Ferrari M, Balestreri F, Baratieri S, et al. Evidence of the rapid protective effect of formoterol dry-powder inhalation against exercise-induced bronchospasm in athletes with asthma. Respiration (Herrlisheim) 2000;67:510–3.

[45] Iikura Y, Hashimoto K, Akasawa A, et al. Serum theophylline concentration levels and preventative effects on exercise-induced asthma. Clin Exp Allergy 1996;26:38–41.

[46] Expert panel report 2: guidelines for the diagnosis and management of asthma. Bethesda (MD): National Institutes of Health; 1997. Pub. No. 98-4051.

[47] Ahmed T, Gonzalez BJ, Danta I. Prevention of exercise-induced bronchoconstriction by inhaled low-molecular-weight heparin. Am J Respir Crit Care Med 1999;160:576–81.

[48] Mickleborough T, Murray R, Ionescu A, et al. Fish oil supplementation reduces severity of exercise-induced bronchoconstriction in elite athletes. Am J Respir Crit Care Med 2003;168: 1181–9.

ELSEVIER
SAUNDERS

Immunol Allergy Clin N Am
25 (2005) 45–66

IMMUNOLOGY
AND ALLERGY
CLINICS
OF NORTH AMERICA

Infectious triggers of asthma

Ana L. MacDowell, MD, Leonard B. Bacharier, MD*

*Department of Pediatrics, Division of Allergy and Pulmonary Medicine,
Washington University School of Medicine and St. Louis Children's Hospital,
One Children's Place, St. Louis, MO 63110, USA*

The rise in the incidence of atopic disease, including asthma, over the past several decades has not been limited to a particular geographic area and has occurred in developed and developing countries. Several factors influence the development and severity of asthma, including atopy, environmental exposures, genetic predisposition, gene–environment interactions, stress, obesity, diet, socio-economic status, and infection. The "Hygiene Hypothesis" [1,2] has focused attention on the role of infection in the development of allergic disease. This hypothesis suggests that infections in early life can have a protective effect on the development of asthma and atopy. Other researchers have suggested, however, that infection may be a cause for the onset and persistence of asthma. In this "Hit and Run Hypothesis," a pathogen promotes dysregulation of the immune system, leading to prolonged inflammatory responses even after the pathogen has been cleared [3]. Thus, the role of infectious agents in the development of asthma is complex: Evidence implicates infections as causal and protective with respect to asthma development.

In addition to the potential role of infection in the inception of asthma, infection has been implicated as the most common precipitant of asthma exacerbations. Several clinical observations have indicated that most asthma episodes are precipitated by factors other than allergen exposure. Many asthma episodes are preceded by upper respiratory tract symptoms and may last several days to weeks, in contrast with allergen-induced asthma exacerbations, where exposure often leads to a rapid onset of symptoms with a recovery time of approximately 24 hours [4,5]. Infections have been linked to asthma exacerbations since the 1950s, and over the past several decades there has been extensive investigation

* Corresponding author.
E-mail address: Bacharier_L@kids.wustl.edu (L.B. Bacharier).

0889-8561/05/$ – see front matter © 2005 Elsevier Inc. All rights reserved.
doi:10.1016/j.iac.2004.09.011

of infectious agents as they relate to asthma development and exacerbations. In this article, we examine infections as triggers of asthma, with a focus on asthma exacerbations.

Epidemiology of respiratory infections leading to asthma exacerbations

Respiratory tract infections (RTIs) are the most common cause of acute illness in adults and children, with upper respiratory infections (URIs) constituting the majority of such illnesses [6]. Adults typically experience two to four URIs per year, and children may have up to 12 URIs per year [7]. RTIs are the major cause of visits to primary care physicians [8] and are associated with significant work and school absenteeism, with an estimated 150 million lost workdays annually. Consequently, RTIs have great economic impact, with an estimated cost of $40 billion annually in the United States [9]. Numerous viruses produce URIs (Table 1), and because the symptom patterns are common between many viruses, it is difficult to determine clinically the specific viral etiology of an acute illness (Table 2).

Viral infections commonly trigger asthma exacerbations, having been noted in nearly half of asthma exacerbations in adults [10] and in an even greater percentage of exacerbations in children. This was demonstrated in a 13-month study investigating the role of viral infections in asthma exacerbations in 114 children 9 to 11 years of age with asthma [11]. Peak expiratory flow (PEF) rate was performed twice daily, and upper and lower respiratory tract symptoms were recorded daily. Virologic samples were obtained within 48 hours of an increase in upper or lower respiratory symptoms, a fall in PEF by more than 50 L/min from the child's baseline, or if the parent subjectively felt that the child was developing a cold. Evidence of a viral infection was detected in 80% to 85% of episodes with respiratory tract symptoms, fall in PEF, or both. The highest detection rate occurred during reported episodes of wheeze, cough, and upper respiratory tract symptoms, together with a decline in PEF. In addition, the severity of a respiratory illness may influence the outcome of a URI because more severe viral infections seem more likely than mild infections to lead to exacerbations of asthma [5]. Viral infection has been noted more often during severe exacerbations of asthma than during milder exacerbations [12].

The advent of more sensitive diagnostic tools to detect specific infectious pathogens, such as detection of microbial DNA or RNA using the polymerase chain reaction (PCR), has strengthened the evidence for viruses as a primary triggering factor in asthma exacerbations [13]. A recent study confirmed a significant increase in the weighted average viral identification in patients of all ages with asthma exacerbation in studies that used PCR when compared with the pre-PCR studies [14]. The same study suggests that viral recovery occurs more often in asthmatic patients who are having an acute exacerbation than in asymptomatic asthmatics or nonasthmatic individuals.

Table 1
Characteristics of infectious agents associated with asthma exacerbations

Pathogen	Family	Type	Number of serotypes	Seasonality	Frequency of cause of common cold in adults [6]
Rhinovirus	Picornaviridae	RNA virus	100+	Year round with fall and spring peaks	45%
Coronavirus	Coronaviridae	Enveloped RNA virus	3	Year round with winter peak. Summer outbreaks have been described.	25%
Influenza virus	Orthomyxoviridae	Enveloped RNA virus	3	Annual epidemic in winter in temperate climates. In tropical climates there may be multiple outbreaks.	14%
Adenovirus	Adenoviridae	Double-stranded, non-enveloped DNA virus	49	Sporadic. Epidemics and endemic disease are more prevalent in the late winter, spring, and summer.	5%
Parainfluenza virus	Paramyxoviridae	Enveloped RNA virus	4	Winter peaks for Parainfluenza 1 and 2; summer peaks for Parainflunza 3	5%
Respiratory syncytial virus	Paramyxoviridae, but lacks neuraminidase and hemagglutinin surface glycoproteins	Enveloped RNA virus	2 (A and B)	Epidemics are mainly in winter and early spring but may be sporadic throughout the year.	1%
Human metapneumovirus	Paramyxoviridae	RNA virus	2	It was initially thought that epidemics occurred between December and April; however, it has been extended to all year round.	Unknown
Mycoplasma pneumoniae	Smallest free-living microorganisms		1	Pleomorphic and ubiquitous in animals and plants; prone to outbreaks throughout the world, at any season	
Chlamydia pneumoniae	Antigenically, genetically, and morphologically distinct from other Chlamydia species. A new name has been proposed: Chlamydophila pneumoniae	All isolates seem to be closely related serologically.	1	Worldwide distribution, with no evidence of seasonality or known animal reservoir	

Table 2
Clinical characteristic of infectious agents triggering asthma

Pathogen	Clinical symptoms	Mode of transmission	Specific immunity
Rhinovirus	Most common virus causing upper respiratory illnesses (40% to 50%)	Person-to-person contact	Some type-specific immunity; of variable degree and brief duration; generally offers little protection against other serotypes
Coronavirus	A common cause of URI in adults and children; also implicated in lower respiratory tract infections. The superficial layers of the nasal mucosa temperature (32°–33°C) yields optimal growth.	Person-to-person via aerosol or fomites	Cellular and humoral immunity are required for virus clearance. Re-infections seem to occur throughout life (implying multiple serotypes [at least four are known] or antigenic variation).
Influenza virus	Systemic involvement differentiates from other viral illness, with fever being almost always present. The onset is abrupt with marked malaise and myalgias.	Person-to-person via droplets, direct contact or contaminated nasopharyngeal secretions	Specific antibodies confer immunity. Antigenic serotypes (A, B, and C) are subclassified by the presence of two surface antigens, hemaglutinin (HA) and neuroaminidase (NA). Antigenic shifts are determined by major changes in HA or NA with emergence of new virus strains, leading to epidemics or pandemics. Antigenic drifts are minor changes with variations within subtype, continuously resulting on variant viruses and leading to seasonal epidemics.
Adenovirus	Adenovirus most commonly causes respiratory illness, but, depending on the infecting serotype, other illnesses may occur; half of infections are asymptomatic.	Via respiratory secretions through person-to-person contact or via the oral-fecal route	There is a worldwide distribution, with a higher prevalence in developing countries and in lower socioeconomic groups. Generally, by school age, most children have been exposed to various serotypes.
Parainfluenza virus	Major cause of laryngotracheobronchitis (croup). Commonly causes URI, pneumonia, and bronchiolitis. Exacerbates symptoms of chronic lung disease.	Person-to-person via direct contact or contaminated nasopharyngeal secretions through respiratory tract droplets and fomites	Reinfection usually causes a mild illness limited to the upper respiratory tract. Most people have exposure to all serotypes by 5 y of age.

Respiratory syncytial virus	Causes acute respiratory illness in patients of all ages. It is the most common cause of bronchiolitis and pneumonia in infants.	Humans are the only source of infection. Transmission occurs by direct or close contact with contaminated secretions. Good hygiene habits are important because the virus may persist in environmental surfaces for many hours and on the hands for 30 min or more.	Almost 100% of children are infected with RSV by 2 y of age.
Human metapneumovirus	Varied — includes cough, coryza, fever, irritability, anorexia, wheezing, pharyngitis, vomiting, or diarrhea	Unknown	By 5 y of age nearly 100% individuals have been infected
Mycoplasma pneumoniae	Most commonly causes respiratory illnesses such as acute bronchitis, including pharyngitis, and occasionally otitis media, which may be bullous. Ten percent of infected individuals develop pneumonia within a few days that may last for 3–4 wk.	Causes disease only in humans; it is highly transmissible by droplets. The long incubation period (ranging from 1–4 wk) along with long asymptomatic carriage (for weeks to months) facilitates familial spread, which may continue for months.	Epidemics occur every 4–7 y because immunity is not long lasting.
Chlamydia pneumoniae	Responsible for a variety of respiratory diseases including pneumonia, acute bronchitis, and, less commonly, pharyngitis, laryngitis, otitis media, and sinusitis. Many infected patients are asymptomatic or mild to moderately ill. A prolonged illness may be present with cough persisting for 2–6 wk, sometimes with a biphasic course.	Assumed transmission is person-to-person, via infected respiratory secretions.	Recurrent infection is common, especially in adults. In tropical, less-developed areas, infection seems to occur earlier in life. In the United States, 50% of adults have antibodies by 20 y of age, with initial infection peaking between 5 and 15 y of age.

Another important observation that links viral infection with asthma exacerbation is the seasonal pattern of distribution of viral infections and asthma exacerbations, especially severe cases requiring hospitalization. In a 2-year study comparing asthma exacerbations due to seasonal allergens, other environmental triggers, and viral infections, a strong relationship was found between the seasonal incidence of asthma and viral infection, although there was no correlation with pollen and spore counts [15]. Similarly, viral infections were the major identifiable risk factor for autumnal asthma exacerbations [16].

In addition to viral infections, RTIs with atypical organisms, such as *Mycoplasma pneumoniae* and *Chlamydia pneumoniae*, precipitate a significant proportion of acute episodes of wheezing, contribute to the severity and persistence of asthma, and may serve as the initial insult that leads to development of asthma [17–19].

Specific infectious agents associated with asthma exacerbations

Rhinovirus

Human rhinovirus (RV) causes nearly half of all upper respiratory illnesses. Although RV infection was initially believed to be limited to the upper airways [20], lower airway epithelial RV infection has been demonstrated [21]. Although infection of the lower respiratory tract may occur, the mechanisms through which viral infections, including RV, provoke asthma are unclear but may include direct extension of upper RTIs to the lower respiratory tract. The mechanism may be indirect and involve effects on airway responsiveness independent of the direct epithelial damage and inflammation associated with lower RTIs (LRTIs). RV infection can enhance the immediate and late-phase responses to allergen [22], potentially augmenting the allergic inflammation within the airway and precipitating asthma exacerbations.

RV infection can lead to profound exacerbation of asthma and is responsible for the majority of hospitalizations for childhood asthma, although less so in adults [20]. RV infections are associated with declines in lung function in asthmatics compared with normal subjects within 2 days after development of a RV infection [23]. RV infection augments airways hyper-responsiveness 4 days after experimental RV infection, an effect that was more pronounced in those with a severe cold [24]. The rise in airways hyper-responsiveness was accompanied by an increase in nasal interleukin (IL)-8 in the RV-infected group at days 2 and 9; the increase in nasal IL-8 at day 2 correlated significantly with the change in airway responsiveness at day 4.

Coronavirus

Coronavirus is the second most common virus associated with asthma episodes in children and adults. Infections due to coronavirus may be associated with less severe lower respiratory tract symptoms than infections with other viruses. This is suggested by the finding that coronavirus-associated asthma episodes in asthmatic school-age children were associated with smaller median declines in PEF (56 L/min) compared with episodes triggered by other viruses (85.5 L/min) [11]. In a study of elderly adults, coronavirus was associated with lower respiratory illness in more than 40% of patients, and one quarter of patients consulted a medical practitioner and received antibiotics. More impressive was the observation that coronavirus infection produced a greater disease burden value than influenza or respiratory syncytial virus [25].

Influenza virus

Influenza virus triggers asthma exacerbations in all age groups [11,26]. In addition, asthmatic individuals seem to be more susceptible to death associated with influenza infections, as observed in the Asian pandemic in 1957 [27]. The time course of influenza-induced asthma exacerbations was examined retrospectively in 20 asthmatic children 8 to 12 years of age with acute respiratory symptoms [28]. Fifteen of 20 patients had decreases in FEV_1 >20% from baseline during the acute stage, beginning from onset of symptoms in all but one subject, whose FEV_1 decreased during the incubation period. FEV_1 decreased maximally on the second day of illness by an average of 30%. Improvement began on the third day, and FEV_1 returned to within 10% of normal between the seventh and tenth day.

Adenovirus

The rate of adenoviral infection declines with age until 9 years and then increases. The exception to this pattern is infection with serotype 7, whose infection rate increases with age [29]. Infection is frequently associated with wheezing, as demonstrated in a retrospective chart review study [30] where wheezing was noted in 58.3% of nonasthmatic children under 2 years of age admitted to an intensive care unit with adenoviral acute LRTI. In this study, the mortality rate was 16.7%, generally in the setting of infection with adenoviral serotype 7. Adenoviral infection has been demonstrated during acute asthma episodes, but the frequency of adenoviral infection is substantially lower that the frequency for rhinovirus and coronavirus [31].

Latent adenoviral infection may have a role in the genesis of asthma. Furthermore, adenoviral shedding may be prolonged, lasting up to 906 days. When nasopharyngeal swabs from 50 asymptomatic asthmatic children and 20 healthy control subjects were examined by PCR, adenovirus DNA was found in 78.4% of asthmatic children, compared with only 5% of healthy control subjects [32]. Adenovirus has been recovered from bronchoalveolar lavage (BAL) in children with asthma 12 months or more after acute infection [33]. In this study, BAL was performed in 34 children (mean age of 5 years) with unfavorable responses to standard corticosteroid and bronchodilator therapy. Adenoviral antigens were detected in BAL fluid (BALF) from 94% of subjects. Repeat studies within 1 year showed that six of eight subjects were positive for adenovirus on two occasions and that three were positive when sampled three times. Cultures of the BALF were positive for adenovirus in all cultures performed, indicating that the virus was capable of replication. Similar studies performed in control patients without persistent asthma failed to detect evidence of adenovirus.

Respiratory syncytial virus

Respiratory syncytial virus (RSV) infects almost 100% of children by 2 years of age and is the most common cause of bronchiolitis and pneumonia in infants [34]. In addition to causing acute LRTI, RSV serves as a trigger for exacerbations of asthma and other chronic lung diseases.

Infants who experience severe RSV bronchiolitis seem to have increased frequencies of wheeze and asthma later in life. A comparison of several retrospective studies of children admitted for bronchiolitis found that the post-bronchiolitis group had a significantly higher frequency of bronchial obstructive symptoms 2 to 10 years later and, when pulmonary function studies were performed, diminished FEV_1 or increased bronchial reactivity compared with healthy control subjects [35]. These findings were confirmed in a prospective study when children hospitalized with confirmed RSV bronchiolitis were evaluated at 7.5 years of age and compared with age- and gender-matched control subjects [36]. By 7.5 years of age, the cumulative prevalence of asthma was 30% in the RSV group versus 3% in the control group, and current asthma was present in 23% of the RSV group versus 2% of the control group. However, the duration of the effect of RSV infection on asthma-related symptoms appears to be limited. In a prospective study of 1246 children enrolled at birth, 207 developed an RSV LTRI not requiring hospitalization during the first 3 years of life [37]. When compared with a control group of children with no LRTI documented during the first 3 years of life, the group with mild RSV LRTI had a substantially increased risk of frequent wheeze at 6 years of age (odds ratio [OR] 4.3), and the risk for frequent wheeze remained significantly increased at 11 years of age (OR 2.4), at which time prebronchodilator FEV_1, but not postbronchodilator FEV_1, was significantly lower in the RSV group. By age 13 years, there were no significant between-group differences in terms of increased risk for frequent or infrequent wheezing. These studies demonstrate that RSV bronchiolitis is a significant independent risk factor for subsequent frequent wheezing, although this effect seems to decrease with age and may be dependent upon the severity of the RSV infection.

Similar to adenoviral infection, the persistence of RSV may underlie in part the sequelae of severe RSV disease. Infection may lead to alteration in the patterns of local interferon, chemokine, and cytokine production [38], potentially leading to chronic inflammation [39]. Furthermore, the age at first viral infection may direct the pattern of disease later in life by generating a Th2-biased memory response to RSV, which may direct responses to other antigens in the lung toward an allergic phenotype. This is suggested by a study in which mice infected with RSV at different ages (1, 7, 28, or 56 days) demonstrated stronger Th2 responses in the group primed at the youngest age when reinfected with RSV at 12 weeks of age [40].

Parainfluenza virus

The parainfluenza viruses (PIV) cause a spectrum of respiratory illness similar to that caused by RSV but result in fewer hospitalizations [41,42]. Most illnesses are limited to the upper respiratory tract [41], although approximately 15% involve the lower respiratory tract, and 2.8 of every 1000 children with such infections required hospitalization [42]. Although less common than RV or coronavirus infection, PIV was detected in 14% of episodes of increased symptoms or decreased PEF in school-aged children [11]. More frequent and severe wheezing has been correlated with elevated levels of IgE antibody to RSV and PIV in nasal secretions of children with bronchiolitis due to RSV and PIV [43].

Human metapneumovirus

Human metapneumovirus (hMPV) was identified in 2001 in respiratory samples from children with respiratory disease in the Netherlands [44]. The clinical symptoms experienced by infected individuals are diverse and may consist of upper or lower respiratory tract symptoms ranging from otitis media to bronchiolitis, croup, pneumonia, and possibly exacerbations of asthma [45]. hMPV is responsible worldwide for community-acquired acute RTIs affecting children and other age groups, with a mean age of illness of 11.6 months and a male predominance (male/female ratio 1.8:1). The broad epidemic seasonality and the evidence of genetic variability suggest that there may be more than one serotype of hMPV [44].

Wheezing is part of the clinical symptomatology associated with hMPV infection. More than half of otherwise healthy children presenting with acute respiratory illness and evidence of hMPV infection experienced wheezing in one study [45]. In series of 19 children with evidence of hMPV infection, bronchiolitis was the most common diagnosis, and 50% of patients had wheezing [46]. Both of these studies evaluated specimens collected from previously healthy children during an acute respiratory illness during which no other pathogen was identified and detected evidence of hMPV in 6.4% [46] and 20% [45] of the previously negative samples.

Although hMPV infection is often accompanied by wheezing, there have been conflicting reports linking hMPV infections and asthma exacerbations [47,48]. Nevertheless, bronchiolitis is a common cause for hospitalization, and given the increasing hospitalization rates over the past two decades [49], it is possible that hMPV may be responsible for a portion of hospitalizations in children with bronchiolitis and wheezing unrelated to RSV infection [46]. Furthermore, co-infection with RSV and hMPV may augment the severity of bronchiolitis [47].

M pneumoniae *and* C pneumoniae

Initial evidence suggested that infection with *M pneumoniae* and *C pneumoniae* was associated with asthma chronicity. Several case reports suggest associations between infections with atypical organisms with decreased expiratory flow rates and increased airway hyper-responsiveness in nonasthmatic individuals [50] and the onset of asthma symptoms in previously healthy nonasthmatic adults [51,52]. Most of these individuals present with complaints of malaise, shortness of breath of gradual onset, and wheezing, which typically resolve after treatment with macrolide antibiotics or oral corticosteroids [51]. Symptoms may progress and persist, as illustrated by an adult male with fever, severe cough, shortness of breath, consolidation on chest radiograph, and evidence of *M pneumoniae* infection based on a rise in serum antibody titers who subsequently developed wheezing episodes with reversible airway obstruction and airway reactivity to methacholine [52]. Infections with these organisms can persist for months, and animal studies show that *M pneumoniae* can be detected by PCR for up to 200 days after infection, even though the animals become antibody and culture negative by 70 days [53]. These reports suggest that *M pneumoniae* may serve as a cause of acute wheezing and a triggering factor for the onset of asthma.

The most comprehensive evaluation of the role of *M pneumoniae* and *C pneumoniae* infections in patients with chronic asthma evaluated 55 adult patients with chronic asthma and 11 control subjects by using PCR, culture, and serology to detect *M pneumoniae* species, *C pneumoniae* species, and viruses from the nasopharynx, lung, and blood [54]. Fifty-six percent of the asthmatic patients had positive PCR studies for *M pneumoniae* ($n = 25$) or *C pneumoniae* ($n = 7$), which were mainly found in BALF or biopsy samples. Only 1 of 11 control subjects had a positive PCR finding for *M pneumoniae*. Cultures for these organisms were negative in all patients. A distinguishing feature between PCR-positive and PCR-negative patients was a significantly greater number of tissue mast cells in the group of patients who were PCR positive.

Of additional significance is the link of atypical infectious organisms with asthma exacerbations. In a serologically based prospective study, 100 adult patients hospitalized with exacerbations of asthma were compared with hospitalized surgical patients with no history of lung disease at any time or URI in the month before admission [55]. In this series, *M pneumoniae* was identified more often than any other pathogen in the asthmatic group (18 *M pneumoniae*, eight *C pneumoniae*, 11 Influenza A, five Influenza B, three PIV-1, two PIV-2, one PIV-3, six adenovirus, two RSV, three *S. pneumoniae*, and five *Legionella* spp.) and in the control group (three *M pneumoniae*). However, only 8 of the 18 patients had *M pneumoniae* identified as the sole infectious agent, making it difficult to ascertain the culpability of *M pneumoniae* as the cause of hospitalization. A study of 71 children with acute wheezing and 80 age-matched healthy children detected *M pneumoniae* in 22.5% and *C pneumoniae* in 15.5% of children with wheezing compared with 7.5% and 2.5%, respectively, in healthy control subjects [56]. When the children who were infected with either organism were treated with clarithromycin, improvement in the course of the disease was observed, further supporting the role of these atypical organisms in the exacerbation of asthma. These findings were recently confirmed in a French series, where *M pneumoniae* infection was found in 20% and *C pneumoniae* infection was found in 3.4% of children during an acute asthma exacerbation [19]. Acute *M pneumoniae* infection was confirmed in 50% and *C pneumoniae* in 8.3% of patients experiencing their first wheezing episode. Further studies are needed to confirm the association between infection and asthma exacerbation, to determine the prevalence of such infections in patients with acute exacerbations of asthma, and to examine if infection with these organisms modifies the severity of the exacerbation or the response to therapy.

Phenotypes of wheezing associated with respiratory tract infections

Viral-induced wheeze (VIW) is characterized by brief episodes of lower respiratory symptoms and decreased pulmonary function in the setting of an acute viral URI, interspersed with longer asymptomatic periods with normal pulmonary function [11,57]. This differs from classic childhood asthma, which is characterized by chronic symptoms, with atopy being a major risk factor [58]. Classic asthma and VIW were considered two different entities until 1969, when a report suggested that the two groups have similar characteristics [59] and benefited similarly from the same prophylactic treatment [60]. In the 1990s, there was a division of the wheezing phenotypes, especially in children [58]. Patients with VIW alone seem to outgrow the symptoms by age 6; however, in some patients, the pattern of VIW may continue into adulthood with less severe symptoms, negative methacholine challenges, and pulmonary functions that remain normal [61]. The inability to reliably differentiate between VIW and asthma, especially in young children, complicates the evaluation of the influence of viral infections on exacerbations of wheezing. Furthermore, this heterogeneity in wheezing phenotypes has implications in terms of the efficacy of therapies used to treat such episodes.

Immunopathology and mechanism of disease

Viruses typically enter the body through contact with mucosal surfaces. The cell-specific distribution of viral receptors determines the viral tropism. Once the viral particles are internalized, nucleic acids are released, and transcription and production of viral proteins starts. The viral genome is replicated, and virions are released, propagating the infection. The immune system is activated through several mechanisms when a viral infection is noted: (1) through cell surface receptor (ie, EBV activates B cells by stimulating CD21), (2) viral proteins may interact with intracellular proteins and signaling molecules activating the host cell, and (3) activation of epithelial cells leading to production of cytokines (interferon [IFN]-α and -β) and chemokines (IL-8; RANTES; MIP-1, -2, and -3; and MCP-3). This culminates in the generation of responses in an attempt to control infection.

One of the earliest responses to viral infection is the production of IFNs by different cell types; IFN-α is produced by leukocytes, IFN-β is produced by fibroblasts, and INF-γ is produced by Th1 cells and natural killer (NK) cells. IFNs induce transcription of many genes, including two with direct antiviral activity, and lead to increased expression of MHC class I and II genes. Interferons are potent activators of antiviral effector cells such as NK cells, CD8 T lymphocytes, and macrophages.

Although the inflammatory process generated by virus infection is generally viewed as a TH1 pattern with a predominance of interferons, especially INF-γ, in atopy there is a predominance of the TH2 cytokine profile. However, viral infections promote increased cytokine-mediated inflammation through direct induction of specific cytokines produced by different viral agents [62]. The ability of certain pathogens to stimulate the production of TH2 cytokines [63] may explain why certain pathogens are more strongly associated with asthma exacerbation than others.

Viruses have been implicated in the inception of asthma because viral infections with a propensity for lower airway involvement during infancy have been associated with chronic lower respiratory tract symptoms and asthma [64]. This seems to be particularly relevant to RSV bronchiolitis, which has been demonstrated to be a significant independent risk factor for subsequent frequent wheezing [37]. The sequelae of severe RSV disease could be explained in part by viral persistence [39]. This has been supported by a recent study demonstrating the persistence of viral genomic and messenger RNA in lung homogenates of BALB/c mice up to 100 days post RSV infection, whereas virus could no longer be detected in BALF after day 14 post-infection [65].

Another possible mechanism by which a virus could promote asthma is by generating changes in patterns of pro-inflammatory cytokine production, which could facilitate virus persistence, as demonstrated with RSV [38]. Viral infection may exert direct effects on airway cells. An increase in the production of IL-10 by nonspecifically stimulated peripheral blood mononuclear cells during acute and convalescent phases of RSV infection requiring hospitalization has been demonstrated [66]. In animal studies, it was suggested that IL-10 may have a direct effect in airway smooth muscle and in the regulation of airway tone [67].

Although there is evidence supporting the role of viral infections in the development of asthma, further investigation is necessary to confirm this hypothesis because the mechanisms that could allow persistency or latency of viral infection are poorly understood.

Interactions between infectious agents and allergy

It has been hypothesized that asthmatic individuals have increased susceptibility to viral infections. Some researchers have found an increased incidence of viral infections in asthmatic children when compared with nonasthmatics [14,26], a pattern that could be explained by the increased expression of ICAM-1, the receptor for RV, in asthmatics subjects [68]. However, this finding was not confirmed in a study that followed cohabitating couples consisting of an atopic asthmatic and a healthy nonatopic, nonasthmatic individual [23]. In this study, subjects completed daily diary cards of upper and lower respiratory tract symptoms and measured PEF twice daily. Nasal aspirates were taken and examined for rhinovirus every 2 weeks. Rhinovirus was detected in 10.1% of samples from the asthmatics and 8.5% of samples from the nonasthmatic participants. After adjustment for confounding factors, asthma did not significantly increase the risk of infection with rhinovirus in asthmatic individuals (OR 1.15).

The effect of atopic status on the rate of viral infection is unclear; evidence exists suggesting no difference between the rate of viral infection between atopic and nonatopic individuals [69] or an even lower rate of viral infections among atopic individuals [15,70], although these studies did not have adequate statistical power to confirm this trend. There is an increased risk of acute wheezing when atopy is combined with viral infection when compared with atopy or virus infection alone [70], and infants with a family history of atopy seem more likely to develop bronchiolitis with a higher rate of hospitalization [71].

Even if asthmatics do not experience more frequent infections than nonasthmatics, it is possible that asthmatics have a higher incidence of symptoms when experiencing viral infections. During rhinoviral infection, there is a greater incidence of symptoms in asthmatics compared with nonasthmatics [72]. This is further suggested by a report that asthmatics experienced seroconversion to influenza A virus at the time of asthma exacerbation even in the absence of signs of respiratory infection [5].

Although there is evidence supporting the role of infection in the genesis of asthma and allergy, a protective effect of infections in the development of atopy has also been postulated. An inverse relationship between infection and allergy was first noted when a study comparing white families with Native Americans reported that IgE levels and the prevalences of asthma and eczema were higher in the white population, whereas helminthic, viral, and bacterial infections were more prevalent in the Native Americans [1]. It was observed that increased family size, often associated with more frequent infections in early childhood, had an inverse relationship with the prevalence of allergic rhinitis [2] and asthma [73]. This was further supported by studies reporting an inverse relationship between the age of day care entry and the diagnosis of asthma [74,75]. One potential explanation for this pattern is that at birth there is a predominant TH2 response, and, as exposure to infections occurs, there is a gradual shift toward a TH1-dominant response. However, if the skewing of the immune response to TH1, which regulates response to viral infection, is impaired, a TH2 response would predominate, favoring the development of allergy. Ex vivo studies have shown that asthmatics exposed to viral infections lack the capacity to mount a strong TH1 response [76,77].

Treatment

There is no clinically effective treatment for the common cold. As the mechanisms of viral-induced wheezing and asthma are elucidated, new forms of treatment may emerge. The involvement of many inflammatory pathways suggests that antiviral and anti-inflammatory therapies have potential roles for intervention after onset of symptoms; however, a combination of both therapeutic approaches may have the greatest impact. Prophylaxis for the acquisition of viral infections, in the form of vaccination or pharmacologic therapy, offers the best hope of disease control.

The major obstacle for treatment is the wide variety of organisms associated with URIs, including viral and bacterial agents (Table 2). In addition, accurate and timely diagnosis is essential for the appropriate targeting of specific anti-infective therapies. The rapid rate of mutation of viruses leads to the emergence of resistant strains. In addition, there are difficulties with the delivery, expense, and efficacy of drugs [78]. Treatment for viral RTIs remains symptomatic, although future approaches will likely be directed toward reducing the inflammatory response elicited by the virus.

Vaccination remains the mainstay of prophylaxis against infections. However, with the exception of influenza, vaccine development for respiratory viruses has been slow and disappointing. Influenza vaccine contains three strains (two A and one B) of inactivated virus, one or two of which are modified yearly based upon predictions of the upcoming viral strains. They are produced in embryonated hen eggs and are highly immunogenic, conferring protection in 70% to 80% of the vaccine recipients with minimal adverse effects. Whole-cell influenza vaccine is no longer available, and the current vaccines consist of subvirion (prepared by disrupting the lipid membrane) or purified surface antigen. Recently, a live-attenuated, cold-adapted, trivalent, intranasal influenza vaccine (FluMist) has been introduced, but it is contraindicated in asthmatics [79].

A long-standing concern that influenza vaccination may trigger exacerbations of asthma was addressed in a multicenter, randomized, double-blind, placebo-controlled, crossover trial in 2032 patients with asthma (age range 3–64 years). This study confirmed the safety of the influenza vaccine in asthmatics by demonstrating that the frequency of exacerbations of asthma was similar in the 2 weeks after vaccination with the active influenza vaccine or placebo (28.8% and 27.7%, respectively) [80].

Although yearly influenza vaccination is recommended as a routine element of asthma management [81], a recent study generated concern about the usefulness of influenza vaccine in preventing influenza-related asthma exacerbations. This randomized, double-blind, placebo-controlled trial showed that the number, severity, and duration of influenza-related asthma exacerbation was similar between the group receiving influenza vaccination and the group receiving placebo over the course of one influenza virus season [82]. Vaccinated children tended to have shorter exacerbations (by approximately 3 days) than nonvaccinated children.

Antiviral therapy targets the source of infection directly, decreasing the number of infectious agents and therefore reducing inflammatory process. The only licensed antiviral therapies are directed against influenza A (amantadine and rimantadine), influenza A and B (zanamivir and oseltamivir), and RSV (ribavirin). The neuraminidase inhibitors, zanamivir and oseltamivir, have an advantage over adamantanes, amantadine, and rimantadine because they have a broader spectrum and are effective against the A and B strains of influenza virus. The inhibition of neuraminidase, whose active site consists of 11 amino acids conserved in all naturally occurring influenza virus [83], prevent cleavage of sialic acid from newly acquired membrane, leaving emerging virus inactive and thereby decreasing infectivity [84]. Both neuraminidase inhibitors improve respiratory outcomes in patients with asthma and acute influenza infections [78] and have the added benefit of being effective in the prophylaxis against influenza infections [85]. Although it is generally well tolerated, there are case reports of bronchospasm after treatment with inhaled zanamivir [86]; however, it is difficult to separate these symptoms from the effects of the influenza infection. The disadvantage of current antiviral therapy is the specificity for influenza and the need for initiation of treatment within 48 hours of onset of infection. The toxicity profile of ribavirin, approved for use in severe RSV infections, limits its clinical use except in settings of severe illness in immunocompromised hosts.

Antibiotic use is appropriate if there is evidence of bacterial infection contributing to asthma exacerbations, although pyogenic lung infections rarely exacerbate asthma and are rarely associated with wheezing. Although some macrolide antibiotics have been reported to have antiviral effects in vitro against rhinoviruses [87], these effects have not been confirmed in vivo, and a recent Cochrane review does not support the use of antibiotics for the treatment of the common cold [88]. The anti-inflammatory effects of macrolide antibiotics are not limited to their ability to interfere with corticosteroid metabolism [89], as evidenced by inhibition of the neutrophil oxidative burst [90], reduction of cytokine formation [91], and reduction of ICAM-1 production [92]. Asthmatic patients infected with *M pneumoniae* or *C pneumoniae* may benefit from prolonged treatment with clarithromycin, as evidenced by significant improvement in FEV_1 [18,93]. Furthermore, in a double-blind, randomized, crossover study, 17 patients with stable mild or moderate asthma not evaluated for *M pneumoniae* or *C pneumoniae* received 200 mg of clarithromycin or placebo twice daily for 8 weeks. Methacholine responsiveness improved in all the patients after 8 weeks of clarithromycin treatment [94]. Improvement in airway hyperresponsiveness after 8 weeks of clarithromycin treatment was confirmed in a group of patients with asthma receiving concomitant therapy with inhaled corticosteroids who were not selected on the basis of infection with *M pneumoniae* or *C pneumoniae* [95]. It remains unclear as to the mechanism by which macrolide antibiotics improve airway hyper-responsiveness in patients with asthma, but possibilities may include treatment of occult or chronic infection, interference with steroid metabolism, or the anti-inflammatory properties of this class of antimicrobials.

Although there are international guidelines for the management of asthma [81,96], there is a relative paucity of evidence regarding therapeutic strategies specifically for VIW in asthmatics or healthy subjects. Because most acute exacerbations of asthma are induced by viral infections and because many forms of asthma therapy, especially inhaled corticosteroids, reduce the frequency and severity of exacerbations, one would presume that the current treatment for chronic asthma would be efficacious in preventing VIW. However, the varying phenotypes of wheezing, especially in childhood, seem to respond differently to such management approaches. This is particularly true for RSV-associated wheezing, which does not consistently respond to medications often used to treat asthma exacerbations, including bronchodilators and corticosteroids [97]. Thus, despite the efficacy of inhaled corticosteroids in the control of asthma and reduction of exacerbations, patients continue to experience exacerbations, particularly in the setting of viral RTIs.

Several treatment approaches have been investigated in an attempt to reduce the morbidity associated with wheezing associated with RTIs. Brunette et al [98] examined the effect of a short course of oral corticosteroid administered in an unblinded manner at onset of URI symptoms in a group of children with histories of recurrent wheezing in the setting of viral infections. Over a 1-year period, the group receiving oral corticosteroids at the early signs of RTIs experienced reductions in the frequencies of wheezing, emergency room visits, and hospitalizations. However, a recent double-blind, placebo-controlled trial evaluating the use of parent-initiated oral corticosteroids at the early signs of an episode of presumed viral-induced wheezing did not detect a difference between oral corticosteroid therapy and placebo in terms of symptom scores and rate of hospitalization [99]. Thus, the role for the use of oral corticosteroids at the early signs of illness in children with recurrent viral wheezing is unclear, and additional investigation is required to determine the efficacy of this approach in the management and attenuation of wheezing episodes.

The repeated use of systemic corticosteroids for such episodes remains a clinical concern. Given the efficacy of inhaled corticosteroids (ICS) in the daily management of asthma and their favorable safety profile when compared with systemic corticosteroids, the use of ICS in the management of VIW has been explored. Although ICS are effective in the management of persistent asthma, current evidence suggests a lack of efficacy in the regular use of ICS in patients with mild VIW [100,101]. A recent meta-analysis concluded that the use of ICS episodically for viral-triggered wheezing in children not using them as maintenance may decrease the rate of oral corticosteroid requirement [101]. In patients receiving daily ICS therapy, the common clinical practice of doubling the dose of ICS at the onset of an asthma exacerbation has been shown to be ineffective in preventing symptom progression [102]. However, a recent study in adults demonstrated the valuable effects of quadrupling the ICS dose with acute asthma exacerbations [103]. These data suggest that corticosteroids, taken orally or inhaled, may be used as treatment and preventive therapy for asthma exacerbations in the setting of RTIs.

The cysteinyl leukotrienes (cysLTs) have been identified as important mediators in the complex pathophysiology of asthma. CysLTs are detectable in the blood, urine, nasal secretions, sputum, and BALF of patients with chronic asthma. Elevated cysLTs have been detected in respiratory secretion of children with viral induced wheezing [104]. Similar to elevated levels in asthmatics, 20 infants with prolonged or persistent wheeze (mean 14.9 months) and a history of viral illness at wheeze onset had significant elevations of leukotrienes in BAL despite the fact that 12 of 20 infants were receiving daily ICS therapy (≤ 450 μg/d) [105]. These findings suggest that, similar to asthma pathophysiology, cysLTs play a role in the pathophysiology of viral-induced wheeze. Additionally, based on the above study, the cysLTs are not fully suppressed by the preferred standard anti-inflammatory therapy, inhaled corticosteroids. Thus, antagonism of the effects of cysLT using the leukotriene receptor antagonists may provide clinical benefit to patients with VIW.

The relative efficacies of these intervention strategies aimed at reduction of wheezing and asthma in the setting of RTIs depend upon the wheezing phenotype and probably the timing of the initiation of therapy. Investigation of other therapeutic approaches to VIW is ongoing and may provide insight as to the optimal treatment approach for this challenging condition.

Summary

Infections have been implicated in asthma exacerbations and in the inception of asthma. Several studies support the concept that viruses and atypical infectious agents may induce asthma exacerbations and contribute to the chronicity of asthma. The further elucidation of the mechanisms that underlie the interaction between infectious agents and asthma will lead to improvements in treatment and prevention of such exacerbations. Studies are needed to explore the vast domain of infectious triggered asthma exacerbations.

References

[1] Gerrard J, Geddes C, Regin P, et al. Serum IgE levels in white and metis communities in Saskatchewan. Ann Allergy 1976;37:91–100.
[2] Strachan D. Hay fever, hygiene, and household size. BMJ 1989;299:1259–60.
[3] Walter MJ, Morton JD, Kajiwara N, et al. Viral induction of a chronic asthma phenotype and genetic segregation from the acute response. J Clin Invest 2002;110:165–75.
[4] Mertsola J, Ziegler T, Ruuskanen O, et al. Recurrent wheezy bronchitis and viral respiratory infections. Arch Dis Child 1991;66:124–9.

[5] Roldaan A, Masural N. Viral respiratory infections in asthamtic children staying in a mountain resort. Eur J Respir Dis 1982;63:140–50.

[6] Myint S. Microbiology and epidemiology of upper respiratory tract infections. In: Johnson SL, Papadopoulos NG, editors. Respiratory infections in allergy and asthma. 1st edition. New York: Marcel Decker; 2003. p. 13–41.

[7] Monto AS, Sullivan KM. Acute respiratory illness in the community: frequency of illness and the agents involved. Epidemiol Infect 1993;110:145–60.

[8] Davey P, Rutherford D, Graham B, et al. Repeat consultations after antibiotic prescribing for respiratory infection: a study in one general practice. Br J Gen Pract 1994;44:509–13.

[9] Fendrick AM, Monto AS, Nightengale B, et al. The economic burden of non-influenza-related viral respiratory tract infection in the United States. Arch Intern Med 2003;163:487–94.

[10] Nicholson KG, Kent J, Hammersley V, et al. Risk factors for lower respiratory complications of rhinovirus infections in elderly people living in the community: prospective cohort study. BMJ 1996;313:1119–23.

[11] Johnston SL, Pattemore PK, Sanderson G, et al. Community study of role of viral infections in exacerbations of asthma in 9–11 year old children. BMJ 1995;310:1225–9.

[12] Beasley R, Coleman E, Hermon Y, et al. Viral respiratory tract infections and exacerbations of asthma in adult patients. Thorax 1988;43:679–83.

[13] Pattermore P, Johnston S, Bardin P. Viruses as precipitants of asthma symptoms. I: epidemiology. Clin Exp Allergy 1992;22:325–36.

[14] Pattermore P. Epidemiology and diagnosis of virus-induced asthma. In: Johnston S, Papadopoulos N, editors. Respiratory infections in allergy and asthma. New York: Marcel Dekker; 2003. p. 43–89.

[15] Carlsen K, Orstavik I, Leegard J, et al. Respiratory virus infections and aeroallergens in acute bronchial asthma. Arch Dis Child 1984;59:310–5.

[16] Dales R, Schweitzer I, Toogood J, et al. Respiratory infections and the autumn increase in asthma morbidity. Eur Respir J 1996;9:72–7.

[17] Cunningham AF, Johnston SL, Julious SA, et al. Chronic Chlamydia pneumoniae infection and asthma exacerbations in children. Eur Respir J 1998;11:345–9.

[18] Kraft M, Cassell GH, Henson JE, et al. Detection of Mycoplasma pneumoniae in the airways of adults with chronic asthma. Am J Respir Crit Care Med 1998;158:998–1001.

[19] Biscardi S, Lorrot M, Marc E, et al. Mycoplasma pneumoniae and asthma in children. Clin Infect Dis 2004;38:1341–6.

[20] Johnston S, Holgate S. Epidemiology of viral respiratory tract infections. In: Myint S, Taylor-Robinson D, editors. Viral and other infections of the human respiratory tract. London: Chapman & Hall; 1996. p. 1–38.

[21] Papadopoulos NG, Bates PJ, Bardin PG, et al. Rhinoviruses infect the lower airways. J Infect Dis 2000;181:1875–84.

[22] Lemanske Jr RF, Dick EC, Swenson CA, et al. Rhinovirus upper respiratory infection increases airway hyperreactivity and late asthmatic reactions. J Clin Invest 1989;83:1–10.

[23] Corne JM, Marshall C, Smith S, et al. Frequency, severity, and duration of rhinovirus infections in asthmatic and non-asthmatic individuals: a longitudinal cohort study. Lancet 2002;359:831–4.

[24] Grunberg K, Timmers MC, Smits HH, et al. Effect of experimental rhinovirus 16 colds on airway hyperresponsiveness to histamine and interleukin-8 in nasal lavage in asthmatic subjects in vivo. Clin Exp Allergy 1997;27:36–45.

[25] Nicholson K, Kent J, Hammersley V, et al. Acute viral infections of upper respiratory tract in the elderly people living in the community: comparative, prospective, population based study of disease burden. BMJ 1997;315:1060–4.

[26] Minor T, Dick E, DeMeo A, et al. Viruses as precipitants of asthmatic attacks in children. JAMA 1974;227:292–8.

[27] Quarles van Ufford W, Savelberg P. Asiatic influenza in allergic patients with bronchial asthma. Int Arch Allergy Appl Immunol 1959;227:292–8.

[28] Kondo S, Abe K. The effects of influenza virus infection on FEV1 in asthmatic children: the time-course study. Chest 1991;100:1235–8.

[29] Fox J, Hall C, Cooney M. The Seattle Virus Watch. VIII: observations of adenovirus infections. Am J Epidemiol 1977;105:362–86.

[30] Carballal G, Videla C, Misirlian A, et al. Adenovirus type 7 associated with severe and fatal acute lower respiratory infections in Argentine children. BMC Pediatr 2002;2:6–12.

[31] Tan WC, Xiang X, Qiu D, et al. Epidemiology of respiratory viruses in patients hospitalized with near-fatal asthma, acute exacerbations of asthma, or chronic obstructive pulmonary disease. Am J Med 2003;115:272–7.

[32] Marin J, Jeler-Kacar D, Levstek V, et al. Persistence of viruses in upper respiratory tract of children with asthma. J Infect 2000;41:69–72.

[33] Macek V, Sorli J, Kopriva S, et al. Persistent adenoviral infection and chronic airway obstruction in children. Am Rev Respir Dis 1994;150:7–10.

[34] Mufson M, Levine H, Wasil R, et al. Epidemiology of respiratory syncytial virus infection among infants and children in Chicago. Am J Epidemiol 1973;98:88–95.

[35] Sigurs N. Epidemiologic and clinical evidence of a respiratory syncytial virus-reactive airway disease link. Am J Respir Crit Care Med 2001;163:S2–6.

[36] Sigurs N, Bjarnason R, Sigurbergsson F, et al. Respiratory syncytial virus bronchiolitis in infancy is an important risk factor for asthma and allergy at age 7. Am J Respir Crit Care Med 2000;161:1501–7.

[37] Stein RT, Sherrill D, Morgan WJ, et al. Respiratory syncytial virus in early life and risk of wheeze and allergy by age 13 years. Lancet 1999;354:541–5.

[38] Guerrero-Plata A, Ortega E, Gomez B. Persistence of respiratory syncytial virus in macrophages alters phagocytosis and pro-inflammatory cytokine production. Viral Immunol 2001;14:19–30.

[39] Southern P, Oldstone MB. Medical consequences of persistent viral infection. N Engl J Med 1986;314:359–67.

[40] Culley FJ, Pollott J, Openshaw PJ. Age at first viral infection determines the pattern of T cell-mediated disease during reinfection in adulthood. J Exp Med 2002;196:1381–6.

[41] Knott AM, Long CE, Hall CB. Parainfluenza viral infections in pediatric outpatients: seasonal patterns and clinical characteristics. Pediatr Infect Dis J 1994;13:269–73.

[42] Reed G, Jewett PH, Thompson J, et al. Epidemiology and clinical impact of parainfluenza virus infections in otherwise healthy infants and young children < 5 years old. J Infect Dis 1997;175:807–13.

[43] Welliver RC. Immunologic mechanisms of virus-induced wheezing and asthma. J Pediatr 1999;135:14–20.

[44] Van den Hoogen B, De Jong J, Groen J, et al. A newly discovered human pneumovirus isolated from young children with respiratory tract disease. Nat Med 2001;7:719–24.

[45] Williams J, Harris P, Tollefson S, et al. Human metapneumovirus and lower respiratory tract disease in otherwise healthy infants and children. N Engl J Med 2004;350:443–50.

[46] Esper F, Boucher D, Weibel C, et al. Human metapneumovirus infection in the United States: clinical manifestations associated with a newly emerging respiratory infection in children. Pediatrics 2003;111:1407–10.

[47] Greensill J, McNamara P, Dove W, et al. Human metapneumovirus in severe respiratory syncytial virus bronchiolitis. Emerg Infect Dis 2003;9:372–5.

[48] Rawlinson W, Waliuzzaman Z, Carter I, et al. Astma exacerbations in children associated with rhinovirus but not with human metapneumovirus infections. J Infect Dis 2003;187:1313–8.

[49] Shay D, Holman R, Newman R, et al. Bronchiolitis-associated hospitalizations among US children, 1980–1996. JAMA 1999;282:1440–6.

[50] Sabato AR, Martin AJ, Marmion BP, et al. Mycoplasma pneumoniae: acute illness, antibiotics, and subsequent pulmonary function. Arch Dis Child 1984;59:1034–7.

[51] Shee CD. Wheeze and Mycoplasma pneumoniae. J R Soc Med 2002;95:132–3.

[52] Yano T, Ichikawa Y, Komatu S, et al. Association of Mycoplasma pneumoniae antigen with initial onset of bronchial asthma. Am J Respir Crit Care Med 1994;149:1348–53.

[53] Marmion BP, Williamson J, Worswick DA, et al. Experience with newer techniques for the laboratory detection of Mycoplasma pneumoniae infection: Adelaide, 1978–1992. Clin Infect Dis 1993;17(Suppl 1):S90–9.

[54] Martin RJ, Kraft M, Chu HW, et al. A link between chronic asthma and chronic infection. J Allergy Clin Immunol 2001;107:595–601.

[55] Lieberman D, Printz S, Ben-Yaakov M, et al. Atypical pathogen infection in adults with acute exacerbation of bronchial asthma. Am J Respir Crit Care Med 2003;167:406–10.

[56] Esposito S, Blasi F, Arosio C, et al. Importance of acute Mycoplasma pneumoniae and Chlamydia pneumoniae infections in children with wheezing. Eur Respir J 2000;16:1142–6.

[57] Doull I, Lampe F, Smith S, et al. The effect of inhaled corticosteroid on episodes of viral associated wheezing in school age children. BMJ 1997;315:858–62.

[58] Martinez F, Wright A, Taussig L, et al. Asthma and wheezing in the first six years of life. N Engl J Med 1995;332:133–8.

[59] Williams H, McNicol K. Prevalence, natural history and relationship of wheezy bronchitis and asthma in children: an epidemiologic study. BMJ 1969;iv:321–5.

[60] Speight A, Lee D, Hey E. Underdiagnosis and treatment of asthma in childhood. BMJ 1983;286:1253–6.

[61] Godden D, Ross S, Abdalla M, et al. Outcome of wheeze in childhood: symptoms and pulmonary function 25 years later. Am J Respir Crit Care Med 1994;149:106–12.

[62] Noah T. Cytokine network in virus infection and asthma. In: Johnson SL PN, editor. Respiratory infections in allergy and asthma. New York: Marcel Dekker; 2003. p. 173–97.

[63] Bendelja K, Gagro A, Bace A, et al. Predominant type-2 response in infants with respiratory syncytial virus (RSV) infection demonstrated by cytokine flow cytometry. Clin Exp Immunol 2000;121:332–8.

[64] Castro-Rodriguez JA, Holberg CJ, Wright AL, et al. Association of radiologically ascertained pneumonia before age 3 yr with asthma-like symptoms and pulmonary function during childhood: a prospective study. Am J Respir Crit Care Med 1999;159:1891–7.

[65] Schwarze J, O'Donnell DR, Rohwedder A, et al. Latency and persistence of respiratory syncytial virus despite T cell immunity. Am J Respir Crit Care Med 2004;169:801–5.

[66] Bont L, Heijnen CJ, Kavelaars A, et al. Monocyte IL-10 production during respiratory syncytial virus bronchiolitis is associated with recurrent wheezing in a one-year follow-up study. Am J Respir Crit Care Med 2000;161:1518–23.

[67] Makela MJ, Kanehiro A, Dakhama A, et al. The failure of interleukin-10-deficient mice to develop airway hyperresponsiveness is overcome by respiratory syncytial virus infection in allergen-sensitized/challenged mice. Am J Respir Crit Care Med 2002;165:824–31.

[68] Gern J, Busse W. Association of rhinovirus infection with asthma. Clin Microbiol Rev 1999;12:9–18.

[69] Huhti E, Mokka T, Nikoskelainen J, et al. Association of viral and mycoplasma infections with exacerbations of asthma. Ann Allergy 1974;33:145–9.

[70] Rakes G, Arruda E, Ingram J, et al. Rhinovirus and respiratory syncytial virus in wheezing children requiring emergency care. IgE and eosinophil analyses. Am J Respir Crit Care Med 1999;159:785–90.

[71] Trefny P, Stricker T, Baerlocher C, et al. Family history of atopy and clinical course of RSV infection in ambulatory and hospitalized infants. Pediatr Pulmonol 2000;30:302–6.

[72] Horn M, Gregg I. Role of viral infection and host factors in acute episodes of asthma and chronic bronchiolitis. Chest 1973;63(Suppl):44S–8S.

[73] Rona RJ, Duran-Tauleria E, Chinn S. Family size, atopic disorders in parents, asthma in children, and ethnicity. J Allergy Clin Immunol 1997;99:454–60.

[74] Ball T, Castro-Rodriguez J, Griffith K, et al. Siblings, day care attendance and the risk of asthma and wheezing during childhood. N Engl J Med 2000;343:538–43.

[75] Kramer U, Heinrich J, Wjst M, et al. Age of entry to day nursery and allergy in later childhood. Lancet 1999;353:450–4.

[76] Papadopoulos NG, Stanciu LA, Papi A, et al. A defective type 1 response to rhinovirus in atopic asthma. Thorax 2002;57:328–32.

[77] Gern JE, Vrtis R, Grindle KA, et al. Relationship of upper and lower airway cytokines to outcome of experimental rhinovirus infection. Am J Respir Crit Care Med 2000;162:2226–31.

[78] Creer D, Gelder C, Johnston S. Treatment of common colds. In: Sebastian L, Johnston NGP, editors. Respiratory infections in allergy and asthma. New York: Marcel Dekker; 2003. p. 675–710.

[79] American Academy of Pediatrics Committee on Infectious Diseases. Recommendations for influenza immunization of children. Pediatrics 2004;113:1441–7.

[80] American Lung Associations Asthma Clinical Research Centers. The safety of inactivated influenza vaccine in adults and children with asthma. N Engl J Med 2001;345:1529–36.

[81] National Asthma Education and Prevention Program. Expert Panel Report II: guidelines for the diagnosis and management of asthma. Bethesda (MD): US Department of Health and Human Services; 1997.

[82] Bueving HJ, Bernsen RM, de Jongste JC, et al. Influenza vaccination in children with asthma: randomized double-blind placebo-controlled trial. Am J Respir Crit Care Med 2004; 169:488–93.

[83] Govorkova EA, Leneva IA, Goloubeva OG, et al. Comparison of efficacies of RWJ-270201, zanamivir, and oseltamivir against H5N1, H9N2, and other avian influenza viruses. Antimicrob Agents Chemother 2001;45:2723–32.

[84] Klenk HD, Rott R. The molecular biology of influenza virus pathogenicity. Adv Virus Res 1988;34:247–81.

[85] Hayden F, Gubareva L, Monto A, et al. Inhaled zanamivir for the prevention of influenza in families. Zanamivir Family Study Group. N Engl J Med 2000;343:1282–9.

[86] Williamson J, Pegram P. Respiratory distress associated with zanamivir. N Engl J Med 2000;342:661–2.

[87] Suzuki T, Yamaya M, Sekizawa K, et al. Erythromycin inhibits rhinovirus infection in cultured human tracheal epithelial cells. Am J Respir Crit Care Med 2002;165:1113–8.

[88] Arroll B, Kenealy T. Antibiotics for the common cold. Cochrane Database Syst Rev 2002;3:CD000247.

[89] Shimuzu T, Kato M, Mochizuki H, et al. Roxithromycin reduces the degree of bronchial hyperresponsiveness in children with asthma. Chest 1994;106:458–61.

[90] Anderson R. Erythromycin and roxithromycin potentiate human neutrophil locomotion in vitro by inhibition of leukoattractant activated superoxide generation and autooxidation. J Infect Dis 1989;5:966–72.

[91] Takizawa H, Desaki M, Ohtoshi T, et al. Erythromycin supresses interleukin 6 expression by human bronchial epithelial cells: a potential mechanism of its anti-inflammatory action. Biochem Biophys Res Commun 1995;210:781–6.

[92] Khair O, Devalia J, Abdelaziz M, et al. Effect of erythromycin on Hemophilus influenzae endotoxin-induced release of IL-6, IL-8, and sICAM-1 by cultured human bronchial epithelial cells. Eur Respir J 1995;8:1451–7.

[93] Kraft M, Cassell GH, Pak J, et al. Mycoplasma pneumoniae and Chlamydia pneumoniae in asthma: effect of clarithromycin. Chest 2002;121:1782–8.

[94] Amayasu H, Yoshida S, Ebana S, et al. Clarithromycin suppresses bronchial hyperresponsiveness associated with eosinophilic inflammation in patients with asthma. Ann Allergy Asthma Immunol 2000;84:594–8.

[95] Kostadima E, Tsiodras S, Alexopoulos EI, et al. Clarithromycin reduces the severity of bronchial hyperresponsiveness in patients with asthma. Eur Respir J 2004;23:714–7.

[96] National Heart, Lung, and Blood Institute. Global Initiative for Asthma: global strategy for asthma management and prevention. Bethesda (MD): National Institutes of Health; 2002.

[97] Milner AD. The role of corticosteroids in bronchiolitis and croup. Thorax 1997;52:595–7.

[98] Brunette MG, Lands L, Thibodeau LP. Childhood asthma: prevention of attacks with short-term corticosteroid treatment of upper respiratory tract infection. Pediatrics 1988;81:624–9.

[99] Oommen A, Lambert PC, Grigg J. Efficacy of a short course of parent-initiated oral pred-nisolone for viral wheeze in children aged 1–5 years: randomised controlled trial. Lancet 2003; 362:1433–8.

[100] Wilson N, Sloper K, Silverman M. Effect of continuous treatment with topical corticosteroid on episodic viral wheeze in preschool children. Arch Dis Child 1995;72:317–20.

[101] McKean M, du Charme F. Inhaled steroid for episodic viral wheeze of childhood. In: Review C, editor. Cochrane Library. Oxford: Update Software; 2000.

[102] Garrett J, Williams S, Wong C, Holdaway D. Treatment of acute asthmatic exacerbations with an increased dose of inhaled steroid. Arch Dis Child 1998;79:12–7.

[103] Foresi A, Morelli MC, Catena E. Low-dose budesonide with the addition of an increased dose during exacerbations is effective in long-term asthma control. Chest 2000;117:440–6.

[104] van Schaik SM, Tristram DA, Nagpal IS, et al. Increased production of IFN-gamma and cysteinyl leukotrienes in virus-induced wheezing. J Allergy Clin Immunol 1999;103:630–6.

[105] Krawiec ME, Westcott JY, Chu HW, et al. Persistent wheezing in very young children is asso-ciated with lower respiratory inflammation. Am J Respir Crit Care Med 2001;163:1338–43.

ELSEVIER
SAUNDERS

Immunol Allergy Clin N Am
25 (2005) 67–82

IMMUNOLOGY
AND ALLERGY
CLINICS
OF NORTH AMERICA

Rhinosinusitis and pediatric asthma

Brian A. Smart, MD[a],*, Raymond G. Slavin, MD[b]

[a]*Asthma and Allergy Center, DuPage Medical Group, 454 Pennsylvania Ave. Glen Ellyn,
IL 60137, USA*
[b]*Division of Allergy and Immunology, Saint Louis University School of Medicine,
1402 South Grand Blvd., St. Louis, MO 63104, USA*

Rhinosinusitis, defined as inflammation of the sinus and nasal mucosa, is commonly referred to as sinusitis, but most experts agree that rhinosinusitis is a superior term [1]. Because the sinus and nasal mucosa are contiguous, inflammation with or without infection in the sinuses usually implies inflammation in the nose as well. Furthermore, nasal symptoms such as congestion are also common features of sinusitis. This distinction between rhinosinusitis and sinusitis may seem to be unnecessary, but it points to an important theme: the tremendous influence localized inflammation with or without infection has upon other areas of the body. An excellent example of such a relationship is the influence rhinosinusitis has upon asthma. This article reviews this relationship, with emphasis upon the pediatric population.

Rhinosinusitis is not exclusively a disease of adult patients. Many young physicians in training are taught that infants and small children do not have paranasal sinuses and therefore cannot have sinusitis. This statement is not true. The maxillary and ethmoid sinuses are present at birth and are visible on radiographs during infancy [2]. The frontal sinuses are visible radiographically between 3 and 7 years of age, and the sphenoid sinuses are visible radiographically by 9 years of age [2]. Although these ages are generally useful guidelines for the radiographic presence of the sinuses, there is a great deal of variation between individuals [2]. Therefore, rhinosinusitis needs to be considered even in very young patients who have persistent rhinitis symptoms.

---

* Corresponding author.
E-mail address: Brian.Smart@Dupagemd.com (B.A. Smart).

Diagnosis

Rhinosinusitis is often difficult to diagnose. Acute rhinosinusitis may be suspected if typical upper respiratory infection symptoms, such as nasal congestion and rhinorrhea, do not resolve after 7 to 10 days [3]. Additional symptoms often include purulent nasal discharge, maxillary facial pain, maxillary dental pain, and, sometimes, fever and chills (Box 1) [3]. Acute rhinosinusitis is defined as 3 to 4 weeks of symptoms. If not treated (or sometimes even if appropriately treated), a patient with acute rhinosinusitis may develop chronic rhinosinusitis, which is defined as inflammation of the nasal and paranasal sinus mucosa for at least 12 weeks. Symptoms in chronic rhinosinusitis may be similar to acute rhinosinusitis but often also include purulent postnasal drip, sore throat, foul breath, fatigue, and malaise [3]. Physical examination often reveals edematous and hyperemic nasal mucosa surrounded by purulent mucus [3]. When a patient first presents with these symptoms, most experts empirically treat with 2 to 3 weeks of antibiotics appropriate for the typical flora (*Streptococcus pneumoniae*, *Haemophilus influenzae*, and *Moraxella catarrhalis* in acute rhinosinusitis, add *Pseudomonas aeruginosa*, Group A streptococcus, *Staphylococcus aureus*, and anaerobes such as *Bacteroides* spp., Fusobacteria, and *Propionibacterium acnes* in chronic rhinosinusitis) [4]. Patients with a poor response to management or recurrent rhinosinusitis may be best evaluated with a coronal noncontract sinus CT. The sinus CT is superior to plain films (Water's

---

Box 1. Diagnostic criteria for rhinosinusitis

Major criteria

- Nasal obstruction
- Post-nasal discharge
- Purulent rhinorrhea
- Anosmia or hyposmia
- Pain or pressure over sinuses
- Headache

Minor criteria

- Halitosis
- Fatigue
- Dental pain
- Cough
- Fever
- Ear congestion

---

view) of the sinuses and to MRI for diagnosis and assessment of rhinosinusitis because of the detailed information it provides about soft tissue inflammation, air-fluid levels, obstruction of the ostiomeatal complex, and other structural abnormalities in all of the paranasal sinuses [3].

Chronic rhinosinusitis is often subtle in presentation. For example, in a recent study, 30% of patients with asthma without any symptoms of nasal congestion, headache, facial pain, or hyposmia had extensive sinus disease on sinus CT [5]. Rhinosinusitis is common and should be considered early in patients with persistent upper respiratory symptoms. It affects 14.1% of the population and is the most commonly reported chronic disease in the United States [6]. Rhinosinusitis accounts for 11.6 million physician office visits per year and is the fifth most common reason for the prescription of antibiotics [7].

Mechanisms of development of rhinosinusitis

Various mechanisms have been advanced for the development of rhinosinusitis. The "infectious rhinosinusitis" mechanism involves the development of obstruction of normal drainage from the sinus ostia. This obstruction is created by inflamed tissue in acute viral rhinosinusitis or in allergic rhinitis or by anatomic abnormalities such as polyps and severe deviation of the nasal septum. Obstructed drainage creates stasis of mucus in the paranasal sinuses, which creates an ideal culture media for bacteria. The growth of bacteria promotes further inflammation and creates a self-perpetuating chronic process.

In contrast to infectious rhinosinusitis, the inflammatory rhinosinusitis mechanism states that chronic rhinosinusitis is primarily an inflammatory process with infection usually being a secondary process. Numerous investigators have reported evidence for this inflammatory process. For example, in the presence or absence of demonstrable allergy, TH_2 cytokines typical of an allergic response have been demonstrated in the sinus mucosa in chronic rhinosinusitis. Riccio et al [8] showed, in a group of 20 allergic and 15 nonallergic children with chronic rhinosinusitis and asthma, that the allergic subjects had increased interleukin (IL)-4 and tumor necrosis factor (TNF)-α, with decreased IL-12 and IFN-γ, whereas nonallergic subjects had increased IL-4 and decreased IFN-γ. The similarity between sinus mucosa specimens in allergic and nonallergic patients with chronic rhinosinusitis also extends to the cellular infiltrate. For example, the sinus mucosa of allergic patients with chronic rhinosinusitis contains elevated numbers of eosinophils, T cells, and B cells, whereas in nonallergic patients with chronic rhinosinusitis (who represent the majority of patients with chronic rhinosinusitis) there is prominent infiltration of eosinophils, but numbers of T lymphocytes are not elevated [9]. The eosinophils in the sinus mucosa may create tissue damage, such as epithelial denudation [10]. Bacteria may superinfect areas of damaged sinus mucosa, leading to the purulent discharge, foul breath, and other features typical of chronic rhinosinusitis [11]. This inflammatory model may explain why many patients with chronic sinusitis seem to respond to extended courses of antibiotics only to experience periodic exacerbations of their disease because the underlying disease is difficult to control. The inflammatory model may also explain why surgical treatment of chronic rhinosinusitis, which relieves obstruction, has mixed success because the inflammatory process responsible for the obstruction is not relieved.

Because chronic rhinosinusitis may be described as a primarily infection-driven or as a primarily inflammation-driven process, any relationship between chronic rhinosinusitis and asthma may operate by disparate mechanisms. Because sharp distinctions are artificially drawn between infection-driven and inflammation-driven chronic rhinosinusitis, there is considerable overlap between these two processes. For example, Tosca et al [12] showed, in a group of pediatric patients, a reduction of inflammatory cell numbers in nasal scrapings and a reduction in levels of IL-4 in rhinosinusal lavage 1 month after treatment with antibiotics, nasal corticosteroids, and a 10-day course of oral corticosteroids in allergic and nonallergic patients. This finding suggests that bacterial infection in the sinuses may help create or help perpetuate the TH_2 inflammation that has been described in chronic rhinosinusitis in allergic and nonallergic individuals.

Evidence of the relationship between rhinosinusitis and asthma

There are numerous examples of the relationship between chronic rhinosinusitis and asthma. Evidence for this relationship dates back to the 1920s and 1930s with studies that identified rhinosinusitis as a trigger for asthma [13,14]. More recent examinations of this relationship include a study by Bresciani et al [15], who reported that 100% of severe steroid-dependent patients with asthma had abnormal sinus CT scans, whereas 88% of patients with mild to moderate asthma had abnormal sinus CT scans. A report from Finland found that, in adult patients with asthma exacerbations, 87% had abnormal sinus radiographs [16]. Similarly, a study from the Netherlands showed that 84% of adult patients with severe asthma had abnormalities on sinus CT [5]. This relationship has been demonstrated in the pediatric population in a study that showed that 27% of pediatric patients admitted with status asthmaticus had abnormal sinus radiographs as defined by two thirds or greater opacification of the paranasal sinuses on sinus x-ray [17]. Another recent study has shown that about 50% of children with asthma, examined by endoscopy, have rhinosinusitis [18]. These examples and others point to the strong association between rhinosinusitis and asthma.

Is there a causal relationship (ie, can rhinosinusitis trigger asthma), or is this association an epiphenomenon (ie, are rhinosinusitis and asthma manifestations of the same underlying disease process)? More evidence is needed to fully answer this question, but there are numerous reports that the medical or surgical management of rhinosinusitis improves coexisting asthma. This improvement in asthma after treatment for rhinosinusitis implies a role for rhinosinusitis as a trigger for asthma [3].

Medical management

One way to prove a possible causal relationship between rhinosinusitis and asthma is to demonstrate improvement in asthma after medical treatment of rhinosinusitis. Rachelefsky et al [19] performed such as study in pediatric patients with concomitant rhinosinusitis and asthma. Rhinosinusitis in these patients was identified with sinus radiographs, and asthma was diagnosed by the presence of 3 months or more of respiratory symptoms such as cough or wheeze during the day and at night and abnormal pulmonary function tests. In this study, 79% of children with asthma were able to discontinue bronchodilators after their rhinosinusitis was medically treated. In this same study, pulmonary function tests normalized in 67% of patients treated medically for sinusitis. Similar results were reported by Friedman et al [20], who showed, in a group of pediatric patients with sinusitis and asthma who received medical treatment for sinusitis, improvement in asthma symptoms in the five patients who kept symptom diary cards and improvement in pulmonary function tests in five of the seven patients measured. Another study showed that 54% of 55 children with asthma and abnormal sinus x-rays had improvement in their asthma with antibiotics, and 67% improved with nasal corticosteroids [21]. Richards et al [22] showed that 12 of 15 children with asthma had asthma exacerbations after acute sinusitis as identified by history, physical examination, and sinus x-rays. These patients demonstrated improvement in their asthma after antibiotic treatment. Another group demonstrated, in 18 children with moderate asthma and chronic rhinosinusitis, significant improvement in asthma symptoms and respiratory function 1 month after treatment with antibiotics, nasal corticosteroid, and a 10-day burst of oral steroids [23]. A study of pediatric patients with sinusitis looked at improvement in bronchial hyper-responsiveness [24]. In this study, methacholine challenges were done before and after documented sinusitis was treated with nasal saline; antibiotics, antihistamine, or decongestant; and 5 days of oral steroids. The patients who had opacified maxillary sinuses at entry and who had normal sinus x-rays after 30 days showed a decrease in their sensitivity to methacholine, whereas a control group of patients with rhinitis who received the same treatment but had normal sinus x-rays at entry or patients with abnormal sinus x-rays that did not improve after treatment did not show decreased sensitivity to methacholine. In another study of children with mild asthma, medical treatment of rhinosinusitis resulted in a significant decrease of bronchial hyper-responsiveness to methacholine [25]. An earlier study showed a similar but less impressive outcome after medical treatment of rhinosinusitis [26]. In this study, 42 children with moderate to severe asthma and abnormal sinus x-rays were treated with ampicillin, oral decongestants, and intranasal steroids and showed improvement in asthma symptom scores and a trend toward less bronchial hyper-reactivity but no change in sinus x-rays compared with control subjects. A group from Croatia has recently reported that endosinusal treatment for chronic rhinosinusitis in patients with asthma results in improvement in asthma [27]. In this study, 18 patients with mild to moderate asthma received maxillary endosinusal treatment with dexamethasone and gentamicin for 7 days. Thirty days after treatment, eosinophil cationic protein and tryptase levels were decreased in the serum and sinus lavage fluid, and FEV_1 and subjective sinusitis scores improved. In patients with rhinosinusitis and asthma, specific medical treatment of rhinosinusitis improves asthma.

Surgical management

Surgical management of chronic rhinosinusitis has been shown to result in improvement of lower airway disease. For example, in a recent study, 15 adult patients with chronic rhinosinusitis who required inhaled steroids and at least intermittent oral prednisone to control asthma showed an improvement in asthma symptoms and a decline in total dosage of steroids and number of days of steroid use in the first year post-surgery [28]. Another study showed improvement in asthma symptoms and peak expiratory flow measurements after endoscopic sinus surgery [29]. In a study of 20 patients 16 to 72 age years of with asthma and chronic rhinosinusitis, functional endoscopic sinus surgery (FESS) resulted in an improvement in asthma [30]. After the procedure, 70% had less frequent asthma, and 65% had less severe asthma, with a 75% reduction in hospitalizations and an 81% reduction in acute care visits in the year after the surgery [30]. Another perspective on the relationship between chronic rhinosinusitis and asthma was provided by a study by Okayama et al [31] of 42 patients with chronic rhinosinusitis, 50 patients with stable asthma, 50 patients with chronic bronchitis, and 40 patients with allergic rhinitis in whom bronchial hyper-reactivity (BHR) to methacholine was studied [31]. This study demonstrated that BHR in patients with chronic rhinosinusitis was less than that of patients with asthma but was similar to patients with chronic bronchitis or allergic rhinitis. After endoscopic surgery for chronic rhinosinusitis, the subjects had a significant decrease in BHR and improvement in nasal symptoms and sinus pathology.

Similar improvements after FESS have been shown in pediatric patients with chronic rhinosinusitis and asthma. For example, in a trial of 52 children age 7 months to 17 years, there was an 89% reduction in chronic cough and a 96% decrease in asthma symptoms by retrospective interview an average of 21.8 months after FESS [32]. This study showed a reduction in monthly asthma exacerbations from 6.7 to 2.5 and a 79% reduction in emergency room visits. In study by Manning et al [33], 14 steroid-dependent children with asthma and chronic sinusitis were studied. After FESS, 11 of these children showed improvement in their asthma.

The data supporting an improvement in asthma after sinus surgery have not all been supportive. A study of 50 patients with asthma who had endoscopic surgery for sinusitis demonstrated that only 20% of the patients had a reduction in the amount of inhaled steroids required to control their asthma [34]. However, this same study showed significant decreases in the use of oral steroids and of hospitalizations in the year after the surgery [34]. In a study by Dhong et al [35] of 19 patients who underwent endoscopic surgery for sinusitis, there were significant improvements in diurnal and nocturnal asthma symptoms and in asthma medication scores but no changes in pulmonary function tests. Goldstein et al [36] performed a retrospective analysis of medical records of 13 patients with asthma who underwent FESS for chronic rhinosinusitis and found no significant change in group mean asthma symptoms, the use of asthma medications, pulmonary function test results, number of emergency room visits, or number of hospitalizations.

Although the evidence for improvement in asthma symptoms and pulmonary function after treatment for concomitant rhinosinusitis is more robust for medical than for surgical treatment, rhinosinusitis has a tremendous influence on asthma. It is possible that some of the medical treatment used, such as oral antibiotics and oral steroids, had pulmonary effects. Furthermore, the investigators cited here have used a variety of different definitions of rhinosinusitis and asthma, which creates further confusion in understanding their results. Nonetheless, it seems clear from the weight and variety of studies of medical and surgical treatment of rhinosinusitis that this disease influences asthma independent of other disease processes. Numerous mechanisms for this relationship have been advanced.

Mechanisms for a causal relationship between rhinosinusitis and asthma

Because the medical treatment of rhinosinusitis results in improvement in concomitant asthma, a direct causative relationship between rhinosinusitis and asthma is an attractive idea. There are a number of hypotheses to explain how this relationship might exist (Box 2). One hypothesis is that naso-pharyngo-bronchial reflexes may be involved in the association between upper and lower airways. These naso-bronchial reflexes have been demonstrated in human and animal models after nasal stimulation with a variety of substances, including silica particles, sulfur dioxide, cold air, mechanical irritation, and fumes [37–41]. These reflexes can be blocked by anticholinergics, lidocaine, resection of neural connections, and ganglionic blockade [39–42]. A postulated neuroanatomic pathway that may reflexly connect the paranasal sinuses to the lungs is as follows: receptors in the nose, pharynx, and possibly in the sinuses give rise to afferent fibers that form part of the trigeminal nerve [3]. The trigeminal nerve connects in the brainstem via the reticular formation with the dorsal vagal

---

Box 2. Proposed mechanisms for a causal relationship between rhinosinusitis and asthma

- Naso-pharyngo-bronchial reflexes
- Drainage of inflammatory cells and mediators into the lungs
- Inhalation of dry, cold air and environmental pollutants
- Local upper respiratory inflammation leading to pulmonary inflammation

nucleus, which sends parasympathetic efferent fibers via the vagus nerve to the bronchi [3]. The parasympathetic nervous system plays a role in maintaining bronchial muscle tone and in mediating acute bronchospastic responses [3]. For example, in a study of 106 patients with chronic sinusitis, histamine challenges to the lower airway were performed before and after medical treatment of sinusitis [43]. FEV_1 was measured as an index of bronchial narrowing, and midinspiratory flow was measured as an index of extrabronchial airway narrowing. After medical treatment of sinusitis, intrabronchial and extrabronchial hyperreactivity decreased, with a greater and earlier reduction in extrabronchial hyperreactivity than intrabronchial hyper-reactivity. The changes in intrabronchial and extrabronchial reactivity were strongly associated with pharyngitis, which was diagnosed by history, physical examination, and nasal lavage. Based upon these results, the authors proposed that airway hyper-responsiveness in rhinosinusitis might depend on pharyngo-bronchial reflexes, which are triggered by the drainage of inflammatory mediators and infected material from infected sinuses into the pharynx. These same authors, in a later study, demonstrated damage of the pharyngeal mucosa in patients with chronic rhinosinusitis in the form of epithelial thinning and an increase in pharyngeal nerve fiber density [44]. These findings support a mechanism of increased exposure of submucosal nerve endings to irritants, leading to the release of sensory neuropeptides via axon reflexes with activation of a neural arc, which result in reflex airway constriction. Another study demonstrated that the local stimulation of irritant receptors by inflammatory mediators may trigger bronchospasm [45]. These investigators looked at the fluid obtained from maxillary sinus lavage in patients undergoing surgery for chronic sinusitis compared with the nasal lavage fluid of patients with allergic rhinitis [45]. This study showed that levels of inflammatory mediators, such as leukotrienes, prostaglandin D_2, and histamine, were significantly elevated in patients with chronic rhinosinusitis and were in a range of concentration that was felt to be consistent with local inflammation and the stimulation of irritant receptors [45]. The evidence, therefore, supports a naso-pharyngo-bronchial reflex as one possible mechanism for a causal relationship between infectious chronic rhinosinusitis and asthma.

Another possible mechanism for a causal relationship between infectious chronic rhinosinusitis and asthma is postnasal drip or drainage of inflammatory cells and mediators into the lungs. These inflammatory cells and mediators create increased airway reactivity and inflammation. This possible mechanism is controversial. In 1990, Bardin et al [46] reported that there was no pulmonary aspiration of sinus contents in patients with concomitant asthma and sinusitis. This group showed, after placement of radionuclide into the maxillary sinuses, that the radionuclide was visible over a 24-hour period in the maxillary sinus, nasopharynx, esophagus, and lower gastrointestinal tract but not in the lungs. In contrast to this report, Ozcan et al [47] reported pulmonary aspiration of radionuclide-labeled nasal secretions during sleep. This study included one group of patients with sinusitis and asthma and a healthy control group. There was no difference in degree of aspiration of nasal secretions between the two groups.

Brugman et al [48] used a rabbit model to show, in sterile sinusitis, an increase in airway responsiveness that seemed, based upon the positioning of the animals, to be related to the postnasal drainage of inflammatory cells or mediators into the lower airway. More evidence is needed to support the hypothesis that postnasal drainage triggers asthma.

Abnormal breathing has been advanced as a possible causal link between rhinosinusitis and asthma. Because the nose warms and humidifies air and traps particles, oral breathing may lead to inhalation of dry, cold air and environmental pollutants. Griffin et al [49] demonstrated evidence for such a relationship in patients with asthma. In this study, nine patients with asthma and five healthy control subjects inhaled subfreezing air through their mouths or their noses. In the patients with asthma, there was better warming of air with nasal respiration and a linear relationship between the degree of air cooling and the drop in FEV_1. Although in this study oral inhalation of cold air impaired lung function, this was probably not the cause of these patients' asthma because the normal control subjects showed no decrease in lung function with similar inspiration of cold air.

Another causal relationship between rhinosinusitis and asthma is suggested by recent research that points to the possibility that local upper respiratory inflammation may lead to pulmonary inflammation through a variety of mechanisms. Mechanisms for this relationship include increases in cell adhesion receptors and release of chemotactic factors, leading to release of leukocytes from storage pools in the bone marrow and differentiation of the progenitors of these inflammatory cells into mature inflammatory cells in the bone marrow and locally in inflamed tissues [50]. For example, in a Dutch study, nasal allergen provocation in a group of nonasthmatic patients with allergic rhinitis resulted in an influx of eosinophils into the nasal epithelium, nasal and bronchial lamina propria, and bronchial epithelium [51]. This influx of eosinophils was mediated at least in part by local adhesion molecules because the number of mucosal eosinophils correlated with the local expression of ICAM-1, E-selectin, and VCAM-1 in nasal and bronchial tissue.

Systemic chemokines are released after nasal allergen challenge. For example, in a murine model of allergic rhinitis, specific nasal challenge with allergen promoted a local inflammatory response in the nasal mucosa and increases in eosinophils, basophils, and $CD34^+$ cells (hemopoietic stem cells) in the bone marrow [52,53]. This response was mediated at least in part by the cytokine IL-5 because nasal eosinophilia was blocked and IL-5–responsive leukocytes in the bone marrow were reduced in IL-5–deficient mice [53]. In a study involving nonasthmatic patients with allergic rhinitis, inhaled allergen challenge resulted in an increase in sputum eosinophil cationic protein and a rise in IL-5 in the plasma [54]. In addition to IL-5, granulocyte/macrophage colony-stimulating factor (GM-CSF), and eotaxin are implicated as important mediators of communication between the airways and the bone marrow and systemic circulation [55]. These mediators are not likely to act as hormones but instead exert local effects promoting the differentiation and maturation of eosinophils, basophils, and mast cells [56]. Other cytokines, such as IL-4 and IL-13, recruit inflammatory cells into nasal and sinus tissue [57]. TH$_2$ lymphocytes from the nasal and sinus tissue probably migrate to the bone marrow, where they stimulate the production and maturation of inflammatory cells [57]. It has been demonstrated, for instance, that the numbers of IL-5–producing T cells in the bone marrow increase after inhalation challenge with allergen [58]. The activated inflammatory cells that are produced in the bone marrow may migrate into the pulmonary tissue [57]. It is possible that activated inflammatory cells may migrate from inflamed sinus tissue into the circulation and directly into pulmonary tissue [57].

Although there are numerous possible mechanisms whereby rhinosinusitis may trigger lower airway responses, such as naso-pharyngo-bronchial reflexes, postnasal drainage of inflammatory cells and mediators, abnormal air warming and filtration, and increases in cell adhesion receptors and release of inflammatory cytokines after upper airway allergen challenge, there is a great deal of evidence to support the concept that rhinosinusitis and asthma are simply local manifestations of systemic inflammatory disease. It seems likely that the true nature of the relationship between rhinosinusitis and asthma is not a triggering phenomenon or a systemic disease but is a complex interplay between dynamic local and systemic pathology.

Chronic rhinosinusitis and asthma as manifestations of a single disease

In recent years, there has been growing interest in the "one airway hypothesis," which states that the relationship between upper and lower airway disease is not necessarily causal but reflects common histopathology between the two areas. Ponikau et al [11] recently studied 22 patients with refractory chronic rhinosinusitis to determine if typical histopathologic features of asthma, such as eosinophilic inflammation, epithelial damage, and basement membrane thickening, are present in chronic rhinosinusitis. Sinus specimens from all 22 subjects showed heterogenous eosinophilic inflammation, epithelial shedding, and thickening of the basement membrane. The damage and inflammation were similar in allergic and nonallergic subjects. It is likely that eosinophils were important effectors of the damage because it has been demonstrated that there is an association between the presence of the extracellular deposition of major basic protein (which is produced by eosinophils) and damage to sinus mucosa [59]. These features, which are similar to asthma, suggest a common process underlying at least some types of chronic rhinosinusitis and asthma [3]. An example of this relationship is a study by Harlin et al [10], who examined tissue from the patients undergoing surgery for chronic rhinosinusitis. In this study it was shown that, although sinus tissue from patients with sinusitis and concomitant asthma, allergic rhinitis, or both had a large number of eosinophils infiltrated in the sinus tissue, sinus tissue patients with a history of chronic rhinosinusitis alone did not. Further evidence for the common change in the sinuses and the lungs is the report of 84% of patients with severe asthma with evidence of abnormality on sinus

CT [5]. In this study, there was a significant correlation between CT scores, eosinophils in peripheral blood and induced sputum, and the level of exhaled nitric oxide, which is a marker of lower airway inflammation. An earlier study demonstrated a similar relationship [60]. In this study, 104 patients with asthma who were undergoing sinus surgery had assessment of sinus CT scans, total serum IgE, specific IgE to common inhalant antigens, and peripheral blood eosinophil count. This group found extensive sinus disease in 39% of the patients and showed that the level of disease correlated well with severity of asthma, presence of specific IgE antibodies, and presence of eosinophilia. The researchers found that 87% of patients with extensive sinus disease by CT had peripheral eosinophilia. There is evidence that rhinosinusitis and asthma may be different manifestations of a common disease.

Bone marrow may provide the link that connects upper and lower airway inflammatory disease into "one airway" [50]. Similar to the pathway of local allergen challenge and inflammation in the upper airway stimulating bone marrow to produce inflammatory cells that have effects upon other tissues (such as the lower airways), allergen-induced inflammation in the lower airways can induce upper airway responses [55]. An example of this is provided by Braunstahl et al [61], who studied patients with nonasthmatic allergic rhinitis. After segmental bronchial allergen challenge, an increase was demonstrated in eosinophils, basophils, and IL-5 in nasal tissue, along with increased numbers of eosinophils in the blood [61,62]. Bone marrow, rather than simply being a conduit of cross-talk between different parts of the airway, seems to take an active role as a source of inflammatory cells that can infiltrate various areas of the body that are affected by allergic disease [55]. In support of this view is a report of transfer of allergic disease into nonallergic individuals after bone marrow transplant [63]. One of the mechanisms whereby bone marrow may maintain an active role in creating systemic allergic disease is the creation in bone marrow of progenitor and mature eosinophils and basophils that autostimulate by producing their own growth factors, such as IL-5 and GM-CSF [55].

Redefining chronic rhinosinusitis

One of the weaknesses of research on chronic rhinosinusitis has been the lack of uniform definitions of this disease. This has led to a variety of different techniques being used (eg, flexible rhinoscopy, sinus x-ray, sinus CT) to establish the presence or absence of chronic rhinosinusitis and to follow response to treatments that have not been uniform (eg, antibiotics, nasal corticosteroids, systemic corticosteroids, nasal saline irrigation, and various surgical techniques). Many investigators have limited themselves to radiographic and symptomatic measures to follow response to treatment, whereas other investigators have looked at cellular infiltrates and biochemical features of rhinosinusitis, such as adhesion molecule expression and levels of cytokines. The heterogeneity of definitions and techniques in investigations of chronic rhinosinusitis has led to the tendency to lump together all chronic rhinosinusitis as though it is a single disorder. Steinke and Borish [57], in a recent review, have attempted to divide chronic rhinosinusitis into four different disorders: infectious rhinosinusitis, chronic inflammatory rhinosinusitis, chronic hyperplastic eosinophilic sinusitis, and allergic fungal sinusitis (Table 1).

According to the definitions of Steinke and Borish [57], infectious rhinosinusitis and chronic inflammatory rhinosinusitis are related to infectious processes. Chronic inflammatory rhinosinusitis represents the smallest subset of patients with chronic rhinosinusitis and typically involves patients with impaired capacity to resist bacterial infection, such as in humoral immunodeficiency and cystic fibrosis. In contrast, infectious rhinosinusitis is related to obstructed drainage from the sinuses, leading to recurrent bacterial infection. This recurrent bacterial infection leads to damage of the sinus epithelium and inflammatory infiltrate of mononuclear cells but not eosinophils. Infectious rhinosinusitis and chronic inflammatory rhinosinusitis, as defined by Steinke and Borish, seem to represent truly infectious processes. It is likely that the relationship between these disorders and asthma is related to such causal mechanisms as naso-pharyngo-bronchial reflexes and postnasal drainage leading to bronchoconstriction rather than to different manifestations of a common process.

Steinke and Borish [57] have defined chronic hyperplastic eosinophilic sinusitis and allergic fungal sinusitis as inflammation-driven processes. Chronic hyperplastic eosinophilic sinusitis, for instance, involves infiltrate of eosinophils, nasal polyposis, allergy, asthma, and aspirin sensitivity. Allergic fungal sinusitis may represent a severe variant of chronic hyperplastic eosinophilic sinusitis with colonization of fungi within the sinuses. These conditions may represent the TH_2-like process with prominent roles for eosinophils and IL-5. As such, the link between chronic hyperplastic eosinophilic sinusitis or allergic fungal sinusitis and asthma may be causal (naso-pharyngo-bronchial reflexes and local inflammation leading to stimulation of bone marrow) and different manifestations of a common disease. It may be useful to understand chronic hyperplastic eosinophilic sinusitis as "asthma of the upper airways" [64]. Venarske and deShazo [65] have recently defined a syndrome called "sinobronchial allergic mycosis," in which coexistent allergic fungal sinusitis and allergic bronchopulmonary mycosis represent a common process of fungal hypersensitivity in the sinuses and the lungs.

Table 1
Subtypes of chronic rhinosinusitis

Subtype	Mechanism
Infectious rhinosinusitis	Obstructed drainage
Chronic inflammatory rhinosinusitis	Impaired resistance to infection
Chronic hyperplastic eosinophilic sinusitis	TH_2-like inflammation
Allergic fungal sinusitis	TH_2-like inflammation and fungal growth

Summary

Rhinosinusitis is common and deserves consideration even in young pediatric patients. This disorder is also often difficult to diagnose. Rhinosinusitis, by a variety of mechanisms, may influence the clinical course of asthma. Therefore, clinicians should consider the possible presence of rhinosinusitis in any patient that presents with chronic rhinitis or asthma. This is particularly true for patients with asthma that is severe or is difficult to manage with asthma medications. Many allergy and asthma specialists empirically treat difficult asthmatics with rhinitis symptoms for rhinosinusitis.

Effective long-term treatment for chronic rhinosinusitis remains an enigma. Because there are different etiologies for chronic rhinosinusitis in different patients with cross-over between different groups (such as bacterial super-infection of inflammatory rhinosinusitis) and because it is often difficult to define the type of chronic rhinosinusitis a patient may have, it is difficult to tailor the ideal treatment. The mainstay of medical treatment for chronic rhinosinusitis, therefore, remains extended courses of oral antibiotics with such adjunctive treatment as oral and nasal corticosteroids. There is a recent report that intensive medical treatment (the cornerstone of which was 1 month of antibiotics) resulted in sustained prevention of relapse of rhinosinusitis, as defined by symptomatic and radiographic measures [66]. When more is learned about chronic rhinosinusitis, there may be possible future roles, in properly selected patients, for such medications as leukotriene inhibitors, antihistamines, and anti-IgE [57].

References

[1] Kaliner MA, Osguthorpe JD, Fireman P, Anon J, Georgitis J, Davis ML, et al. Sinusitis: bench to bedside. Current findings, future directions. J Allergy Clin Immunol 1997;99:S829–48.

[2] Corren J, Rachelefsky GS, Shapiro GG, Slavin RG. Sinusitis. In: Bierman CW, Pearlman DS, Shapiro GG, Busse WW, editors. Allergy, asthma, and immunology from infancy to adulthood. 3rd edition. Philadelphia: WB Saunders; 1996. p. 428–35.

[3] Copilevitz C, Slavin R. Sinusitis and asthma. In: Kaliner MA, editor. Current review of asthma. 1st edition. Philadelphia: Current Medicine LLC; 2003. p. 61–5.

[4] Joint Task Force on Practice Parameters. Parameters for the diagnosis and management of sinusitus. J Allergy Clin Immunol 1998;102:S107–44.

[5] ten Brinke A, Grootendorst DC, Schmidt JT, De Bruine FT, van Buchem MA, Sterk PJ, et al. Chronic sinusitis in severe asthma is related to sputum eosinophilia. J Allergy Clin Immunol 2002;109:621–6.

[6] Benson V, Marano MA. Current estimates from the National Health Interview Survey, 1995. Vital Health Stat 1998;199:1–428.

[7] McCaig LF, Hughes JM. Trends in antimicrobial drug prescribing among office-based physicians in the United States. JAMA 1995;273:214–9.

[8] Riccio AM, Tosca MA, Cosentino C, Pallestrini E, Ameli F, Canonica GW, et al. Cytokine pattern in allergic and non-allergic chronic rhinosinusitis in asthmatic children. Clin Exp Allergy 2002;32:422–6.

[9] Christodoulopoulos P, Cameron L, Durham S, Hamid Q. Molecular pathology of allergic disease. II: upper airway disease. J Allergy Clin Immunol 2000;105:211–23.

[10] Harlin SL, Ansel DG, Lane SR, Myers J, Kephart GM, Gleich GJ. A clinical and pathologic study of chronic sinusitis: the role of the eosinophil. J Allergy Clin Immunol 1988;81:867–75.

[11] Ponikau JU, Sherris DA, Kephart GM, Kern EB, Gaffey TA, Tarara JE, et al. Features of airway remodeling and eosinophilic inflammation in chronic rhinosinusitis: is the histopathology similar to asthma? J Allergy Clin Immunol 2003;112:877–82.

[12] Tosca MA, Cosentino C, Pallestrini E, Riccio AM, Milanese M, Canonica GW, et al. Medical treatment reverses cytokine pattern in allergic and nonallergic chronic rhinosinusitis in asthmatic children. Pediatr Allergy Immunol 2003;14:238–41.

[13] Gottlieb MJ. Relation of intranasal disease in the production of bronchial asthma. JAMA 1925; 85:105–7.

[14] Bullen SS. Incidence of asthma in 400 cases of chronic sinusitis. J Allergy 1932;4:402–7.

[15] Bresciani M, Paradis L, Des Roches A, Vernhet H, Vachier I, Godard P, et al. Rhinosinusitis in severe asthma. J Allergy Clin Immunol 2001;107:73–80.

[16] Rossi OV, Pirila T, Laitinen J, Huhti E. Sinus aspirates and radiographic abnormalities in severe attacks of asthma. Int Arch Allergy Immunol 1994;103:209–13.

[17] Fuller CG, Schoettler JJ, Gilsanz V, Nelson Jr MD, Church JA, Richards W. Sinusitis in status asthmaticus. Clin Pediatr 1994;33:712–9.

[18] Tosca MA, Riccio AM, Marseglia GL, Caligo G, Pallestrini E, Ameli F, et al. Nasal endoscopy in asthmatic children: assessment of rhinosinusitis and adenoiditis incidence, correlations with cytology and microbiology. Clin Exp Allergy 2001;31:609–15.

[19] Rachelefsky G, Katz R, Siegel SC. Chronic sinus disease with associated reactive airway disease in children. Pediatrics 1984;73:526–9.

[20] Friedman R, Ackerman M, Wald E, Casselbrant M, Friday G, Fireman P. Asthma and bacterial sinusitis in children. J Allergy Clin Immunol 1984;74:185–9.

[21] Businco L, Fiore L, Frediani T, Artuso A, Di Fazio A, Bellioni P. Clinical and therapeutic aspects of sinusitis in children with bronchial asthma. Int J Paediatr Otolaryngol 1981;3: 287–94.

[22] Richards W, Roth RM, Church JA. Underdiagnosis and undertreatment of chronic sinusitis in children. Clin Ped 1991;30:88–92.

[23] Tosca MA, Cosentino C, Pallestrini E, Caligo G, Milanese M, Ciprandi G. Improvement of clinical and immunopathologic parameters in asthmatic children treated for concomitant chronic rhinosinusitis. Ann Allergy Asthma Immunol 2003;91:71–8.

[24] Oliveira C, Sole D. Improvement of bronchial hyperresponsiveness in asthmatic children treated for concomitant sinusitis. Ann Allergy Asthma Immunol 1997;79:70–4.

[25] Tsao CH, Chen LC, Yek KW, Huang JL. Concomitant chronic sinusitis treatment in children with mild asthma: the effect on bronchial hyperresponsiveness. Chest 2003;123:757–64.

[26] Adinoff AD, Cummings NP. Sinusitis and its relationship to asthma. Pediatr Ann 1989;18: 785–90.

[27] Kalogjera L, Vagic D, Baudoin T. Effect of endosinusal treatment on cellular markers in mild and moderate asthmatics. Acta Otolaryngol 2003;123:310–3.

[28] Palmer JN, Conley DB, Dong RG, Ditto AM, Yarnold PR, Kern RC. Efficacy of endoscopic sinus surgery in the management of patients with asthma and chronic sinusitis. Am J Rhinol 2001;15:49–53.

[29] Ikeda K, Tanno N, Tamura G, Suzuki H, Oshima T, Shimomura A, et al. Endoscopic sinus surgery improves pulmonary function in patients with asthma associated with chronic sinusitis. Ann Otol Rhinol Laryngol 1999;108:355–9.

[30] Nishioka GJ, Cook PR, Davis WE, McKinsey JP. Functional endoscopic sinus surgery in patients with chronic sinusitis and asthma. Otolaryngol Head Neck Surg 1994;110:494–500.

[31] Okayama M, Iijima H, Shimura S, Shimomura A, Ikeda K, Okayama H, et al. Methacholine bronchial hyperresponsiveness in chronic sinusitis. Respiration (Herrlisheim) 1998;65:450–7.

[32] Parsons D, Phillips S. Functional endoscopic surgery in children. Laryngoscope 1993;103: 899–903.

[33] Manning S, Wasserman R, Silver R, Phillips DL. Results of endoscopic sinus surgery in pediatric patients with chronic sinusitis and asthma. Arch Otolaryngol Head Neck Surg 1994;120:1142–5.

[34] Dunlop G, Scadding GK, Lund VJ. The effect of endoscopic sinus surgery on asthma: management of patients with chronic rhinosinusitis, nasal polyposis, and asthma. Am J Rhinol 1999; 13:261–5.

[35] Dhong H, Jung YS, Chung SK, Choi DC. Effect of endoscopic sinus surgery on asthmatic patients with chronic rhinosinusitis. Otolaryngol Head Neck Surg 2001;124:99–104.

[36] Goldstein MF, Grundfast SK, Dunsky EH, Dvorin DJ, Lesser R. Effect of functional endoscopic sinus surgery on bronchial asthma outcomes. Arch Otolaryngol Head Neck Surg 1999; 125:314–9.

[37] Kaufman J, Wright GH. The effect of nasal and nasopharyngeal irritation of airway resistance in man. Am Rev Respir Dis 1969;100:636–6.

[38] Speizer FE, Frank NR. A comparison of changes in pulmonary flow resistance in healthy volunteers acutely exposed to sulfur dioxide by mouth and by nose. Br J Int Med 1966;23:75.

[39] Nolte D, Berger B. On vagal bronchoconstriction in asthmatic patients by nasal irritation. Eur J Respir Dis 1983;64:110–5.

[40] Fontanari P, Burnet H, Zattara-Hartmann MC, Jammes Y. Changes in airway resistance induced by nasal inhalation of cold dry, dry, or moist air in normal individuals. J Appl Physiol 1996; 81:1739–43.

[41] Nadel JA, Whiddicome JC. Reflex effects of upper airway irritation on total lung resistance and blood pressure. J Appl Physiol 1962;17:861–5.

[42] Holtzman MJ, Sheller JR, Dimeo M, Nadel JA, Boushey HA. Effect of ganglionic blockade on bronchial reactivity in atopic subjects. Am Rev Respir Dis 1980;122:17–25.

[43] Bucca C, Rolla G, Scappaticci E, Chiampo F, Bugiani M, Magnano M, et al. Extrathoracic and intrathoracic airway responsiveness in sinusitis. J Allergy Clin Immunol 1995;95:52–9.

[44] Rolla G, Colagrande P, Scappaticci E, Bottomicca F, Magnano M, Brussino L, et al. Damage of the pharyngeal mucosa and hyperresponsiveness of airway in sinusitis. J Allergy Clin Immunol 1997;100:52–7.

[45] Georgitis JW, Matthews BL, Stone B. Chronic sinusitis: characterization of cellular influx and inflammatory mediators in sinus lavage fluid. Int Arch Allergy Immunol 1995;106:416–21.

[46] Bardin PG, Van Heerden BB, Joubert JR. Absence of pulmonary aspiration of sinus contents in patients with asthma and sinusitis. J Allergy Clin Immunol 1990;86:82–8.

[47] Ozcan M, Ortapamuk H, Naldoken S, Olcay I, Ozcan KM, Tuncel U. Pulmonary aspiration of nasal secretions in patients with chronic sinusitis and asthma. Arch Otolaryngol Head Neck Surg 2003;129:1006–9.

[48] Brugman SM, Larsen GL, Henson PM, Honor J, Irvin CG. Increased lower airways responsiveness associated with sinusitis in a rabbit model. Am Rev Respir Dis 1993;147: 314–20.

[49] Griffin MP, McFadden ER, Ingram RH. Airway cooling in asthmatic and nonasthmatic subjects during nasal and oral breathing. J Allergy Clin Immunol 1982;69:354–9.

[50] Denburg JA, Sehmi R, Saito H, Pil-Seob J, Inman MD, O'Byrne PM. Systemic aspects of allergic disease: bone marrow responses. J Allergy Clin Immunol 2000;106(Suppl):S242–6.

[51] Braunstahl GJ, Overbeek SE, Kleinjan A, Prins JB, Hoogsteden HC, Fokkens WJ. Nasal allergen provocation induces adhesion molecule expression and tissue eosinophilia in upper and lower airways. J Allergy Clin Immunol 2001;107:469–76.

[52] Saito H, Howie K, Wattie J, Denburg A, Ellis R, Inman MD, et al. Allergen-induced murine upper airway inflammation: local and systemic changes in murine experimental allergic rhinitis. Immunology 2001;104:226–34.

[53] Saito H, Matsumoto K, Denburg AE, Crawford L, Ellis R, Inman MD, et al. Pathogenesis of murine experimental allergic rhinitis: a study of local and systemic consequences of IL-5 deficiency. J Immunol 2002;168:3017–23.

[54] Beeh KM, Beier J, Kornmann O, Meier C, Taeumer T, Buhl R. A single nasal allergen challenge increases induced sputum inflammatory markers in non-asthmatic subjects with seasonal allergic rhinitis: correlation with plasma interleukin-5. Clin Exp Allergy 2003;33:475–82.

[55] Denburg JA, Keith PK. Systemic aspects of chronic rhinosinusitis. Immunol Allergy Clin North Am 2004;24:87–102.

[56] Vancheri C, Ohtoshi T, Cox G, Xaubet A, Abrams JS, Gauldie J, et al. Neutrophilic differentiation induced by human upper airway fibroblast-derived granulocyte/macrophage colony-stimulating factor (GM-CSF). Am J Respir Cell Mol Biol 1991;4:11–7.

[57] Steinke JW, Borish L. The role of allergy in chronic rhinosinusitis. Immunol Allergy Clin North Am 2004;24:45–57.

[58] Wood LJ, Sehmi R, Dorman S, Hamid Q, Tulic MK, Watson RM, et al. Allergen-induced increases in bone marrow T lymphocytes and interleukin-5 expression in subjects with asthma. Am J Respir Crit Care Med 2002;166:883–9.

[59] Hisamatsu K, Ganbo T, Nakazawa T, Murakami Y, Gleich GJ, Makiyama K, et al. Cytotoxicity of human eosinophil granule major basic protein to human nasal sinus mucosa in vitro. J Allergy Clin Immunol 1990;86:52–63.

[60] Newman LJ, Platts-Mills TA, Phillips CD, Hazen KC, Gross CW. Chronic sinusitis: relationship of computed tomographic findings to allergy, asthma, and eosinophilia. JAMA 1994;271:363–7.

[61] Braunstahl GJ, Kleinjan A, Overbeek SE, Prins JB, Hoogsteden HC, Fokkens WJ. Segmental bronchial provocation induces nasal inflammation in allergic rhinitis patients. Am J Respir Crit Care Med 2000;161:2051–7.

[62] Braunstahl GJ, Overbeek SE, Fokkens WJ, Kleinjan A, McEuen AR, Walls AF, et al. Segmental bronchoprovocation in allergic rhinitis patients affects mast cell and basophil numbers in nasal and bronchial mucosa. Am J Respir Crit Care Med 2001;164:858–65.

[63] Agosti JM, Sprenger JD, Lum LG, Witherspoon RP, Fisher LD, Storb R, et al. Transfer of allergen-specific IgE-mediated hypersensitivity with allogeneic bone marrow transplantation. N Engl J Med 1988;319:1623–8.

[64] Borish L. Sinusitis and asthma: entering the realm of evidence-based medicine. J Allergy Clin Immunol 2002;109:606–8.

[65] Venarske DL, deShazo RD. Sinobronchial allergic mycosis: the SAM syndrome. Chest 2002; 121:1670–6.

[66] Subramanian HN, Schechtman KB, Hamilos DL. A retrospective analysis of treatment outcomes and time to relapse after intensive medical treatment for chronic sinusitis. Am J Rhinol 2002; 16:303–12.

ELSEVIER
SAUNDERS

Immunol Allergy Clin N Am
25 (2005) 83–105

IMMUNOLOGY
AND ALLERGY
CLINICS
OF NORTH AMERICA

The relationship of psychologic stress with childhood asthma

Gordon R. Bloomberg, MD[a],*, Edith Chen, PhD[b]

[a]*Division of Allergy and Pulmonary Medicine, Washington University Medical School,
St. Louis Children's Hospital, One Children's Place, St. Louis, MO 63110, USA*
[b]*Department of Psychology, University of British Columbia, BC 2329 West Mall Vancouver, BC,
Canada V6T 1Z4*

Asthma has a long tradition as a "psychosomatic disease" [1]. Previously seen as an episodic, periodic condition, asthma seemed to appear suddenly as exacerbations occurring with little warning and unidentified causes [2]. Asthma, classified as extrinsic or intrinsic depending on whether known factors such as allergens precipitated the acute episode, was considered by many to have strong psychologic causes [3,4]. Emotional causes were commonly sought as explanations for acute exacerbations. Leading physicians in the 1930s and 1940s saw childhood asthma in the context of a mother–child interaction with dependency conflict precipitating or aggravating symptoms as a result of the threat of separation [3]. Studies of the parental interaction during this period indicated a range of parental attitudes, from rejection to over-protection [3].

Later, allergens, upper respiratory infections, and exercise were recognized to be related to bronchial smooth muscle contraction. Biologic processes were identified. Continued investigation emphasized cellular and molecular explanations for the underlying pathophysiology that is responsible for the exacerbations and persistence of asthma activity [5–7], yet there is much interest in the interface and reciprocal interaction between biology of asthma, behavior, stress, and the immune system [1,8,9]. Asthma is considered a symptom complex resulting from the presence of chronic inflammation in the airways, whether it is the result of allergen sensitization, respiratory viral infection, exercise, or other

* Corresponding author. Division of Allergy and Pulmonary Medicine, Department of Pediatrics, St. Louis Children's Hospital, Suite 5 S 30, One Children's Place, St. Louis, MO 63110.
E-mail address: bloomberg@kids.wustl.edu (G.R. Bloomberg).

0889-8561/05/$ – see front matter © 2005 Elsevier Inc. All rights reserved.
doi:10.1016/j.iac.2004.09.001

nonidentified causes. The impact of psychologic factors on the prevalence of asthma does not distinguish between the fundamental mechanisms underlying the chronic inflammation immediately responsible for the expression of asthma. Yet, it is the mind-body paradigm linking psychologic stress to neuroendocrine and immune functioning that provides a framework to explore the relationship. The environment of the allergic child and the child with asthma is of substantial clinical importance. Genetic predisposition, allergens, exposure to respiratory viral infections, air contaminants, residence (ie, city or farm), and family size are important in determining the inception of asthma and its continuing activity. The environment also includes the experiences that result in stressful situations. Stressful experience may result in the inception of asthma, exacerbations, and inadequate control. In this article we explore the relationship between psychologic stress as an exacerbating factor of asthma and the mechanisms through which this relationship may exist.

The impact of asthma upon the child's psychologic adjustment

In 2001, the percentage of children with asthma was 8.7%, or 6.3 million children [10]. This number of children represents a significant degree of physical disability and financial cost, but, additionally, there are psychologic, social and educational consequences that affect the financial burden upon the family, restrict of the child's physical activities, impair of the child's development of social connections and adaptive resources, and cause general disruption in the family [11].

Many children with asthma have no psychologic difficulties as a result of their asthma, and, as a group, children with asthma do not exhibit higher psychologic disturbance than other children [12,13]. This may be related to the level of asthma severity because most asthma can be classified as mild to moderate. The subgroup of children with severe, poorly controlled disease is the group most disposed to increased psychopathology and family dysfunction [14] and poor compliance with prescribed management and in whom the risk of complications, including fatality, is high [12]. Although psychologic and disease risk factors are interactive and no single causal direction exists in the relationship between disease and psychopathology, it is instructive to sort out the effect of psychologic stress and its impact upon childhood asthma.

Stress and asthma

The concept of stress as a disease-causing stimulus was introduced in 1936 by Hans Selye [15]. Although his ideas have been modified, the consideration of stress as disease causing has been explored in many studies in laboratories involving animals and humans and under epidemiologic and clinical conditions. Stressful events occur in various forms. Public disaster, academic examinations, public speaking, marital discord, family dysfunction, neighborhood conditions, and exposure to violence are stressful situations documented to be related to asthma symptoms. Stress may affect the organism through cognitive changes in health behavior and comorbid diseases or may have more direct physiologic effects through the pathways of neuroendocrine and neuroimmune systems.

Definitions of stress

In attempting to understand the effects of stress on health, researchers have used multiple approaches in defining stress. Many of these approaches are common to the studies of stress and asthma as reported in this article. Conceptualizations of stress fall into three primary approaches: (1) objective (or environmental) characteristics, (2) subjective characteristics, and (3) biologic responses [16]. Of the three, probably the most common approach is defining stress by the events that happen to an individual. Events that are judged by consensus to place demands on an individual are labeled as "stressors." This approach labels objective events that occur in individuals' lives as stress.

The second approach argues for the importance of factoring in the individual's subjective reactions to the stressor. This approach states that the amount of stress experienced depends in large part on how an individual interprets, or appraises, a situation and that the same objective event may cause different stress reactions in different individuals depending on their perceived ability to handle the stressor [17].

The third approach relies on the ability to detect a biologic response to stress. This approach acknowledges that the same stressor may cause different reactions in different individuals but relies on biologic indicators of stress rather than an individual's self-report of stress.

How stress is measured

Each of these approaches to conceptualizing stress has its own methods of measuring stress. Studies that define stress based on environmental characteristics often involve querying subjects about the events that have occurred in their lives. For example, life-event checklists ask participants to indicate which of a list of events have happened during a specific time frame (eg, the previous 6 months) [18]. These are typically events that have been judged by raters to be objectively stressful (eg, death of a parent or loss of a job). Researchers can sum the total number of events that have happened or can create weights, meaning that different events count differentially depending on the seriousness of the event. Duration of events and timing of events can be ascertained as factors that may contribute to the association of stress with health.

Another type of stressor-based approach involves the collection of daily diary information [19]. Rather than interviewing subjects once every few months or every year, individuals can be asked to collect data every day about events that happen. Subjects can be prompted multiple times a day to answer questions about whether negative events have occurred over much shorter intervals (eg, several hours). One advantage to the daily-diary approach is that subjects have better recall of events occurring that day (as opposed to trying to remember what has happened over the past 6 months). The disadvantage is that this type of data collection is burdensome and can be done only for short periods of time; thus, one might miss big life events that occur outside of the data collection window.

Measuring the subjective component of stress entails querying subjects about their appraisals of stress. Questionnaire measures of general perceived stress, such as the Perceived Stress Scale [20], assess the degree to which subjects generally find life to be stressful (ie, overloading, uncontrollable, and unpredictable). In addition, more specific appraisal questions can be asked regarding life events by probing subjects about their appraisals of a specific life event (rather than life in general). Last, laboratory-based approaches involve separating appraisals from stressor events by presenting subjects with identical stressors in a laboratory setting and asking for their subjective appraisal of each stressor [21]. By keeping the stressor constant across all subjects, one can test for individual differences in how subjects perceive the stressor.

Biologic approaches to measuring stress include assessing physiologic systems that are responsive to changing demands in the environment [22,23]. Frequently, measured systems in the stress literature include the autonomic nervous system (ANS), the neuroendocrine system, and the immune system [8,16,24]. ANS measures include assessing the activity of the sympathetic and parasympathetic nervous systems. Neuroendocrine measures commonly include the products of two identified stress response systems, the hypothalamic-pituitary-adrenal axis and the sympathetic-adrenal-medullary axis. These products include cortisol, epinephrine, and norepinephrine [16]. Immune measures typically include enumerative assays (measuring the numbers of different types of cells) and functional assays (eg, measuring how effective cells are at killing a target) [8,16]. Biologic measures can be taken at rest as an indicator of basal state or in response to an acute stressor to measure an individual's reactivity to stress. The biologic measures chosen for a study depend on the health outcome of interest. For example, in asthma, research has focused on inflammatory markers and on ANS effects on the airways.

Pathways between stress and illness

The two most commonly discussed pathways through which stress exerts its effects are the direct effects of stress on biologic systems and the effects of stress on behaviors that affect illness. Researchers have proposed that the cumulative wear and tear of stress can result in allostatic load—a detrimental physiologic toll on the body that can predispose one to disease [25–27]. In addition to this general physiologic load, effects of stress on biologic systems that are relevant to specific diseases may have implications for disease. For instance, inflammatory processes that relate to stress and asthma are important to understand. The Th1/Th2 balance may be affected in both situations. Cytokine secretion patterns characteristic of this altered paradigm orchestrate the cellular events that relate to airway in-flammation and hyper-responsiveness [28], and it is generally accepted that the inflammatory response in asthma involves a Th2 mechanism [28–30]. Research into the effects of stress related to asthma and the pathways by which this effect may occur is often directed toward evaluating alterations in the immune response by measuring cytokine changes.

In terms of behavioral pathways, stress could affect illness in at least two ways. One involves the changes in health behaviors that occur during times of stress. For example, individuals experiencing stress are more likely to smoke, have poorer diets, and be physically inactive [31–33]. These changes in health behaviors could place high-stress individuals at risk for developing or exacer-bating illnesses. Second, among individuals with chronic illnesses, stress could affect behaviors such as adherence to medication regimens. For example, higher perceived stress has been associated with nonadherence to antiretroviral medications among HIV-positive women [34]. In addition, psychologic stressors, such as family dysfunction and depression, are associated with greater non-adherence in patients with asthma or HIV [35,36].

Evidence for stress and illness relationships

The objective and subjective components of stress have been linked to in-fectious and inflammatory illnesses. Objective measures refer to the occurrence of specific stressor experiences, such as marital and job-related stressors as exemplified by the relation to clinical exacerbations of multiple sclerosis (MS) [37] and minor stressors in rheumatoid arthritis [38,39]. A stressor may have a delayed effect, with a period of 2 weeks between the occurrence of the stressor and an exacerbation [40]. Cumulative effects have an independent effect, as noted in studies of HIV infections [41–44]. The factors of objective stressors, timing, and cumulative effects are apparent in asthma as related in the studies reviewed in this article.

Subjective, or perceived, stress has been found to be related to infectious and inflammatory illnesses. For example, subjects who reported higher levels of per-ceived stress were more likely to become infected and to develop clinical colds (based on physician examination and antibody titers) after experimental exposure to a virus that causes the common cold [45]. Subjective assessments, such as perceived conflict and disruption in one's routine, have been found to predict the development of new MS-related brain lesions 8 weeks later [46].

Studies in children relating stress and asthma

Asthma has long been a prototype for psychosomatic disease [47]. Stress related to asthma has been studied in the laboratory, by daily diary of life events, and by survey. Changes in airway function, as measured by spirometry, metha-choline challenge, and airway resistance, have been demonstrated in laboratory studies where children with asthma were asked to watch a movie or perform a stressful task. Participants in these studies did not experience overt asthma symptoms [48–51]. Alternatively, a sense of breathlessness that was considered excessive was observed in the asthma group in a study of adolescents, asthmatics, and control subjects experiencing stress induction by a frustrating computer task. The subjects experienced high levels of negative emotion and stress, but no participant developed airways obstruction or reduction in lung function [52]. These investigators previously studied patients with asthma before and after watching an emotional film and performing standardized physical exercise. It was concluded that negative emotions affect subjective rather than objective symptoms of asthma. There was relatively high breathlessness irrespective of the objective symptoms of asthma. They suggested that children in a negative emotional state who are uncertain about the condition of their airways are inclined to interpret exercise-related general sensations, such as fatigue, heart pounding, and sighing, in line with expectations as symptoms of airways obstruction [53].

Daily diary studies of patients with asthma show that life stressors have been associated with lower same-day peak expiratory flow rate and greater self-report of asthma symptoms. Psychosocial variables, such as activities, location, social contacts, mood, and stressors, are strongly related to peak expiratory flow rate (PEFR) and asthma symptoms and are a major contributor to the observed diurnal cycle in PEFR and symptoms [54]. Sandberg [55] used continuous monitoring by diaries and daily peak flow measurements in a prospective study of children with moderate to severe asthma, all receiving inhaled corticosteroid medication. Asthma exacerbations, severely negative life events, and chronic stressors were key measures. The authors interpreted their results as demonstrating that severely negative life events increase the risk of children's asthma attacks over the coming few weeks. This risk is magnified and brought forward in time if the child's life situation is also characterized by multiple chronic stressors. In this group of children, the risk of new exacerbations was significantly greater during the autumn and winter months and lowest in the summer, suggesting a mechanism at least partly explained by reports of the detrimental effect of stress on the resistance to childhood respiratory viral infections [56,57]. In children without high chronic stress, most of the severely negative events were unpredictable and frequently involved loss. However, in the group of children with a high level of background stress, the situation was different. In this group, with backgrounds including poverty, poor housing, parental psychiatric and physical illness, parental alcohol dependence, family discord, and school problems, severe events immediately preceding an acute asthma exacerbation in most instances arose directly from an existing chronic adversity. This clinical study is consistent with laboratory studies showing that when persons who are undergoing chronic life stress are confronted with an acute psychologic challenge, exaggerated psychologic, sympathomedullary reactivity is present and associated with immune changes [58].

Sandberg et al [59] studied the effect of positive experiences in the relation between stress and asthma in children. In the cohort reported previously [55], they assessed whether life events involving substantial positive effects on the child could protect against the increased risk associated with stressful life events. They demonstrated that a life event with a definite positive effect can counteract the increased risk of an asthma exacerbation precipitated by a severely negative life event provided that the chronic stress was of low to medium level, noting that the protective effect did not apply where there was chronic stress.

That stressful life events increase the risk of onset of asthma comes from a large study by postal survey of risk factors for asthma and atopic disease among 10,667 Finnish first-year university students 18 to 25 years of age. Stressful life events, such as severe disease or death of a family member and parental or personal conflicts, were retrospectively recorded during the preceding year and in grouped yearly intervals before the survey response. Concomitant parental and personal conflicts increased the risk of asthma when adjusted by parental asthma, education, and passive smoke exposure at an early age [60].

A link between stress-related immunosuppression and health is demonstrated by studies of first-year medical students during examination periods [45,61]. These studies indicated that an increased susceptibility to upper respiratory infections was mediated by immune suppression as reflected by significant decrements in interferon (IFN)-γ secretions upon mitogen stimulation of lymphocytes. Additional evidence of immune suppression was uncovered by the finding that antibody titers to Epstein-Barr virus (EBV) increased during the examination periods, suggesting that reactivation of latent EBV had occurred, consistent with decreased cellular immune control of latent virus. Concurrently, there was an increase in the incidence of self-reported symptoms of infectious illness [24].

Bronchospasm in asthma may occur through mechanisms involving immune/inflammatory and cholinergic/vagal pathways [62]. Emotions therefore might influence airway function through psychobiologic pathways that are psychoneuroimmunologic and psychophysiologic (the autonomic system) [62]. Emotions have long been considered an exacerbating factor in asthma, with negative emotions exacerbating asthma and resulting from having asthma [63]. One mechanism assumed to relate asthma symptoms triggered by emotion takes place through the ANS: alpha sympathetic activation and parasympathetic activation. It is thought that "individual response stereotypy," a predisposition among patients with asthma to respond to many diverse stressors with bronchoconstriction, is responsible [63].

Altered immune function is considered a pathway by which stress is possibly mediated toward asthma. The changes that occur are consistent with a cytokine milieu that could worsen asthma [30]. This has been studied in several situations where students undergoing academic examinations are evaluated for changes in cytokine patterns, an examination stress model. Marshall [64] demonstrated cytokine alterations occurring in healthy nonasthmatic medical students undergoing examination stress. The effect of examination stress on regulatory cytokines was assessed by measuring Th-1 cytokines (IFN-γ) and Th-2 cytokines (interleukin [IL]-10) from mitogen-stimulated peripheral blood mononuclear cells 4 weeks before and 48 hours after the examination. A decreased IFN-γ and increased IL-10, resulting in a decreased IFN-γ/IL-10 ratio, was demonstrated during examination stress, with significant correlation between cytokine pattern response and the number and degree of subjective adjustment to daily hassles. The authors suggest that the data showed that psychologically stressful situations shift type-1/type-2 cytokine balance toward a type-2 pattern and result in an immune dysregulation rather than overall immunosuppression. The authors state, "This may partially explain the increased incidence of type-2 mediated conditions such as increased viral infections, latent viral expression, allergic/asthmatic reactions, and autoimmunity reported during periods of high stress."

The influence of academic examination stress on cellular immune response has been confirmed in additional studies of asthmatic subjects and healthy control participants. Immunologic responses were found to be similar in both groups [65,66]. Lung function was not changed in the asthmatic subjects. The authors concluded that there is no aggravation of inflammatory disease in well-managed patients with asthma. Further studies by this group of investigators showed that high social support attenuated the magnitude of examination-induced immune changes during times of stress [67]. The importance of social support is noted again in our discussions of the effect of stress related to family, neighborhood, caregiving, and comorbid conditions such as depression.

In addition to studies of cytokine profiles and in contrast to previous studies, evidence of airway inflammation has been found in response to examination stress [68]. Antigen challenge was evaluated in college students with mild asthma during a low-stress phase and a stress phase determined by the timing of the final examination. Questionnaires assessed psychologic state for anxiety and depression. An inhaled antigen challenge was completed, and sputum samples were collected before challenge and at 6 hours, 24 hours, and 7 days postchallenge. Sputum eosinophils and eosinophil-derived neurotoxin levels significantly increased at 6 and 24 hours postchallenge and were enhanced during the stress phase. IL-5 generation from sputum cells was increased at 24 hours during stress and correlated with airway eosinophils. The investigators suggested that stress can act as a cofactor to increase eosinophilic airway inflammation to antigen challenge and in this way enhances asthma severity. However, in this study, as in the other academic examination studies that demonstrated cytokine changes, there was no significant deterioration in lung function or worsening of asthma symptoms.

With regard to the above studies and the notion that stress causes a change in immune balance that might favor asthma activity in susceptible patients, there is a rationale for stress management. In chronically stressed adult populations, stress management intervention has been found to be beneficial for producing changes in immune functioning [69]. Adults with mild to moderate severe asthma were asked to write about the most stressful event of their lives or about emotionally neutral topics. Patients who wrote about stressful life events had clinically relevant changes in health status at 4 months compared with the control group. The asthma patients in the experimental group showed improvement within 2 weeks [70]. Stress management has also been evaluated in a 4-week intervention in young adults with asthma. The treatment group showed significant improvement in measures of lung function compared with a placebo group, but no differences were found in measures of perceived stress [71].

Asthma and socioeconomic status, the neighborhood, and the community

Health problems in general are increasingly recognized as the result of influences operating at several levels, among which the individual, family, and community are included [72]. The influence upon health that socioeconomic status imposes is well recognized. Individuals in lower socioeconomic status (SES) experience higher rates of morbidity and mortality in almost every disease category than those within higher levels [73]. Low social support and high numbers of negative life events are associated with higher rates of morbidity and mortality among adults with asthma [74]. Among younger age groups, there is evidence to support the traditional SES relationship with respect to prevalence of asthma and respiratory illnesses, but among children age 9 and older these health associations are not apparent [75]. Among the older children, SES seems to have a reverse association or no association with the prevalence rates of asthma and respiratory illnesses. This may be important to take note of when assessing the relationship of community and neighborhood stress to asthma events. However, in contrast with prevalence rates, severe asthma does seem to consistently display the traditional SES relationship across all childhood ages [75]. Based on this pattern, there seems to be preliminary support for the persistence model for SES and severe asthma. This is consistent with epidemiologic data reported by Akinbami [76], where prevalence is not increased among African American children as much as in other groups, but morbidity is greatly increased. An association between socioeconomic status and the prevalence of severe asthma has also been reported in German grade-school children. The prevalence of severe asthma was found to be significantly higher in low as compared with the high socioeconomic group. This association could not be explained by established risk factors [77]. This may vary by country because socioeconomic status had no impact on prevalence in a prospective study of a birth cohort in Dunedin, New Zealand [78].

Within American cities, asthma prevalence, morbidity, and mortality are disproportionately increased among children living in central urban areas and low socioeconomic conditions [79]. Among the risk factors present in this environment, psychologic factors need to be considered [72,80]. Neighborhood disadvantage comprises many characteristics that may act individually and collectively to produce chronic stress. Stressful events have been identified among African American and Hispanic children living in urban neighborhoods, with the younger children and those children living in the most disadvantaged neighborhoods experiencing the more stressful events [81–83]. Stress in the context of neighborhood and community life seems to influence the prevalence and exacerbations of asthma. One such instance is the presence of community violence [83–85]. The prevalence of exposure to violence is substantial, with several surveys confirming that children from preschool through elementary school and adolescence have had knowledge or exposure to drug deals, shootings, stabbings, rape, woundings, killings, and dead bodies in their immediate community [86–91]. Many children report psychologic disturbance of depression and anxiety about their own safety, and these feelings are correlated with the degree of stress. Depression is a significant comorbidity for asthma severity possibly as a result of cognitive and behavioral interferences with asthma management.

The association between exposure to violence and asthma is reported in the reports given by the caregivers of children studied within the Inner-City Asthma Study [92]. Increased exposure to violence predicted a higher number of symptom days, and caretakers reported losing sleep on more nights even after controlling for socioeconomic status, housing deterioration, and negative life events. Psychologic stress and caretaker behaviors only partially explained the association between higher exposure to violence and increased asthma morbidity. Although the mechanisms mediating this association are not fully explained, exposure to violence was not considered to be merely a marker for factors of the usual concerns of income, employment status, caretaker education, housing problems, and other life events.

On an individual basis, exposure to violence may have an immediate and proximal effect on asthma exacerbations [93]. Among African American patients with hypertension, the factor of violence in the community may be real or perceived, but it has a profound impact as a barrier to appropriate health care [94]. This continues to be an important issue for children because, although there is an overall decline in violence rates in the United States, homicides, firearm-related mortality, and homicide-related arrests among children and adolescents are increasing [95]. In this regard, the effect of violence may be attenuated by neighbors willing to intervene on behalf of the common good, an example of social support, and by the fact that "collective efficacy" is negatively associated with variations in violence [84].

Stress, as a factor related to childhood asthma, may mediate its effect through the caregiver in the family, as reported in an earlier study of the inner-city environment in relation to childhood asthma (National Cooperative Inner-City Asthma Study) [96]. The caretakers of these children reported elevated levels of psychologic distress, and 50% had symptoms at a level of clinical severity. They also experienced a large number of undesirable life events. High levels of life stress were identified as significant concerns, placing children in inner-city communities at increased risk for problems related to adherence and asthma morbidity. This model assumes that individual or child psychologic variables influence asthma morbidity through asthma management behaviors [97]. However, low socioeconomic status and psychologic stress may be linked through immunologic alterations of the markers implicated in asthma, as noted by Chen et al [73] in a study of adolescents with persistent asthma living in high or low socioeconomic neighborhoods. The authors note that the path through individually encountered stressors, interpretations of stress, and immune markers should be considered among the many possible mechanisms linking socioeconomic disadvantage with disease.

Intervention based on the knowledge that psychosocial factors influence health behavior has recently shown to be effective. Attention to these aspects using a nurse-directed intervention program has been shown to reduce high health care use [98].

Family dysfunction as a stress factor for childhood asthma

A family in turmoil is stressful for all and especially for children, although in the case of an child with asthma, the problem may be bidirectional. Mothers of children with asthma report more perceived parenting stress, and the quality of the mother–child relationship is more problematic than for a comparison group of mothers with healthy children [99]. Noncompliance with prescribed medication is predicted by problems of psychologic adjustment and degree of family conflict [100,101]. This may not be the only pathway by which family stress causes illness. Biologic interaction may also be factor, and family dysfunction, such as marital conflict, has been shown to affect immune functioning [102].

Health care use in relation to asthma is an outcome that is affected by family dysfunction. Among the risk factors examined in relation to prior hospitalization in the Childhood Asthma Management Program, the results of the psychologic evaluations of patients with prior hospitalization demonstrate that family psychologic characteristics may affect the risk of hospitalization. The children without hospitalizations had higher Child Behavior Check List Total Competence scores, indicating greater social and academic capability than that reported by parents of the hospitalized children [103]. This capability may be a modulating factor in withstanding environmental and psychologic stressors. Families with less psychologic resources may have greater difficulty effectively managing the child's illness well enough to avoid hospitalization [103,104]. For instance, caretaker characteristics were found to be associated with a high degree of lifetime hospitalizations and predictive of readmissions over the following year [104]. This emphasizes the bidirectional effects of psychologic stress in asthma whereby poorly managed asthma becomes a stressor for a family with less resources to cope and intensifies asthma complications.

Caregiver stress and the inception of childhood asthma

There is evidence that psychosocial factors such as stress affect patients with existing asthma [55]. There is also evidence that disturbed family interaction and caregiver stress may affect the infant as a predictor of wheezing illness [92, 105–110]. If it is considered that there are critical times of vulnerability for atopic sensitization, the development of allergy may be a function of age and events that modulate asthma or allergy that occur early in life [111]. Wheezing frequently begins in early life [112,113], and the interaction between genetic and environmental factors seems to be an important key in unraveling pathogenic mechanism [114,115]. Among the predictors of repeated wheeze in the first year of life, maternal smoking during pregnancy, lower respiratory illnesses in the first year of life, low birth weight, and cockroach allergen level in the family room are found to be predictors by multivariate analysis [116]. Early problems in the parenting of genetically predisposed children have also been linked to the onset of asthma [117]. The child's immediate environment is first contacted through parental influences. Parenting difficulties include problems with infant caregiving and components of maternal functioning, such as postpartum depression and inadequate marital support [106,118]. Given parental influence upon the predisposition for asthma, environmental factors from birth on determine the expression of symptoms thereon. From the many studies noting that psychologic stress modifies immune function and cytokine production, the relationship of stress in early childhood may be considered an additional factor predisposing to atopy and asthma. Family functioning as an environmental variable may, along with exposure to allergens and respiratory infections, be a contributing factor in the onset of asthma and its persistence into later childhood.

Considering that Th-2–polarized memory to allergens is established in infancy [119], much of the investigation into the effect of stress on the developing immune system is based on the Th-2 paradigm response [120–125]. This work often measures the immune alterations by evaluating cytokine expression as an indication of imbalance in the Th-2/Th-1 activity with augmented Th-2 cell response together with downregulated Th-1 response [28,29]. There is reduced production of the cytokine IFN-γ by T cells from asthmatic patients, and this correlates with disease severity [126]. Defective IFN-γ production may be important in asthma, and this is frequently examined in studies of infants in relation to the impact of psychologic stress and the evaluation of cytokine TNF-α [28,127,128].

If stress can alter the immune system to a Th-2 paradigm response, it is pertinent to ask if stressful experience early in life is related to the appearance of asthma in children of parents who have a history of asthma. Stress in this case would be mediated through the parent's psychologic state measured as parenting problems, maternal coping, and perceived stress. An important aspect of measuring parental stress as a stressful event affecting the infant is how the mother responds to the stressful episode. An infant whose parents experience stressful life events but who are able to manage their own responses and maintain a positive environment of the child would presumably have a different emotional experience than an infant whose parents are not able to provide this buffering [106]. The adult stress literature indicates that social support is a key factor in explaining why some individuals are more adversely affected than others by stressful events [129]; therefore, studies need to take into account paternal support and maternal perception of stress [106].

For infants, the quality of parenting is hypothesized to serve as a mediator between life events that affect the family and the emotional experience of very young infants. The mother is considered an emotional regulator for the infant. Studies include children who are genetically vulnerable to asthma, and evaluations are made early in the infant's life before the onset of wheezing illnesses. Allergic and immune markers are measured as serologic levels of IgE and cytokine patterns. Questionnaires and interviews are used to evaluate caregiver stress, anxiety, depression, and marital tension or support. Mrazek [105] showed that early problems in coping and parenting were associated with the later onset of asthma. Klinnert [106] added that although neither parenting stress nor parenting risk was a significant predictor of asthma onset, the interaction effect between the two was a significant predictor of asthma onset. A further study of this population found that frequent illness, elevated IgE levels, and parenting difficulties entered into a predictive model were independently related to the development of asthma [107]. In another birth cohort, prospectively studied, caregiver stress was shown to influence immunologic function. Caregiver stress was measured repeatedly, and blood was drawn from the children at 21 to 46 months of age. A stimulation index was used as a response of lymphocyte proliferation to mitogen and antigen. Persistently higher household stress levels were observed for high responders, and it was concluded that higher family stress in early childhood may enhance allergen-induced lymphocyte proliferations [130]. The population reported by Klinnert et al [108] was followed to school age with confirmation that parenting difficulties rated in the first year of life were significantly and independently associated with asthma at school age, providing further support for the supposition that psychosocial factors contribute to asthma onset and persistence into childhood. Further studies have confirmed the effect of caregiver stress on early childhood wheeze as independent of caregiver smoking, breast feeding behaviors, allergen exposure, birth weight, and lower respiratory illness [109]. In this study it is significant that caregiver stress prospectively predicted wheeze in infants, whereas wheeze in the children did not predict subsequent caregiver stress.

Wright et al [92], in a prospective birth cohort predisposed to atopy, examined the relationships between caregiver stress on the markers of early immune response (ie, IgE expression, mitogen induced, and allergen-specific proliferative response) and subsequent cytokine expression (INF-γ, TNF-α, IL-10, IL-13). Immune alteration in the direction of atopy was demonstrated. Higher caregiver stress in the first 6 months of life was associated with significant stimulation by dust mite antigen (Df1) and nominally by cockroach antigen (Bla g 2). Higher stress levels between ages 6 and 18 months were associated with a high total IgE level. There was significant association of higher stress with increased production of TNF-α and a trend toward reduced INF-γ production. Although much of the work on the effect of caregiver stress upon immune alterations in infants is based on the Th-2 hypothesis, some researchers have challenged this model, pointing out the role of IFN-γ in asthma [131].

Not all studies are in agreement with the reports noted previously. Some prospective studies do not show these same relationships. Gustafson [132] concluded that dysfunctional family interaction was the result rather than the cause of wheezing in infancy. In a whole population cohort followed from birth through 10 years of age, genetic and environmental risk factors were collected prospectively to determine the role of these factors in whether persistent child-hood wheezing phenotypes had an early or late onset. Low social class, recurrent chest infections at 2 years of age, and parental smoking demonstrated in-dependent significance for early-onset persistent wheeze, but inherited factors showed only independent significance in the development of late-onset persistent wheeze [133]. The authors concluded that inheritance was of prime significance in the cause of persistent childhood wheeze but that environmental factors early in life may combine with genetic predisposition to produce an early onset.

Overall, chronic stress may affect cytokine expression, allergic inflammation, and asthma expression. Dysregulation in the balance of neuroimmunologic mechanisms that occur with chronic stress may alter the immune balance, and the infant's stress response is linked to the level of caregiver stress [92].

Comorbid conditions as exacerbating stress in childhood asthma

Depression can be a significant comorbidity for illness and can lead to behaviors that increase the risk of further disease. For instance, among rural adolescents there is a strong longitudinal relationship between baseline depres-sive symptoms and several important risk behaviors/factors, such as tobacco, substance abuse, depression, and a history of physical/sexual abuse [134]. De-pression is a common comorbid psychiatric diagnosis in children with severe asthma, and the predominant evidence suggests that children with more severe asthma are at higher risk for the development of two types of psychiatric disturbances: depression and anxiety [117,135]. Children with severe asthma and children with asthma plus additional chronic conditions have a significant risk for emotional and behavioral problems. This comes from a national survey of United States in which these two groups were compared with children who did not report chronic conditions and children who had the same chronic conditions but without asthma [136]. Among the subscales scores examined in relation to these groups, anxiety/depression was elevated only for asthma. In a population-based study in Puerto Rico of children with asthma, depression and separation anxiety was common, and children with severe asthma had significant degrees of potential internalizing disorders [137]. These findings are reflected in the child's ability to adjust to school activity. Severely ill children with asthma without comorbid psychiatric illness are able to cope with their increased school absenteeism, but the combination of depression and asthma is associated with problematic school performance [138].

The effect of depression as a comorbidity may be mediated through the caretaker, again bringing up the importance of considering the parental en-vironment of the child. Considering the disparate burden of increased morbidity among inner-city children, mental health of the children and their caretakers was found to be a significant factor among the psychosocial factors in predicting asthma morbidity [139]. Maternal depression is a strong predictor of emergency department visits [140]. Poor mental health in the children or their caretakers had the strongest relationship to asthma morbidity. Although a child with any chronic disease can lead to depression in the caregiver, a depressed caregiver can compound the difficulty of treating a child with a chronic disease [141]. Children whose caregivers have more depressive symptoms are more likely to have higher morbidity [142]. Maternal depression is reported to be associated with a constellation of beliefs and attitudes that significantly influence adherence to asthma management [143].

Although biologic mechanisms may be in play [8,144], the pathway of depression related to higher morbidity seems most likely to be in the area of non-compliance to medications [138,144]. Compared with nondepressed patients, the odds are three times greater that depressed patients will be noncompliant with medical treatment recommendations [145]. Depression involves hopelessness and cognitive problems related to remembering and following through on medications. Research suggests that family support and social network are important in promoting and maintaining the patient's compliance to prescribed medical treatments [145]. An opportunity for intervention is indicated by the finding that social support is associated with reductions in the need for acute care among a low-income Medicaid minority group [146].

Fatal asthma

The occurrence of depressive symptoms in severely asthmatic children is a risk factor for a fatal attack [117]. Psychologic factors implicated in pediatric asthma death are the most serious issues to be considered in patients with severe asthma. Emotional stress, particularly separation and loss, are of special psychologic significance [147], and a common theme of depression, emotional precipitation of attacks, unsupportive families, and a tendency to deny symptoms is present in all samples where psychologic factors have been investigated [148–153].

In a case-controlled study of physiologic and psychologic characteristics associated with deaths due to asthma in childhood, Strunk et al [148,150] identified eight variables that could discriminate cases from control subjects. A subsequent study of patients matched for severity of illness, age, and sex revealed that most of the clinical characteristics previously thought to place patients at greater risk for a fatal attack were equally frequent in the children who died and in control cases. This emphasized the important role of psychologic issues as risk factors for a fatal outcome in severe asthma [149]. A family disturbance, an abnormal reaction to separation or loss, and expressed hopelessness and despair are warning signs that a fatality may be imminent [151]. Many of the psychologic stress factors and comorbid conditions described in the preceding sections are noted in relation to this most dramatic and tragic outcome of childhood asthma. These include patient–staff conflict, patient–parent conflict, deficient self-care, noncompliance with prescribed care, depressive symptoms, emotional or behavioral reactions to separation or loss, and family dysfunction [150]. The vulnerable age groups centered in early or mid-adolescence. This resonates with a study of adolescents considered at risk for adjustment problems secondary to lower economic strata and educational or vocational failure. When examined on multiple measures of psychologic distress, those with asthma had higher scores for anxiety, depression, and global distress than those without asthma [154]. This study suggested that asthma is an additional and significant independent stressor or risk factor among adolescents who already are at high risk for multiple adjustment problems and emphasizes the bidirectional aspects of asthma and psychologic stress. Additional attention to psychologic issues is needed in the child with severe and difficult-to-manage asthma [155].

Summary

Psychologic stress can have a biologic effect upon the immune system, altering cytokine patterns in the direction of Th-2 response. Negative life events represent acute and chronic stresses that can affect asthma, causing symptoms and poor control. The family and neighborhood environment represent significant potential stressors. The mental health of the caregiver is an important mediator in the child's state of asthma and potential inception of asthma expression. Depression is particularly dangerous especially in the context of severe asthma. Social support should be examined as an attenuating factor in children with asthma because this may be a most important adjunct to appropriate medical management.

The National Heart, Lung, and Blood Institute's National Asthma Education Program calls for a number of psychologic components in the comprehensive treatment of asthma [156]. Psychologic stress may be present at every level of the child's interaction with the environment. Especially in the child whose asthma is more severe and in whom management is difficult, attention to the psychologic environment is important and relevant. There are many opportunities for intervention at every level.

Acknowledgments

I thank Kathryn Ray, librarian at St. Louis Children's Hospital, for her help in gathering the references for this article.

References

[1] Creer TL, Stein REK, Rappaport L, Lewis C. Behavioral consequences of illness: childhood asthma as a model. Pediatrics 1992;90:808–15.
[2] Szefler SJ. Asthma: the new advances. Adv Pediatr 2000;47:273–308.

[3] French TM, Alexander F. Pyschogenic factors in bronchial asthma: part I. Washington, DC: National Research Council; 1941.

[4] Rappaport BZ, Hecht R. A discussion of asthma from the point of view of the allergist. In: French TM, Alexander F, editors. Psychogenic factors in bronchial asthma, part I. Manesha (WI): Psychosomatic Medicine Monographs; 1941. p. 1–12.

[5] Busse WW, Lemanske Jr RF. Asthma. N Engl J Med 2001;344:350–62.

[6] Wahn U, von Mutius E. Childhood risk factors for atopy and the importance of early intervention. J Allergy Clin Immunol 2001;107:567–74.

[7] Lemanske Jr RF. Inflammation in childhood asthma and other wheezing disorders. Pediatrics 2002;109(Suppl):368–72.

[8] Herbert R, Cohen S. Stress and immunity in humans: a meta-analytic review. Psychosom Med 1993;55:364–79.

[9] Busse W, Kiecolt J, Coe C, Martin R, Weiss S, Parker S. Stress and asthma. Am J Respir Crit Care Med 1995;151:249–52.

[10] Woodruff TJ, Axelrad DA, Kyle AD, Nweke O, Miller GG, Hurley BJ. Trends in environmentally related childhood illnesses. Pediatrics 2004;113:1133–40.

[11] Annett R, Bender B. Psychology of pediatric asthma. In: Murphy S, Kelly H, editors. Pediatric asthma, lung biology in health and disease. New York: Marcel Dekker; 1999. p. 211–34.

[12] Bender B, Klinnert M. Psychological correlates of asthma severity and treatment outcome in children. In: Kotses H, Harver A, editors. Self-management of asthma. New York: Marcel Dekker; 1998. p. 63–88.

[13] Bender B, Annett R, Ikle D, DuHamel T, Rand C, Strunk R. Relationship between disease and psychological adaptation in children in the childhood asthma management program and their families. Arch Pediatr Adolesc Med 2000;154:706–13.

[14] McNichol K, Williams H, Allan J, McAndrew I. Spectrum of asthma in children-III: psychological and social components. BMJ 1973;4:16–20.

[15] Selye H. A syndrome produced by diverse nocuous agents. Neuropsychiatry Classics 1998;10: 230–1.

[16] Cohen S, Kessler RC, Gordon LU. Strategies for measuring stress in studies of psychiatric and physical disorders. In: Cohen S, Kessler R, Gordon L, editors. Measuring stress: a guide for health and social scientists. New York: Oxford University Press; 1995. p. 3–26.

[17] Lazarus R, Folkma S. Stress, appraisal, and coping. New York: Springer; 1984.

[18] Turner R, Wheaton B. Checklist measurement of stressful life events. In: Cohen S, Kessler RC, Gordon LU, editors. Measuring stress: a guide for health and social scientists. New York: Oxford University Press; 1995. p. 29–58.

[19] Shiffman S, Stone A. Ecological momentary assessment in health psychology. Health Psychol 1998;17:3–5.

[20] Cohen S, Kamarck T, Mermelstein R. A global measure of perceived stress. J Health Soc Behav 1983;24:385–96.

[21] Chen E, Matthews K. Development of the cognitive appraisal and understanding of social events (CAUSE) videos. Health Psychol 2003;22:106–10.

[22] Baum A, Grunberg N. Measurement of stress hormones. In: Cohen S, Kessler RC, Gordon LU, editors. Measuring stress: a guide for health and social scientists. New York: Oxford University Press; 1995. p. 175–92.

[23] Manuck S, Cohen S, Rabin B, Muldoon M, Bachen E. Individual differences in cellular immune response to stress. Psychol Sci 1991;2:111–5.

[24] Glaser R, Rice J, Sheridan J, Fertel R, Stout J, Speicher C, et al. Stress-related immune suppression: health implications. Brain Behav Immun 1987;1:7–20.

[25] McEwen BS, Stellar E. Stress and the individual: mechanisms leading to disease. Arch Intern Med 1993;153:2093–101.

[26] McEwen B. Protective and damaging effects of stress mediators. New Engl J Med 1998; 338:171–9.

[27] Seeman T, Singer B, Rowe J, Horwitz R, McEwen B. Price of adaption: allostatic load and

its health consequences: MacArthur studies of successful aging. Arch Intern Med 1997;157: 2259–68.

[28] Chung K, Barnes P. Cytokines in asthma. Thorax 1999;54:825–57.

[29] Barnes P. Cytokines as mediators of chronic asthma. Am J Respir Crit Care Med 1994; 150:S42–9.

[30] Marshall G, Agarwal S. Stress, immune regulation, and immunity: applications for asthma. Allergy Asthma Proc 2000;21:241–6.

[31] Ng D, Jeffery R. Relationships between perceived stress and health behaviors in a sample of working adults. Health Psychol 2003;22:638–42.

[32] Hellerstedt W, Jeffery R. The association of job strain and health behaviours in men and women. Int J Epidemiol 1997;26:575–83.

[33] Carey M, Kalra D, Carey K, Halperin S, Richards C. Stress and unaided smoking cessation: a prospective investigation. J Consult Clin Psychol 1993;61:831–8.

[34] Murphy D, Greenwell L, Hoffman D. Factors associated with antiretroviral adherence among HIV-infected women with children. Women Health 2002;36:97–111.

[35] Mehta S, Moore R, Graham N. Potential factors affecting adherence with HIV therapy. AIDS 1997;11:1665–70.

[36] Lehrer P, Feldman J, Giardino N, Song H, Schmaling K. Psychological aspects of asthma. J Consult Clin Psychol 2002;70:691–711.

[37] Sibley W. Risk factors in multiple sclerosis. In: Raine C, McFarland H, Tourtellotte W, editors. Multiple sclerosis: clinical and pathogenetic basis. London: Chapman & Hall; 1997. p. 141–8.

[38] Thomason B, Brantly P, Jones G, Dyer H, Morris J. The relation between stress and disease: activity in rheumatoid arthritis. J Behav Med 1992;15:215–20.

[39] Zautra A, Hoffman J, Matt K, Yocum D, Potter P, Castro W, et al. An examination of individual differences in the relationship between interpersonal stress and disease activity among women with rheumatoid arthritis. Arthritis Care Res 1998;11:271–9.

[40] Ackerman K, Martino M, Heyman R, Moyna N, Rabin B. Stress-induced alteration of cytokine production in multiple sclerosis patients and controls. Psychosom Med 1998;60:484–91.

[41] Evans D, Leserman J, Perkins D, Stern R, Murphy C, Zheng B, et al. Severe life stress as a predictor of early disease progression in HIV infection. Am J Psychiatry 1997;154:630–4.

[42] Leserman J, Jackson E, Petitto J, Golden R, Silva S, Perkins D, et al. Progression to AIDS: the effects of stress, depressive symptoms, and social support. Psychosom Med 1999;61:397–406.

[43] Leserman J, Petitto J, Golden R, Gaynes B, Gu H, Perkins D, et al. Impact of stressful life events, depression, social support, coping, and cortisol on progression to AIDS. Am J Psychiatry 2000;157:1221–8.

[44] Leserman J, Petitto J, Gu H, Gaynes B, Barroso J, Gold R, et al. Progression to AIDS, a clinical AIDS condition and mortality: psychosocial and physiological predictors. Psychol Med 2002; 32:1059–73.

[45] Cohen S, Tyrrell D, Smith A. Psychological stress in humans and susceptibility to the common cold. N Engl J Med 1991;325:606–12.

[46] Mohr D, Goodkin D, Bacchetti P, Boudewyn A, Huang L, Marrietta P, et al. Psychological stress and the subsequent appearance of new brain MRI lesions in MS. Neurology 2000;55: 55–61.

[47] Rietveld S, Everaerd W, Creer T. Stress-induced asthma: a review of research and potential mechanisms. Clin Exp Allergy 2000;30:1058–66.

[48] Miller B, Wood B. Psychophysiologic reactivity in asthmatic children: a cholinergically mediated confluence of pathways. J Am Acad Child Adolesc Psychiatry 1994;33:1236–45.

[49] Miller B, Wood B. Influence of specific emotional states on autonomic reactivity and pulmonary function in asthmatic children. J Am Acad Child Adolesc Psychiatry 1997;36:669–77.

[50] McQuaid E, Fritz G, Nassau J, Lilly M, Mansell A, Klein R. Stress and airway resistance in children with athma. J Psychosom Res 2000;49:239–45.

[51] Tal A, Miklich D. Emotionally induced decreases in pulmonary flow rates in asthmatic children. Psychosom Med 1976;38:190–200.

[52] Rietveld S, Van Beest I, Everaerd W. Stress-induced breathlessness in asthma. Psychol Med 1999;29:1350–66.

[53] Rietveld S, Prins P. The relationship between negative emotions and acute subjective and objective symptoms of childhood asthma. Psychol Med 1998;28:407–15.

[54] Smyth J, Soefer M, Hurewitz A, Kliment A, Stone A. Daily psychosocial factors predict levels and diurnal cycles of asthma symptomatology and peak flow. J Behav Med 1999;22:179–93.

[55] Sandberg S, Paton J, Ahola S, McCann D, McGuinness D, Hillary C, et al. The role of acute and chronic stress in asthma attacks in children. Lancet 2000;356:982–7.

[56] Cobb JMT, Steptoe A. Psychosocial influences on upper respiratory infectious illness in children. J Psychosom Res 1998;45:319–30.

[57] Cohen S, Doyle WJ, Skoner DP. Psychological stress, cytokine production, and severity of upper respiratory illness. Psychosom Med 1999;61:175–80.

[58] Pike J, Smith T, Hauger R, Nicassio P, Patterson T, McClintick J, et al. Chronic life stress alters sympathetic, neuroendocrine, and immune responsivity to an acute psychological stressor in humans. Psychosom Med 1997;59:447–57.

[59] Sandberg S, McCann D, Ahola S, Paton J, McGuinness D. Positive experiences and the relationship between stress and asthma in children. Acta Paediatr 2002;91:152–8.

[60] Kilpeläinen M, Koskenvuo M, Helenius H, Terho E. Stressful life events promote the manifestation of asthma and atopic diseases. Clin Exp Allergy 2002;32:256–63.

[61] Cohen S, Frank E, Doyle W, Skoner D, Rabin B. Types of stressors that increase susceptibility to the common cold in healthy adults. Health Psychol 1998;17:214–23.

[62] Miller B, Wood B. Emotions and family factors in childhood asthma: psychobiologic mechanisms and pathways of effect. Adv Psychosom Med 2003;24:131–60.

[63] Lehrer P, Isenberg S, Hochron S. Asthma and emotion: a review. J Asthma 1993;30:5–21.

[64] Marshall G, Agarwal S, Lloyd C, Cohen L, Henninger E, Morris G. Cytokine dysregulation associated with exam stress in healthy medical students. Brain Behav Immun 1998;12:297–307.

[65] Kang D-H, Coe C, McCarthy D. Academic examinations significantly impact immune responses, but not lung function, in healthy and well-managed asthmatic adolescents. Brain Behav Immun 1996;10:164–81.

[66] Kang D-H, Coe C, McCarthy D, Ershler W. Immune responses to final exams in healthy and asthmatic adolescents. Nurs Res 1997;46:12–9.

[67] Kang D-H, Coe C, Karaszewski J, McCarthy D. Relationship of social support to stress responses and immune function in healthy and asthmatic adolescents. Res Nurs Health 1998;21:117–28.

[68] Liu L, Coe C, Swenson C, Kelly E, Kita H, Busse W. School examinations enhance airway inflammation to antigen challenge. Am J Respir Crit Care Med 2002;165:1062–7.

[69] Miller G, Cohen S. Psychological interventions and the immune system: a meta-analytic review and critique. Health Psychol 2001;20:47–63.

[70] Smyth J, Stone A, Hurewitz A, Kaell A. Effects of writing about stressful experiences on symptom reduction in patients with asthma or rheumatoid arthritis. JAMA 1999;281:1304–9.

[71] Hockemeyer J, Smyth J. Evaluating the feasibility and efficacy of a self-administered manual-based stress management intervention for individuals with asthma: results from a controlled study. Behav Med 2002;27:161–72.

[72] Wright R, Fisher E. Putting asthma into context: community influences on risk, behavior, and intervention. In: Kawachi I, Berkman LF, editors. The neighborhoods and health. Oxford (NY): Oxford University Press; 2003. p. 233–62.

[73] Chen E, Fisher E, Bacharier L, Strunk R. Socioeconomic status, stress, and immune markers in adolescents with asthma. Psychosom Med 2003;65:984–92.

[74] Smith A, Nicholson K. Psychosocial factors, respiratory viruses and exacerbation of asthma. Psychoneuroendocrinology 2001;26:411–20.

[75] Chen E, Matthews K, Boyce W. Socioeconomic differences in children's health: how and why do these differences change with age? Psychol Bull 2002;128:295–329.

[76] Akinbami LJ, LaFleur BJ, Schoendorf KC. Racial and income disparities in childhood asthma in the United States. Ambul Pediatr 2002;2:382–7.

[77] Mielck A, Reitmeir P, Wjst M. Severity of childhood asthma by socioeconomic status. Int J Epidemiol 1996;25:388–93.

[78] Hancox RJ, Milne BJ, Taylor DR, Greene JM, Cowan JO, Flannery EM, et al. Relationship between socioeconomic status and asthma: a longitudinal cohort study. Thorax 2004;59: 376–80.

[79] Weiss KB, Gergen PJ, Crain EF. Inner-city asthma: the epidemiology of an emerging US public health concern. Chest 1992;101(Suppl):362S–367.

[80] Wright R, Rodriquez M, Cohen S. Review of psychosocial stress and asthma: an integrated biopsychosocial approach. Thorax 1998;53:1066–74.

[81] Kessler R. Stress, social status, and psychological distress. J Health Soc Behav 1979;20: 259–72.

[82] Tarnowski K. Disadvantaged children and families in pediatric primary care settings. J Clin Child Psychol 1991;20:351–9.

[83] Attar BK, Guerra NG, Tolan PH. Neighborhood disadvantage, stressful life events, and adjustment in urban elementary-school children. J Clin Child Psychol 1994;23:391–400.

[84] Sampson R, Raudenbush S, Earls F. Neighborhoods and violent crime: a multilevel study of collective efficacy. Science 1997;277:918–24.

[85] Wright R, Mitchell H, Visness C, Cohen S, Stout J, Evans R, et al. Community violence and asthma morbidity: the inner-city asthma study. Am J Public Health 2004;94:625–32.

[86] Taylor L, Zuckerman B, Harik V, Groves BM. Witnessing violence by young children and their mothers. J Dev Behav Pediatr 1994;15:120–3.

[87] Schwab-Stone ME, Ayers TS, Kasprow W, Voyce C, Barone C, Schriver T, et al. No safe haven: a study of violence exposure in an urban community. J Am Acad Child Adolesc Psychiatry 1995;34:1343–52.

[88] Hurt H, Malmud E, Brodsky NL, Giannetta J. Exposure to violence: psychological and academic correlates in child witnesses. Arch Pediatr Adolesc Med 2001;155:1351–6.

[89] Osofsky JD, Wewers S, Hann DM, Fick AC. Chronic community violence: what is happening to our children? Psychiatry 1993;56:36–45.

[90] Sheehan K, DiCara JA, LeBailly S, Christoffel KK. Children's exposure to violence in an urban setting. Arch Pediatr Adolesc Med 1997;151:502–4.

[91] Groves BM. Children who see too much: lessons from the child witness to violence project. Boston: Beacon Press; 2002.

[92] Wright R, Finn P, Contreras J, Cohen S, Wright R, Staudenmayer J, et al. Chronic caregiver stress and IgE expression, allergen-induced proliferation, and cytokine profiles in a birth cohort predisposed to atopy. J Allergy Clin Immunol 2004;113:1051–7.

[93] Wright RJ, Steinbach SF. Violence: an unrecognized environmental exposure that may contribute to greater asthma morbidity in high risk inner-city populations. Environ Health Perspect 2001;109:1085–9.

[94] Fong R. Violence as a barrier to compliance for the hypertensive urban African American. J Nat Med Assoc 1995;87:203–7.

[95] Hennes H. A review of violence statistics among children and adolescents in the United States. In: Hennes H, Calhoun AD, editors. Violence among children and adolescents. Philadelphia: WB Saunders; 1998. p. 269–80.

[96] Wade S, Weil C, Holden G. Psychosocial characteristics of inner-city children with asthma. Pediatr Pulmonol 1997;24:263–76.

[97] Klinnert M. Psychosocial influences on asthma among inner-city children. Pediatr Pulmonol 1997;24:234–6.

[98] Castro M, Zimmermann NA, Crocker S, Bradley J, Leven C, Schechtman KB. Asthma intervention program prevents readmissions in high healthcare users. Am J Respir Crit Care Med 2003;168:1095–9.

[99] Carson D, Schauer R. Mothers of children with asthma: perceptions of parenting stress and the mother-child relationship. Psychol Rep 1992;71:1139–48.

[100] Christiaanse M, Lavigne J, Lerner C. Psychosocial aspects of compliance in children and adolescents with asthma. J Dev Behav Pediatr 1989;10:75–80.

[101] Wamboldt FS, Wamboldt MZ, Gavin LA, Roesler TA, Brugman SM. Parental criticism and treatment outcome in adolescents hospitalized for severe, chronic asthma. J Psychosom Res 1995;39:995–1005.

[102] Kiecolt-Glaser J, Malarkey W, Chee M, Newton T, Cacioppo J, May H-Y. Negative behavior during marital conflict is associated with immunological down-regulation. Psychosom Med 1993;55:395–409.

[103] Bacharier L, Dawson C, Bloomberg G, Bender B, Wilson L, Strunk R. Hospitalization for asthma: atopic, pulmonary function, and psychological correlates among participants in the Childhood Asthma Management Program. Pediatrics 2003;112:e85–92.

[104] Chen E, Bloomberg GR, Fischer EBJ, Strunk RC. Predictors of repeat hospitalizations in children with asthma: the role of psychosocial and socio-environmental factors. Health Psychol 2003;22:12–8.

[105] Mrazek D, Klinnert M, Mrazek P, Macey T. Early asthma onset: consideration of parenting issues. J Am Acad Child Adolesc Psychiatry 1991;30:277–82.

[106] Klinnert M, Mrazek P, Mrazek D. Early asthma onset: the interaction between family stressors and adaptive parenting. Psychiatry 1994;57:51–61.

[107] Mrazek D, Klinnert M, Mrazek P, Brower A, McCormick D, Rubin B, et al. Prediction of early-onset asthma in genetically at-risk children. Pediatr Pulmonol 1999;27:85–94.

[108] Klinnert M, Nelson H, Price M, Adinorr A, Leung D, Mrazek D. Onset and persistence of childhood asthma: predictors from infancy. Pediatrics 2001;108:E69.

[109] Wright RJ, Cohen S, Carey V, Weiss ST, Gold DR. Parental stress as a predictor of wheezing in infancy: a prospective birth-cohort study. Am J Respir Crit Care Med 2002;165:358–65.

[110] Jackson B, Wright RJ, Kubzansky LD, Weiss ST. Examining the influence of early life socioeconomic position on pulmonary function across the life span: where do we go from here? Thorax 2004;59:186–8.

[111] McGeady SJ. Immunocompetence and allergy. Pediatrics 2004;113:1107–13.

[112] Martinez FD. Development of wheezing disorders and asthma in preschool children. Pediatrics 2002;109(Suppl):362–7.

[113] Yunginger J, Reed CE, O'Connell J, Melton LI, O'Fallon W, Silverstein M. A community-based study of epidemiology of asthma incidence rates. Am Rev Respir Dis 1992;146:888–94.

[114] Lemanske Jr RF. Issues in understanding pediatric asthma: epidemiology and genetics. J Allergy Clin Immunol 2002;109:S521–4.

[115] Morgan W, Martinez F. Risk factors for developing wheezing and asthma in childhood. Pediatr Clin North Am 1992;39:1185–203.

[116] Gold D, Burge H, Carey V, Milton D, Platts-Mills T, Weiss S. Predictors of repeated wheeze in the first year of life: the relative roles of cockroach, birthweight, acute lower respiratory illness, and maternal smoking. Am J Respir Crit Care Med 1999;160:227–36.

[117] Mrazek D. Psychological aspects in children and adolescents. In: Barnes PJ, Grunstein M, Leff A, Woolcock AJ, editors. Asthma. Philadelphia, New York: Lippincott-Raven; 1997. p. 2177–83.

[118] Mrazek D, Mrazek P, Klinnert M. Clinical assessment of parenting. J Am Acad Child Adolesc Psychiatry 1995;34:272–82.

[119] Yabuhara A, Macaubas C, Prescott SL, Venaille TJ, Holt BJ, Habre W, et al. TH2-polarized immunological memory to inhalant allergens in atopics is established during infancy and early childhood. Clin Exp Allergy 1997;27:1261–9.

[120] Romagnani S. Human T_H1 and T_H2 subsets: doubt no more. Immunol Today 1991;12:256–7.

[121] Romagnani S. Induction of T_H1 and T_H2 responses: a key role for the 'natural' immune response? Immunol Today 1992;13:379–81.

[122] Donovan C, Finn P. Immune mechanisms of childhood asthma. Thorax 1999;54:938–46.

[123] Bjorksten B. The intrauterine and postnatal environments. J Allergy Clin Immunol 1999;104:1119–27.

[124] Mosman T, Sad S. The expanding universe of T-cells subsets: Th1, Th2 and more. Immunol Today 1996;17:138–46.

[125] Romagnani S. Immunologic influences on allergy and the Th1/Th2 balance. J Allergy Clin Immunol 2004;113:395–400.

[126] Barnes P, Chung K, Page C. Inflammatory mediators of asthma: an update. Pharmacol Rev 1998;50:515–96.

[127] Kim M, Agrawal D. Effect of interleukin-1 beta and tumor necrosis factor-alpha on the expression of G-proteins in CD4 + T-cells of atopic asthmatic subjects. J Asthma 2002;39:441–8.

[128] Halasz A, Cserhati E, Magyar R, Kovacs M, Cseh K. Role of TNF-alpha and its 55 and 75 kDa receptors in bronchial hyperreactivity. Respir Med 2002;96:262–7.

[129] Cohen S, Willis T. Stress, social support and the buffering hypothesis. Psychologic Bulletin 1985;46:310–57.

[130] Wright R, Finn P, Boudreau J, Staudenmayer J, Wand M, He H, et al. Allergen-induced lymphocyte proliferation in early childhood: role of stress. Presented at the 2001 Meeting of the American Thoracic Society. San Francisco, May 18–23, 2001.

[131] Holtzman M, Sampath D, Castro M, Look D, Jayaraman S. The one-two of T helper cells: does Interferon-α knock out the Th2 hypothesis for asthma? Am J Respir Cell Mol Biol 1996;14: 316–8.

[132] Gustafsson P, Björkstén B, Kjellman N-I. Family dysfunction in asthma: a prospective study of illness development. J Pediatr 1994;125:493–8.

[133] Kurukulaaratchy RJ, Matthews S, Arshad SH. Does environment mediate earlier onset of the persistent childhood asthma phenotype? Pediatrics 2004;113:345–50.

[134] Burns J, Cottrell L, Perkins K, Pack R, Stanton B, Hobbs G, et al. Depressive symptoms and health risk among rural adolescents. Pediatrics 2004;113:1313–20.

[135] Mrazek D. Psychiatric complications of pediatric asthma. Ann Allergy 1992;69:285–90.

[136] Bussing R, Halfon N, Benjamin B, Wells K. Prevalence of behavior problems in US children with asthma. Arch Pediatr Adolesc Med 1995;149:565–72.

[137] Ortega A, McQuaid E, Canino G, Goodwin R, Fritz G. Comorbidity of asthma and anxiety and depression in Puerto Rican children. Psychosomatics 2004;45:93–9.

[138] Galil N. Depression and asthma in children. Curr Opin Pediatr 2000;12:331–5.

[139] Weil C, Wade S, Bauman L, Lynn H, Mitchell H, Lavigne J. The relationship between psychosocial factors and asthma morbidity in inner-city children with asthma. Pediatrics 1999; 104:1274–80.

[140] Bartlett S, Kolodner K, Butz A, Eggleston P, Malveaux F, Rand C. Maternal depressive symptoms and emergency department use among inner-city children with asthma. Arch Pediatr Adolesc Med 2001;155:347–53.

[141] Wagner CW. The ongoing evaluation of the impact of depression on asthma. Ann Allergy Asthma Immunol 2002;89:540–1.

[142] Shalowitz MU, Berry CA, Quinn KA, Wolf RL. The relationship of life stressors and maternal depression to pediatric asthma morbidity in a subspecialty practice. Ambul Pediatr 2001;1: 185–93.

[143] Bartlett SJ, Krishnan JA, Riekert KA, Butz A, Malveaux F, Rand C. Maternal depressive symptoms and adherence in inner-city children with asthma. Pediatrics 2004;113:229–37.

[144] Herbert TB, Cohen S. Depression and immunity: a meta-analytic review. Psychologic Bulletin 1993;113:472–86.

[145] DiMatteo M, Lepper H, Croghan T. Depression is a risk factor for noncompliance with medical treatment: meta-analysis of the effects of anxiety and depression on patient adherence. Arch Intern Med 2000;160:2101–7.

[146] Fisher Jr EB, Strunk RC, Sussman L, Sykes R, Walker M. Community organization to reduce the need for acute care for asthma among African American children in low-income neighborhoods: The Neighborhood Asthma Coalition. Pediatrics 2004;114:116–23.

[147] Friedman M. Psychological factors associated with pediatric asthma death: a review. J Asthma 1984;21:97–117.

[148] Strunk R, Mrazek D, Fuhrmann G, LaBrecque J. Physiologic and psychological characteristics associated with deaths due to asthma in childhood: a case-controlled study. JAMA 1985; 254:1193–8.

[149] Strunk R, Mrazek D. Deaths from asthma in childhood: can they be predicted? N Engl Reg Allergy Proc 1986;7:454–61.

[150] Strunk R. Asthma deaths in childhood: identification of patients at risk and intervention. J Allergy Clin Immunol 1987;80:472–7.

[151] Miller B, Strunk R. Circumstances surrounding the deaths of children due to asthma: a case-control study. Am J Dis Child 1989;143:1294–9.

[152] Fritz GSR, Lewiston N. Psychological factors in fatal childhood asthma. Am J Orthopsychiatry 1987;57:253–7.

[153] Kravis L. An analysis of fifteen childhood asthma fatalities. J Allergy Clin Immunol 1987; 80:467–72.

[154] Gillaspy SR, Hoff AL, Mullins LL, Van Pelt JC, Chaney JM. Psychological distress in high-risk youth with asthma. J Pediatr Psychol 2002;27:363–71.

[155] Birkhead G, Olfaway N, Strunk R, Townsend M, Teutsch S. Investigation of a cluster of deaths of adolescents with asthma: evidence implicating inadequate treatment and poor patient adherence with medications. J Allergy Clin Immunol 1989;84:484–91.

[156] National Heart Lung and Blood Institute. Practical guide for diagnosis and management of asthma; based on Expert Panel Report 2: guidelines for the diagnosis and management of asthma. Bethesda (MD): National Institutes of Health; 1997.

ELSEVIER
SAUNDERS

Immunol Allergy Clin N Am
25 (2005) 107–130

IMMUNOLOGY
AND ALLERGY
CLINICS
OF NORTH AMERICA

Patient-identified barriers to asthma treatment adherence: responses to interviews, focus groups, and questionnaires

Bruce G. Bender, PhD[a,b,*], Sarah E. Bender, BS[c]

[a]*Division of Pediatric Behavioral Health, National Jewish Medical and Research Center,
1400 Jackson Street, Denver, CO 80206, USA*
[b]*Department of Psychiatry, Division of Psychology, University of Colorado School of Medicine,
Denver, CO 80206, USA*
[c]*Department of Psychology, Pennsylvania State University, State College, PA 16803, USA*

Nonadherence to long-term treatment is a worldwide problem resulting in illness exacerbation and increased health care costs for most chronic conditions, including asthma [1]. In Canada, the estimated economic burden of hospitalization attributable to patient nonadherence with asthma controller therapy, based on national health statistics and adherence estimates, exceeded $1.6 billion in 2000 [2]. In the United States, studies of medication-taking behavior indicate that, on average, only about half of prescribed asthma medications are taken, and the remaining half of medications are often taken at incorrect times or with inhalation techniques that are inconsistent with physician instructions [3].

Nonadherence contributes to asthma exacerbations and increased health care cost. For example, when a nonadherent asthma patient presents with continuing symptoms, the physician may unnecessarily step up therapy because he believes the patient is not responding sufficiently to the original less intensive and less costly therapy. Seeing the patient fail to respond to an apparently appropriate therapy, the physician may feel compelled to order expensive diagnostic tests to

---

* Corresponding author. Division of Pediatric Behavioral Health, National Jewish Medical and Research Center, 1400 Jackson Street, Denver, CO 80206.
E-mail address: benderb@njc.org (B.G. Bender).

try to better understand the patient's poor response to treatment. Although not all nonadherence results in dangerous or costly complications, research across a range of chronic diseases, including asthma, suggests that nonadherence results in excess urgent care and hospitalizations. For example, Milgrom et al [4] have demonstrated that pediatric asthma patients who were the least adherent were more likely to have asthma exacerbations requiring a prednisone burst. On a national level, Isakedjiian et al [2] estimated the economic burden of hospitalization attributable to patient nonadherence with controller therapy in Canada. Using national health statistics and an average admission rate due to nonadherence of 5.2% (based on literature review), they concluded that Canadian hospital expenditures due to nonadherence exceeded $1.6 billion.

Despite apparent recognition of the problem, there is little evidence to indicate that adherence rates have improved in recent decades. Newer, more effective drugs may be somewhat forgiving in the face of partial adherence, but too often nonadherence is so pervasive and extreme that many patients receive minimal benefit. The national trend toward shifting increasing drug costs to patients will almost certainly serve to further decrease adherence. In short, the problem of nonadherence may be getting worse, causing increased disease exacerbations and driving health care costs upward.

It has been hoped that behavioral and educational interventions would improve treatment success and decrease dangerous asthma exacerbations. Numerous studies have introduced adherence interventions, but few have delivered cost-effective or easy distribution across a large population. A review of reports from 16 studies that attempted to improve adherence and outcome with interventions consisting primarily of asthma education and self-management training found that many of the studies failed to change adherence behaviors. Those that did report improved adherence suffered from methodologic shortcomings, including high attrition rates and absence of objective adherence measures [5]. We recommended the funding of new studies developing innovative strategies to improve adherence. To accomplish this, qualitative research exploring the personal world of patients—including perceptions, priorities, preferences, fears, and goals—is essential to identify the reasons why, despite enormous collective effort, asthma health care providers, educators, and behavioral scientists have been unable to greatly affect adherence.

Procedures

Numerous qualitative studies using interviews, questionnaires, and focus groups to assess patient perspectives have been published in recent years. To provide a better understanding of this literature, reports of patient perceptions and attitudes toward their treatment, particularly in relation to taking prescribed inhaled steroids to treat their disease, were reviewed. There were 29 published articles in which adults with asthma or children with asthma and their parents were surveyed. These studies contained 32 separate studies or study phases. These included reports of studies using questionnaires, personal interviews, or focus groups conducted to learn about patients' experiences with asthma, their medication-taking habits, their attitudes toward their disease and its treatment, and other associated factors (Table 1). From this review of the results of past studies, a list of the most common factors reported by adult patients to influence their adherence was compiled. A smaller literature, addressing adherence in children or minority and low-income patients, was similarly reviewed.

The manner in which information was gathered varied considerably. Most interviews were semi-structured (ie, the interviewer used a predetermined set of questions but allowed the interview to explore other topics as they arose). Some interviews were unstructured (ie, no specific set of questions was pre-set). In other cases, the interviewer read a set of questions to the participant face-to-face or over the telephone without exploratory conversation. More typically, questionnaires were completed by the participant alone in a room or with a group of other participants.

Information from each study is included in Table 1. Type of inquiry, question categories, response themes, and conclusions are represented. Response themes were taken from focus groups, open-ended questionnaires, and unstructured or semi-structured interview where the investigators attempted to organize information after the completion of data collection. In each case, the themes described in Table 1 were those interpreted by the author of the article. In the case of close-ended questionnaires, which did not allow for expanded written responses or discussion, no response themes were derived.

Results

Recurring reasons for nonadherence from interviews, questionnaires, and focus groups with adult asthma patients and children with asthma and their parents are listed below. This listing is ordered in estimated degree of emphasis (highest emphasis followed by lower emphasis). Considered in making this dual ranking was frequency with which each reason was reported and the emphasis placed on specific factors by the study's author. The resulting list is not so precise as to indicate that, for example, item 4 was more important to patients than item 3. Rather, the listing separates factors into two levels of emphasis, with the first group broadly receiving more emphasis than the second group. Although many of these patient-report studies have been conducted with adults, some have sought such information from children and their parents. Additionally, the views of low-income, inner-city patients have been specifically sought in a small number of studies. What follows is a listing of patient perceptions of factors interfering with their adherence grouped as (1) adult—high emphasis, (2) adult—lower emphasis, (3) children with asthma and their parents, and (4) low-income subjects.

Table 1
Studies examining causal factors for treatment nonadherence

Publication	Respondents	Inquiry type	Question categories	Response themes
Apter et al (2003) [6]	85 adults with moderate or severe persistent asthma	Individual interview	Modifiable determinants of adherence: 1. Knowledge of inhaled steroids 2. Patient/physician communication 3. Social support 4. Depression 5. Health beliefs (attitude) 6. Self-efficacy Immutable barriers: 1. Sociodemographics 2. Disease severity 3. Past adherence	N/A: Closed-ended questions
Bauman et al (2002) [7]	Parents of 1199 children (4–9 y) with asthma	Questionnaires	1. Admitted nonadherence 2. Risk for nonadherence 3. Indicators of asthma severity 4. Caregiver mental health (Brief Symptom Inventory) 5. Child mental health (Child Behavior Checklist)	N/A: Closed-ended questions
Boulet (1998) [8]	603 late adolescents and adults (16+ y) with asthma in Canada	Individual interview	1. Respiratory symptoms 2. Perceptions of the role of ICS 3. Concerns about ICS	1. Perceptions about ICS: Correct: a. Reduces inflammation/swelling of airways b. Prevents asthma attacks c. Gets asthma symptoms under control Incorrect: a. Opens the airways/relieves constriction b. Relieves an asthma attack c. Builds up/strengthens lungs

| Buston and Wood (2000) [9] | 49 adolescents (14–20 y) with asthma in Glasgow | Individual interview | Not provided | 2. Concerns about ICS:
  a. Fear of side effects
  b. Need for higher doses over time for same effect
  c. May become less effective over time
  d. Weight gain
  e. Building huge muscles
  f. Infections
  g. Making bones brittle/ susceptible to fractures
  h. Stunting growth
  i. Cataracts
  j. Diabetes
Reasons for noncompliance:
1. Forgetfulness
2. Belief that medication is ineffective, not needed
3. Denial of having asthma
4. Difficulty using inhaler
5. Inconvenience
6. Embarrassment
7. Fear of side effects
8. Laziness |
| Chambers et al (1999) [10] | 394 adults with asthma with prescribed ICS | Questionnaire | 1. Demographics
2. General health
3. Experience with asthma
4. Frequency of use of ICS
5. Reasons for noncompliance
6. Attitudes toward ICS
7. Health beliefs
  a. Motivation
  b. Perceived benefits of compliance
  c. Perceived seriousness of condition
  d. Risks of treatment | Most frequent reasons for noncompliance selected:
1. I use it only when I need it.
2. I don't like using medicine unless I feel sick.
3. I don't want to use steroids.
4. I feel fine.
5. I don't like the side effects. |

(continued on next page)

Table 1 (*continued*)

Publication	Respondents	Inquiry type	Question categories	Response themes
Chan and DeBruyne (2000) [11]	170 parents of children (mean = 7.1 y) with chronic asthma requiring inhaled steroids in Malaysia	Questionnaire and interview	Questionnaire: parental concerns about inhaler therapy Interview: how many doses missed in last 2 wk	Most common concerns about inhaled therapy: 1. Associated side effects 2. Dependence/addiction Also selected: 3. Inhaled therapy too costly 4. Inhaled therapy too difficult to administer
Donnelly et al (1987) [12]	128 parents of children with asthma and 110 parents of children without asthma in Australia	Questionnaire administered by interviewer	Parental attitudes toward/perceptions of: 1. Impact of asthma on children 2. Impact of asthma on family	N/A: Closed-ended questions
Erickson et al (2001) [13]	100 adults with asthma	Questionnaire	1. Self-reported compliance 2. Disease characteristics a. Number of years diagnosed with asthma b. Perceived severity c. Evaluated severity	N/A: Closed-ended questions
Fiese and Wamboldt (2003) [14]	80 families with a child (7–14 y) with asthma	Interview and questionnaires	1. Interview about asthma's effect on family, health care use 2. Functional Severity of Asthma scale 3. I Worry Scale 4. Family Ritual Questionnaire (measure of planning in family)	Classification of family management strategies from interview: 1. Reactive (family acts when anxiety is present) 2. Coordinated care (one member of the family handles health issues in a predetermined way) 3. Family partnerships (multiple family members are involved, multiple sources of information are used)

George et al (2003) [15]	15 African American adults with persistent asthma	Focus groups	1. Adherence
			2. Attitudes toward treatment
			3. Relationship with caregiver
			4. Ways to increase research participation
				1. Barriers to ICS use
				  a. "I don't need it everyday" (skipping doses when symptoms not present)
				  b. Difficulty obtaining medicine through managed care plan
				  c. Social interruptions
				  d. Missing a dose and opting not to take it rather than take it late
				  e. Fear of adverse effects
				2. Attitudes toward providers
				  a. Relationship with provider, desire to be seen as a "unique individual"
				  b. Participation in clinical research in order to gain information
				3. Strategies to promote ICS adherence and research participation
				  a. Fewer doses per day
				  b. Make medicating a part of daily routine (standardize times of day, link to other activities)
				  c. More detailed information about side effects at initial prescribing
				  d. Good listening, empathy by provider

Hand and Bradley (1996) — pilot [16]	Eight adults with asthma in England	Unstructured interview	Unstructured interview: Patients asked to consider the advantages and disadvantages of using their inhalers (salbutamol and beclomethasone)	1. Positive attitude toward using inhalers 2. Negative attitude toward using inhalers 3. Satisfaction with the doctor 4. Ease in obtaining inhalers 5. Perceived benefits of inhalers 6. Concern about side effects 7. Uncertainty about inhalers 8. Involvement of others in asthma management

(continued on next page)

Table 1 (*continued*)

Publication	Respondents	Inquiry type	Question categories	Response themes

Hand and Bradley (1996) [16]	40 adults with asthma in England	Structured interview	1. Beliefs about inhaler treatment asked about each:
			  a. Salbutamol
			  b. Beclomethasone
			  c. Inhalers in general
			2. Two inhalers separately
				N/A: Closed-ended questions

Horne and Weinman (1999) [17]	324 adult asthmatic, cardiac, renal, and oncology patients in the UK	Questionnaires	1. Beliefs about Medicines Questionnaires (patients' beliefs about the necessity of and concerns about medication) 2. Self-report scale about medication adherence	
Ireland (1997) [18]	10 children (9–12 y) with asthma in England	Individual interview	Open-ended, flexible questioning First question: "Tell me what having asthma is like for you?"	1. Discontinuity: what makes them feel different from "normal" kids 2. "Normal for me": comparing current states to a personal baseline of what's "normal for me" 3. Paying attention: deliberately problem-solving around effects of asthma 4. Leaving asthma behind: when events can't be changed, use of cognitive/behavioral strategies

Kolbe et al (2002) [19]	77 SLTA patients, 239 controls (acute asthma patients), and 100 community controls in New Zealand	Questionnaire administered by interviewer	1. Demographics
			2. Anxiety and depression
			3. Social support
			4. Life events
			5. Attitudes and beliefs about asthma
			  a. Emotional (adjustment to asthma)
			  b. Doctor–patient relationship
			  c. Stigmatization
			  d. Self-efficacy
				N/A: Closed-ended questions

| Kolbe et al (1998) [20] | 138 late adolescent and adult (age 15+) patients admitted to the hospital for an asthma attack in New Zealand | Questionnaire administered by interviewer | 1. Demographic information
2. Quality of ongoing medical care and usual asthma management
  a. Acquisition of PEF meters
  b. Action plans
  c. Availability of oral steroids
  d. Accessibility of family doctor
3. SES as related to asthma management
  a. Unemployment
  b. Financial dependence on social security benefits
  c. Financial difficulties in the last year
  d. Inability to afford doctor visits or prescription costs
4. Asthma morbidity
  a. ICU admissions
  b. Hospital admissions
  c. Visits to ED
  d. Courses of oral corticosteroids
  e. Need for continuous oral corticosteroids
5. Anxiety and depression
6. Social support
7. Life events
8. Attitudes and beliefs about asthma
9. Patient behavior during attack | Closed-ended questions, but see tables 2 and 3 (pp. 16–17) for most frequent responses |

(continued on next page)

Table 1 (*continued*)

Publication	Respondents	Inquiry type	Question categories	Response themes
Lewith et al (2002) [21]	327 adult asthma patients	Questionnaire and measures of asthma symptoms at baseline and a later point	1. Attitudes towards Alternative Medicine Scale (AAMS) 2. Attitudes toward treatment 3. A belief that the body varies in terms of "a healthy balance"	N/A: Closed-ended questions
Logan et al (2003) [22]	152 adolescents (11–18 y) with asthma	Questionnaire battery	Factors: 1. Disease/regimen/medical systems 2. Cognitive difficulties 3. Social support/lack of self-efficacy 4. Denial/distrust 5. Peer/family issues	N/A: Closed-ended questions

Lozano et al (2003) [23]	Parents of 638 children (3–15 y) with mild to moderate persistent asthma	Questionnaire administered by interviewer	1. Demographics
			2. Medication classes
			3. Reliever dosing in past 4 wk
			4. Controller dosing in past 4 wk
			5. Asthma symptom-days in past 2 wk (5–14 symptom-days/high reliever use: "excess asthma symptoms or high reliever use")
			6. Processes of asthma care
			  a. Specialist visit
			  b. Individualized written care plan
			  c. Health care use
				N/A: Closed-ended questions

McQuaid et al (2003) [24]	106 children with asthma and their parents	Interview and questionnaires	7. Adequacy of control
			  a. Current regimen: controller versus no controller
			  d. Excess symptoms or reliever: yes versus no
			  *adequate control: controller (a) and no (b)
			  *inadequate control: yes (b)
				N/A: Adherence questions closed-ended

Meng and McConnell (2002) [25]	28 children (7–12 y) with moderate to severe asthma and their parents	Focus group interviews with children and parents (separately)	Child: 1. Concepts of Asthma Interview 2. Asthma Knowledge Questionnaire 3. Asthma Responsibilities Questionnaire Parent: 1. Asthma Functional Severity Scale Questions about self-management decisions that parents and children must make	Child themes: 1. Worries 2. Asthma knowledge 3. Medications 4. Parental supports 5. School issues Parent themes: 1. School issues 2. Nocturnal symptoms 3. Early warning signs 4. Triggers 5. Peak flow meters 6. Medications

(continued on next page)

Table 1 (continued)

Publication	Respondents	Inquiry type	Question categories	Response themes

Penza-Clyve et al (2004) [26]	36 children (9–15 years) with asthma	Focus groups guided by semistructured interview	Sample open-ended questions:
			1. What are some annoying things about having asthma?
			2. What gets in the way of taking your regular inhalers?
			3. What advice would you give a kid with asthma who was having a hard time taking his/her medication regularly?
				1. Asthma consequences
				  a. Limitations on well-being
				  b. Unavoidable exposures to triggers
				  c. Medication annoyances
				  d. Benefits of asthma
				2. Barriers to adherence
				  a. Reduced motivation
				  b. Difficulty remembering
				  c. Social barriers
				  d. Limits to accessibility
				3. Child-generated strategies to improve adherence
				  a. Use of reminders
				  b. Implementing social strategies
				  c. Enhancing accessibility
				  d. Increasing motivation
				  e. Adopting a "just-do-it" attitude

Peterson-Sweeney et al (2003) [27]	18 parents of children (2–18 years) with asthma	Individual semi-structured interview	1. Understanding of the nature of asthma 2. How asthma affects the child and family 3. Knowledge about asthma medications 4. Attitudes/beliefs about asthma medications and their administration 5. Partnership and communication with the health care provider	Themes of asthma management and medication use: 1. "I know my child" — mothers usually take responsibility for management 2. "Trial and error" — approach to management 3. "Partnership" — variety in amount of perceived collaboration with provider 4. "Need for education" — knowledge about medication by providers

			5. "Negotiating responsibility"— communication between parent and child 6. "Hassles with medication administration"— includes resistance by children and forgetting 7. "Preferences" — types of medication 8. "The benefits outweigh the risks of side effects" N/A: Closed-ended questions (except for single question on compliance)

Put et al (2000) [28]	85 adult asthma patients in Belgium	Questionnaires and structured interview	1. Asthma symptoms
			  a. Asthma Quality of Life Questionnaire
			  b. Asthma Symptom Checklist
			2. Psychologic variables
			  a. Hospital Anxiety and Depression Scale
			  b. Negative Emotionality Scale
			3. Compliance — interview
			  a. Compliance
			  b. Side effects
			  c. Therapeutic effect

Schmaling et al (2000) [29]	53 adult patients with asthma	Questionnaires	Asthma Decisional Balance Questionnaire: pros and cons of regular asthma medication use 1. Gains and losses expected for self 2. Gains and losses expected for others 3. Self-approval and disapproval of the target behavior 4. Approval and disapproval of the behavior by others N/A: Closed-ended questions

(continued on next page)

Table 1 (*continued*)

Publication	Respondents	Inquiry type	Question categories	Response themes
			Asthma Readiness to Change Questionnaire 1. Stage of change of optimal medicine use 2. Consistency of medication-related behavior Readiness and Confidence Rulers 1. Readiness to be compliant 2. Confidence in ability to be compliant	N/A: Closed-ended questions
Thomas et al (1996) [30]	1386 adults who had been to the ED for one of five complaints, including asthma	On-site questionnaire and questionnaire administered by phone interview (10 d later)	Phone questionnaire: 1. Patient's intervening use of health care services 2. Patient's satisfaction with ED care 3. Self-reported problems with the process of care and discharge instructions 4. Compliance with follow-up instructions 5. Self-reported health status at time of follow-up 6. Compliance with follow-up appointments and medications	
Wade et al (1999) [31]	789 inner-city children (4–9 y) with asthma and their parents	Individual interview	1. Identification of everyone who helps care for child's asthma	N/A: Closed-ended questions

Study	Sample	Method	Measures	Results
Wroe (2002) [32]	173 adults with asthma (104 hospital patients, 67 nonpatients)	Questionnaire	2. Level of responsibility assumed by each caregiver in the following domains: a. Medication use b. Attack prevention and trigger avoidance c. Use of medical care 1. Nonadherence 2. Reasons for/against taking medication as prescribed 3. Consultation first received about medication	1. Intentional nonadherence 2. Unintentional nonadherence
Van Es et al (1998) [33]	14 adolescents (12–16 y) with asthma in the Netherlands	Focus group interviews	1. Self-management behavior a. Prevention b. Attack management c. Social skills 2. Feelings about having asthma 3. Opinion of health care provided by pediatrician	1. Actions to prevent/relieve symptoms a. Use of medication only when symptoms are severe b. Forgetting to take medicine c. Participants often reporting smoking, and few knew the harmfulness of smoking to asthmatics 2. Relationships to others a. Most not hesitant to tell others about their asthma, take medicine in others' presence b. Fear of being assertive (eg, asking someone to put out a cigarette) 3. Feelings about having asthma a. Most not ashamed of their asthma b. All sometimes frustrated with asthma, especially when physically limited by it

(continued on next page)

Table 1 (*continued*)

Publication	Respondents	Inquiry type	Question categories	Response themes
				4. Participant-pediatrician contact 　a. All trusted pediatrician and his/her ability to treat asthma 　b. Some felt pediatrician's explanation of medicine too complex to be understood 　c. Most afraid to tell pediatrician how they managed asthma 　d. Want more information about asthma and treatment 5. Recommendations for treatment/education 　a. Give practical information about symptom prevention 　b. Explain how medication works 　c. Give information personally (versus in leaflets) 　d. Use drawings, pictures, films 　e. Provide pictures of lungs of persons with and without asthma 　f. Provide film with peers explaining asthma management 　g. Provide forum for peer discussion of asthma
Yoos et al (2003) — phase 1 [34]	Eight experts in care of children with asthma	Group discussion	Unstructured discussion about factors affecting anti-inflammatory use	1. Nature of the disease 2. Knowledge of the function of anti-inflammatories 3. Benefits/costs of anti-inflammatory therapy 4. Patient-health care provider communication

Yoos et al (2003) — phase 2 [34]	21 parents of children with asthma	Semi-structured face-to-face interview	1. Understanding of the nature and causes of asthma 2. Symptoms 3. Effect of asthma on child and family 4. Expectations about outcomes of the disease 5. Knowledge, attitudes, and beliefs about treatment (especially anti-inflammatories)	1. Nature of asthma 2. Uncertainty related to symptom evaluation and willingness to tolerate a high level of symptoms 3. Medication issues 4. Dispersion of responsibility for managing asthma 5. Relationship with health care provider
Yoos et al (2003) — phase 4 [34]	109 parents of children (2–19 y) with asthma	Questionnaire administered by telephone	1. Nature of the disease and symptoms 2. Cause/triggers 3. Treatment expectations 4. Ideas about medications a. Attitudes toward anti-inflammatories b. Child's reaction to medications c. Knowledge about how medications work 5. Parent–health care provider relationship	N/A: Closed-ended questions

Abbreviations: ED, emergency department; ICS, inhaled corticosteroids; SES, socioeconomic status.

Adults—high emphasis factors

1. *Fear of adverse effects of medication.* Many patients expressed concerns about negative side effects of inhaled steroids or fears that the potential health costs outweigh the benefits of following their prescribed treatment regime. Patients often reported the wish to take the least amount of medication necessary and to reduce their medication use when symptoms improve.

2. *Belief that the medication does not help or is not necessary.* Some patients believed that there was no real positive effect of their medication, such as better control of their asthma or improvement in their quality of life. In some cases this was related to the fact that many of the inhaled steroids used to treat asthma do not show immediate effects.

3. *Sense of only an intermittent need for medication.* Related to the last theme, adults with asthma often noted that they took their inhaled steroids only when their symptoms were noticeable or bothersome. This pattern of intermittent use contrasts with practice guidelines under which inhaled steroids are to be used daily to control underlying inflammation.

4. *Inconvenience of medication use.* Many patients indicated that they faced a number of difficulties related to using their medications, including having to take several different medications or multiple doses per day, inconvenience of carrying medications around, and difficulty using their inhalers. All of these factors contributed to their nonadherence.

5. *Cost of medication.* Patients sometimes indicated that the cost of their inhalers added to the likelihood that they would not fill a prescription.

6. *Dislike of provider.* The importance of having an asthma care provider who was sensitive and empathetic, listened well to patient concerns, and provided sufficient and comprehendible information about the disease and treatment was raised by some patients. Patients were more likely to follow their physician's directives if they liked and trusted the physician and felt that the physician had taken the time to understand their asthma.

Adults—lower emphasis factors

The following less common themes related to nonadherence emerged in patients' responses:

7. *Stigmatization.* Some patients indicated that they were less likely to take their medication because of stigma associated with having a chronic illness, especially when medication brought their asthma to light in the presence of others.

8. *Inadequate knowledge.* Nonadherence was linked to a feeling of not having enough knowledge about the disease or its treatment and so being less likely to take medication as prescribed.

9. *Forgetfulness.* A small number of patients noted that they forgot to take their medication at least some of the time.
10. *Belief that their asthma is not serious.* Some individuals revealed that they did not believe that their asthma was serious enough to warrant the inconvenience of taking inhaled steroids daily, sometimes because of the mildness of their symptoms.
11. *Worry about diminishing effectiveness of medication over time.* Certain patients expressed concern that if they took their medication daily for a long period of time, their body would adapt to the constant exposure to the drug and the medication would no longer be effective.
12. *Fear of addiction/dependence.* Worry about becoming addicted to or dependent on controller medication was expressed by a number of patients.
13. *Lack of social support.* Some individuals indicated that a lack of social support made it more difficult to be adherent with their asthma treatment. On the other hand, having social support, family, or friends who were supportive or even helped with the patient's experience with and treatment of asthma promoted adherence.

Children with asthma and their parents

Although the factors listed above apply to most individuals with asthma, there are subgroups of individuals with the disease for whom the strongest influences on adherence may be different. One such subgroup is children with asthma. Across the studies examined, children with asthma and their parents indicated that the following factors were most important:

1. *Stigmatization.* The children noted that taking their medication is often undesirable when it reminds them that they are different from "normal" children and when it reveals their illness to other children, such as at school. Stigmatization seems to be a more important influence on children with asthma than on adult patients.
2. *Fear of side effects.* Parents of children with asthma noted worrying that inhaled steroids might have adverse affects on their children, such as shorter height or increased irritability.
3. *Fear of addiction/dependence.* Like adult patients, parents of children with asthma expressed fear that their children would become addicted to or dependent on their inhaled steroids over time.
4. *Difficulty with administration of medication.* Some parents indicated that it was difficult to administer their children's asthma medication, due in part to children's resistance.
5. *Dividing responsibility for treatment among children and caregivers.* Treatment adherence for children's asthma is different from that of adults because it often depends on several people, including the child, the parent(s), and other caregivers (eg, baby-sitters, teachers, and grandparents) taking on different levels of responsibility for different aspects of treatment.

Parents indicated that the challenge of sharing these responsibilities and communicating about these tasks clearly and accurately sometimes contributes to nonadherence.

Low-income patients

Another subgroup that may indicate a different list of factors affecting adherence is low-income patients (including minority patients) with asthma. This group often indicated the following reasons for nonadherence:

1. *Difficulty/cost of obtaining medication.* Some low socioeconomic status patients face a large number of hassles in obtaining medication, including difficulty getting to appointments, difficulty obtaining prescriptions through managed care plans, and prohibitive costs of medication.
2. *Fear of adverse effects of medication.* Concerns often focused upon the safety of steroids and the notion that potential side effects may not be revealed to the public even when they are know by manufacturers and medical researchers.
3. *Interference of life hassles.* Urban, poor individuals are more likely to report that a large percentage of their efforts on maintaining basic needs, such as paying bills, obtaining food, and maintaining personal safety, with the consequence that nonurgent medical care is often ignored.
4. *Distrust of medical establishments.* Patients in this subgroup are more likely to be wary of information and instructions given by hospitals and doctors and therefore may be less likely to comply with prescribed treatments.

Discussion

Asthma may be unstable because patients do not adhere to their treatment plan. Many patients with asthma do not easily accept the belief that daily use of controller medications is essential to controlling their asthma, and some are concerned that the risks or inconveniences of these medications may exceed their benefits. Several studies identified patients who reported that they possessed insufficient information about their asthma or its treatment, but across studies neither inadequate information nor forgetfulness emerged among the primary reasons why patients did not consistently take their medication.

Patients in numerous studies expressed concerns about the safety of their medications, particularly inhaled steroids. These concerns, likely in combination with the often-expressed doubt that the medications are helpful or necessary, undermine patient willingness to use their medications as prescribed. Further, patients often seem to perceive their illness as a series of events requiring inter-mittent rather than daily treatment. Many are willing to use controller medications during exacerbations but prefer to avoid them when symptoms are not apparent.

Some of these patients concluded that their illness is not serious enough to require daily medications. Indeed, many patients underestimate the seriousness of their asthma [35]. In short, patients frequently are reluctant to take large amounts of medication that they view as potentially unsafe, that they do not perceive as necessary on a daily basis, or that do not promptly make them feel better. A study of the personal beliefs of 324 patients with chronic illness revealed that many patients were concerned that the side-effect risk of their medication might outweigh the benefits. This perceived risk/benefit gap was greater among asthma or cardiac patients than oncology or dialysis patients [17]. For many patients, the apparent logic of taking medications only when symptoms are present is additionally supported by the cost savings realized when patients take less medication and therefore extend the lifespan of each container of medication.

Subpopulations of patients, including children and low-income patients, may identify a different set of factors interfering with willingness to use daily asthma medications. Parents of children with asthma express some of the same concerns and doubts as those reported by adults with asthma, including worry about side effects. However, children and their parents additionally expressed concerns about long-term dependence on medication, stigmatization occurring when medications are used in front of peers, and the ongoing struggle between parent and child over the child's willingness to take medication and, as they grow older, to assume greater responsibility for remembering to take the medication independently from the parent. Low-income and minority patients share concern about side effects but additionally note specific barriers to adherence, including the difficulty and cost of obtaining medication and a general distrust of medications and medical institutions.

That these special patient populations may not use their medications for reasons that are not identical to those of the general adult population suggests that specific interventions may need to be designed for them. However, the exact nature of interventions likely to succeed is not clear. It is difficult to know from these studies whether the factors patients identify as undermining their willingness to use daily prescribed asthma medications are remediable. If inadequate knowledge about controller medication were the primary factor, basic patient education might change adherence behavior. However, attempts to improve asthma self-management through brief or extensive educational programs seem in most cases to result in little change in medication-related behavior or asthma control [1]. Patients dissatisfied with their caregiver might change caregivers. Reducing the cost of medications or providing supplemental sources of payment could benefit those who state that medication cost undermines their adherence, although there is no evidence that reducing cost increases adherence. Indeed, low-income families exempt from most medication costs are often among those who are least adherent [6]. Apter et al [6] have shown that, although numerous factors influencing the adherence of minority patients with asthma cannot practically be changed (eg, race, gender, education), some of the greatest influences on adherence—negative attitude toward the medication [6] and communication with the caregiver [36]—can be improved with intervention.

The body of information obtained from patients' perspectives indicates the need to reappraise current approaches to the management of asthma. The evidence reviewed here casts doubts on whether expert guidelines dictating that daily treatment of asthma is necessary for optimal control are attainable. Until now, the collective opinion of medical caregivers and patient educators has been that patient behavior should be conformed to match the requirements of the guidelines. Although patients should be educated about their disease and its treatment, the bulk of information indicates that no amount of education has been able to convince most patients with asthma to take their medications every day. In short, the expert guidelines [37] may be unattainable for many asthma patients not because of pharmacologic shortcomings but because of behavioral limitations.

Resolution of the incompatibility between behavioral capability and pharmacologic requirement is essential if greater control of asthma and decreased morbidity, mortality, and cost are to be achieved. The reformulation of expert guidelines for asthma treatment must include consideration of what has been learned from adherence research. Requiring patients to engage in treatment regimens that they are unwilling or unable to follow is a formula for failure. On the other hand, effective treatments for asthma cannot be abandoned. Many pharmaceutical firms, understanding that patients are more predisposed to take medications that are easy to use, have developed drugs that are more widely accepted by patients because they combine two drugs into one inhaler, are required only once per day, or are taken in tablet form. Although patients are sometimes more willing to take such simplified medications, adherence with these products still falls well below their prescribed frequency [38,39]. The most promising answer to the pharmacologic versus behavioral efficacy debate is found in the emergence of the Shared Decision Making Model of health caregiving [40,41]. The model requires that the doctor-knows-best model be replaced with collaboration between the physician and patient. The patient is encouraged to voice his or her preferences and values, and the physician brings expertise and communicates information about the disease, possible treatments, and risks. Discussion of risks includes the risk of under-treatment and risks brought by the medications. For example, for patients with asthma, the interaction may include discussion of side effects of inhaled steroids considered against risk of poorly controlled illness. Cost, difficulty in obtaining the medication, and risk of dependence on the medication may enter into the discussion. The Shared Decision Making Model requires the physician to allow some flexibility into the decision-by-algorithm approach in which the physician, following expert guidelines, chooses the treatment, which the patient is then required to take. Instead, physician and patient negotiate the best match of effective treatment and patient preference. Physician and patient must agree on the treatment goal. The objective of this collaboration is to arrive at a treatment that the physician and the patient will embrace, producing a partnership in which the two work together to gain control of the illness rather than accepting the authoritative hierarchy in which the physician attempts to convince the patient to take his medicine.

There are limitations to the Shared Decision Making Model. Some patients still wish to be told by their health care provider which medicine to take. Some physicians may not feel comfortable relinquishing some of their authority or spending more time communicating with the patient. Some diseases have little room for treatment negotiation. Nonetheless, when the physician is willing to share decision-making with the patient and when the patient understands that he will be able to exercise choice in planning the treatment, the possibility greatly increases that the patient will accept responsibility for deciding how to take care of his illness. When this occurs, greater adherence and increased asthma control are likely to follow [42].

References

[1] Bender B, Boulet L-P, Chaustre I, et al. In adherence to long-term therapies: evidence for action. Geneva, Switzerland: World Health Organization; 2003.

[2] Iskedjiian M, Addis A, Einarson T. Estimating the economic burden of hospitalization due to patient nonadherence in Canada. Value Health 2002;5:470–1.

[3] Bender B, Creer T. Promoting adherence and effective self-management in patients with asthma. In: Leung D, Sampson H, Geha R, Szefler S, editors. Pediatric asthma: principles and practice. St. Louis: Mosby; 2003. p. 457–64.

[4] Milgrom H, Bender B, Ackerson L, et al. Noncompliance and treatment failure in children with asthma. J Allergy Clin Immunol 1996;98:1051–7.

[5] Bender B, Milgrom H, Apter A. Adherence intervention research: what have we learned and what do we do next? J Allergy Clin Immunol 2003;112:489–94.

[6] Apter A, Boston R, George M, et al. Modifiable barriers to adherence to inhaled steroids among adults with asthma: it's not just black and white. J Allergy Clin Immunol 2003;111:1219–26.

[7] Bauman LJ, Wright E, Leickly FE, et al. Relationship of adherence to pediatric asthma morbidity among inner-city children. Pediatrics 2002;110:1–7.

[8] Boulet L-P. Perception of the role and potential side effects of inhaled corticosteroids among asthmatic patients. Chest 1998;113:587–92.

[9] Buston K, Wood S. Non-compliance amongst adolescents with asthma: listening to what they tell us about self-management. Fam Pract 2000;17:134–8.

[10] Chambers C, Markson L, Diamond J, et al. Health beliefs and compliance with inhaled corticosteroids by asthmatic patients in primary care practices. Respir Med 1999;93:88–94.

[11] Chan P, DeBrune J. Parental concern towards the use of inhaled therapy in children with chronic asthma. Pediatr Int 2000;42:547–51.

[12] Donnelly J, Donnelly W, Thong Y. Parental perceptions and attitudes toward asthma and its treatment: a controlled study. Soc Sci Med 1987;24:431–7.

[13] Erickson S, Coombs J, Kirking D, et al. Compliance from self-reported versus pharmacy claims data with metered-dose inhalers. Ann Pharmacother 2001;35:997–1003.

[14] Fiese B, Wamboldt F. Tales of pediatric asthma management: family-based strategies related to medical adherence and health care utilization. J Pediatr 2003;143:457–62.

[15] George M, Freedman T, Norfleet A, et al. Qualitative research-enhanced understanding of patients' beliefs: results of focus groups with low-income, urban, African American adults with asthma. J Allergy Clin Immunol 2003;111:967–73.

[16] Hand C, Chir B, Bradley C. Health beliefs of adults with asthma: toward an understanding of the difference between symptomatic and preventive use of inhaler treatment. J Asthma 1996;33:331–8.

[17] Horne R, Weinman J. Patients' beliefs about prescribed medicines and their role in adherence to treatment in chronic physical illness. J Psychosom Res 1999;47:555–67.

[18] Ireland L. Children's perceptions of asthma: establishing normality. Children's Nursing 1997; 6:1059–64.

[19] Kolbe J, Fergusson W, Vamos M, et al. Case-control study of severe life-threatening asthma (SLTA) in adults: psychological factors. Thorax 2002;57:317–22.

[20] Kolbe J, Vamos M, Fergusson W, et al. Determinants of management errors in acute severe asthma. Thorax 1998;53:14–20.

[21] Lewith G, Hyland M, Shaw S. Do attitudes toward and beliefs about complementary medicine affect treatment outcomes? Am J Public Health 2002;92:1604–6.

[22] Logan D, Zelikovsky N, Labay L, et al. The illness management survey: identifying adolescents' perceptions of barriers to adherence. J Pediatr Psychol 2003;28:323–33.

[23] Lozano P, Finkelstein J, Hecht J, et al. Asthma medication use and disease burden in children in a primary care population. Arch Pediatr Adolesc Med 2003;157:81–8.

[24] McQuaid E, Kopel S, Klein F, et al. Medication adherence in pediatric asthma: reasoning, responsibility, and behavior. J Ped Psychol 2003;28:323–33.

[25] Meng A, McConnell S. Decision-making in children with asthma and their parents. J Am Acad Nurse Pract 2002;14:363–71.

[26] Penza-Clyve S, Mansell C, McQuaid E. Why don't children take their asthma medications? A qualitative analysis of children's perspectives on adherence. J Asthma 2004;41:189–97.

[27] Peterson-Sweeney K, McMullen A, Yoos H, et al. Parental perceptions of their child's asthma: management and medication use. J Pediatr Health Care 2003;17:118–25.

[28] Put C, Van den Bergh O, Demedts M, et al. A study of the relationship among self-reported noncompliance, symptomatology, and psychological variables in patients with asthma. J Asthma 2000;37:503–10.

[29] Schmaling K, Afari N, Blume A. Assessment of psychological factors associated with adherence to medication regimens among adult patients with asthma. J Asthma 2000;37:335–43.

[30] Thomas E, Burstin H, O'Neil A, et al. Patient noncompliance with medical advice after the emergency department visit. J Ann Emerg Med 1996;27:49–55.

[31] Wade S, Islam S, Holden G, et al. Division of responsibility for asthma management tasks between caregivers and children in the inner city. J Dev Behav Pediatr 1999;20:93–8.

[32] Wroe A. Intentional and unintentional nonadherence: a study of decision making. J Behav Med 2002;25:355–71.

[33] van Es SM, le Coq EM, Brouwer AI, et al. Adherence-related behavior in adolescents with asthma: results from focus group interviews. J Asthma 1998;35:637–46.

[34] Yoos H, Kitzman H, McMullen A. Barriers to anti-inflammatory medication use in childhood asthma. Ambul Pediatr 2003;3:181–90.

[35] Bich-Phyong N, Wilson S, German D. Patients' perceptions compared with objective ratings of asthma severity. Ann Allergy Asthma Immunol 1996;77:209–15.

[36] Apter A, Reisine S, Affleck G, et al. Adherence with twice-daily dosing of inhaled steroids. Am J Respir Crit Care Med 1998;157:1810–7.

[37] National Heart, Lung, and Blood Institute. Guidelines for the diagnosis and management of asthma, highlights of the expert panel report II, February, 1997. Bethesda (MD): National Heart, Lung, and Blood Institute; 1997.

[38] Jones C, Santanello N, Boccuzzi S, et al. Adherence to prescribed treatment for asthma: evidence from pharmacy benefits data. J Asthma 2003;40:93–101.

[39] Sherman J, Patel P, Hutson A, et al. Adherence to oral montelukast and inhaled fluticasone in children with persistent asthma. Pharmacotherapy 2001;21:1464–7.

[40] Charles C, Gafni A, Whelan T. Decision-making in the physician-patient encounter: revisiting the shared treatment decision-making model. Soc Sci Med 1999;49:651–61.

[41] Godolphin W. The role of risk communication in shared decision making. BMJ 2003;327:692–3.

[42] O'Connor A, Drake E, Fiset V, et al. Annotated bibliography: studies evaluating decision-support interventions for patients. Can J Nurs Res 1997;29:113–20.

ELSEVIER
SAUNDERS

Immunol Allergy Clin N Am
25 (2005) 131–148

IMMUNOLOGY
AND ALLERGY
CLINICS
OF NORTH AMERICA

Gastroesophageal reflux: a potential asthma trigger

Susan M. Harding, MD

Division of Pulmonary, Allergy and Critical Care Medicine, University of Alabama at Birmingham,
1900 University Blvd, THT Rm 215, Birmingham, AL 35294, USA

Gastroesophageal reflux (GER), the retrograde movement of gastric contents into the esophagus, afflicts millions of Americans. A population-based survey of randomly selected adults shows that the prevalence rate of heartburn or regurgitation at least weekly approaches 20% [1]. Sir William Osler formally recognized GER as a potential trigger of asthma and stated "...attacks may be due to direct irritation of the bronchial mucosa or indirectly, too, by reflex influences from stomach..." [2]. Since Osler's time, we have gained significant insight into the association between asthma and GER [3].

Gastroesophageal reflux prevalence and epidemiologic considerations in asthmatics

GER symptoms are common in adults and children with asthma. Field et al [4] examined 109 asthmatics and 135 subjects in two control groups and found that heartburn was present in 77% of asthmatics compared with 50% of subjects in the control groups. Furthermore, 41% of asthmatics noted GER-associated respiratory symptoms, and 28% used their inhalers while experiencing GER symptoms. These data verify that GER symptoms are more prevalent in asthmatics compared

---

This work was supported by NHLBI grant no. HL75614-01 from the National Institutes of Health. Dr. Harding has received grant funding and is a consultant for AstraZeneca LP.

E-mail address: sharding@uab.edu

with control populations and that asthmatics associate GER symptoms with their asthma symptoms. This high prevalence was verified by Perrin-Fayolle et al [5], who found that 65% of consecutive asthmatics had GER symptoms. Asthma symptoms also correlated with esophageal acid events on 24-hour esophageal pH testing. Our laboratory noted that of 151 respiratory symptoms reported during 24-hour esophageal pH testing, 119 (79%) were associated with esophageal acid [6]. Approximately 50% of children with asthma have GER symptoms [7].

GER may be clinically "silent" in asthmatics. In difficult-to-control asthmatics who did not have GER symptoms, Irwin et al [8] found that 24% had GER-responsive asthma. Our laboratory observed in consecutive asthmatics without GER symptoms that 62% of them had abnormal esophageal pH tests [9]. Demographic variables did not identify asthmatics with clinically silent GER. In children, GER was detected by scintigraphy in 23% of asthmatics who did not have GER symptoms [10].

Biopsy-proven esophagitis was found in 43% of consecutive adult asthmatics [11]. In children, esophagitis was present in 8.5% of asthmatics who had abnormal esophageal pH tests [12]. Sontag et al [13] performed esophageal pH tests in consecutive asthmatics and reported abnormal esophageal acid contact times in 82%. Compared with control subjects, asthmatics had more frequent reflux episodes and higher esophageal acid contact times. Our laboratory showed that 72% of asthmatics with GER symptoms had abnormal esophageal acid contact times [6]. Abnormal esophageal acid contact times are prevalent in children. Cinquetti et al [12] examined 77 asthmatic children age 39 to 170 months and reported abnormal esophageal acid contact times in 47 (61%). Asthma severity was proportional to esophageal acid amounts, and nocturnal GER was more frequently found in the moderate and severe asthmatics compared with the mild asthmatics [12]. Tucci et al [14] noted that 75% of asthmatic children had abnormal esophageal acid contact times.

Although many of the above studies used selected populations, asthmatics, compared with control subjects, have a higher frequency of GER symptoms and higher esophageal acid contact times. In general, approximately 50% to 80% of adults and children with asthma have GER (Table 1).

Table 1
Prevalence of gastroesophageal reflux in asthmatics

Findings	Prevalence	
	Adults	Children
Heartburn	77%	50%
Reflux-associated respiratory symptoms	41%	—
Clinically silent GER	62%	23%
Esophagitis	43%	5.85%[a]
Abnormal esophageal pH	82%	75%

[a] Children with abnormal esophageal pH tests.
Data from Refs. [4,7,9–14].

Epidemiologic considerations also give insight as to how GER may affect asthma. A case-control study examined more than 101,000 veterans discharged with esophagitis or esophageal stricture from 172 Veterans Administration hospitals and compared them with randomly selected veterans without esophageal disease. The veterans with significant esophageal disease had a 1.51 odds ratio (OR) of having asthma [15]. Gislason et al [16] examined the association between respiratory symptoms and nocturnal GER in a population-based study of more than 2600 young adults from three European countries. Subjects with nocturnal GER, compared with those without nocturnal GER, had a higher likelihood of wheezing (adjusted OR 2.5, 95% confidence interval [CI] 1.6–3.9) and physician-diagnosed asthma (adjusted OR 2.2, 95% CI 1.0–4.7). Asthmatics with nocturnal GER had greater peak expiratory flow rate (PEF) variability. These data support the hypothesis that GER during sleep has the potential to alter pulmonary function during the night. In a large prospective cohort study of more than 6500 asthmatics, Diette et al [17] noted that asthmatics over 65 years of age had higher heartburn prevalence compared with younger asthmatics and that GER was a risk factor for asthma hospitalizations. That GER was a risk factor for asthma hospitalization was verified by Shireman et al [18], who performed a retrospective cross-sectional analysis of Ohio Medicaid claims over 12 months involving 11,000 asthmatics. GER was predictive for a higher number of oral corticosteroid bursts ($P < 0.001$) and for an increased risk of asthma-related hospitalizations ($P < 0.007$).

There also are epidemiologic studies examining children. El-Serag [19] performed a case-control study in 10,000 children without neurologic defects (1980 subjects with GER and 7920 control subjects without GER) and reported that children with GER had a higher asthma prevalence compared with control subjects (13% versus 7%, $P < 0.001$). Even after adjusting for differences in age, gender, and ethnicity, GER remained a significant risk factor for asthma, with an OR of 1.9 (95% CI 1.6–2.3, $P < 0.001$). All of these studies show that GER prevalence is high in children and adults with asthma and that the two diseases may interact.

Predisposing factors to gastroesophageal reflux development in asthmatics

Under normal conditions in the stomach, the angle of His acts as a flap valve to prevent material from leaving the stomach. The lower esophageal sphincter (LES) is the major anti-reflux barrier and has an intrinsic basal tone along with augmentation by crural diaphragm contractions [20]. If GER occurs, a swallow initiates peristalsis that clears gastric contents from the esophagus. Saliva neutralizes the acid pH and rinses the refluxate from the esophageal mucosa. GER disease is a multifactorial process resulting from three potential motility abnormalities, including an incompetent LES, inefficient esophageal clearance of refluxed material, and delayed gastric emptying. Transient LES relaxations are LES relaxations not associated with swallows and are responsible for approximately 75% of GER episodes in adults [20]. Specific predisposing factors for GER development in asthmatics include an increased pressure gradient between the thorax and the abdominal cavity (over-riding the LES pressure), autonomic dysregulation, and the high prevalence of hiatal hernia and obesity found in asthmatics. Asthma medications may promote GER [3].

Asthmatics can have an increased pressure gradient between the thorax and the abdominal cavity. At the end of expiration, the pressure gradient between the stomach and esophagus is 4 to 5 mm Hg [20]. Therefore, a normal LES pressure of 10 to 35 mm Hg is sufficient to counteract this pressure gradient. However, with airflow obstruction, especially during asthma exacerbations, a more negative pleural pressure is produced that may overcome the LES pressure, thus promoting GER.

Autonomic dysregulation may potentiate GER because transient LES relaxations are vagally triggered [20,21]. Our laboratory showed that asthmatics with GER have heightened vagal responsiveness [22]. Heightened vagal tone can result in a decreased LES pressure and stimulate transient LES relaxations [20,21].

Another factor is alteration in crural diaphragm function. The crural diaphragm contributes to LES pressure generation, especially during inspiration [20]. Hyperinflation associated with bronchospasm places the crural diaphragm at a functional disadvantage because of geometric flattening [23].

Hiatal hernias also predispose to GER and are common in asthmatics. Mays et al [24] noted that 64% of asthmatics, compared with 19% of control subjects, had hiatal hernia. Sontag et al [11] performed endoscopies in 186 consecutive asthmatics and reported the presence of hiatal hernia in 58%. Obesity contributes to GER, and GER is associated with an increased body mass index (BMI) and asthma symptoms as noted in the European Community Respiratory Health Survey [16,25].

Finally, medications including theophylline, albuterol, and oral corticosteroids may predispose to GER development. Theophylline increases gastric acid secretion and lowers LES pressure [26]. Ekström et al [27], in a placebo-controlled trial, noted that GER symptoms increased 170% and daytime reflux increased 24% with theophylline. However, there are conflicting data about the importance of theophylline [28]. Crowell et al [29] performed a prospective randomized double blind, placebo-controlled, crossover trial evaluating the effects of sequential doses of nebulized albuterol (2.5–10 mg) on esophageal manometry. Nebulized albuterol produced a dose-dependent reduction in LES pressure from 17 to 8.9 mm Hg. Furthermore, the amplitude of esophageal contractions at 5 cm and 10 cm above the LES was compromised [29]. Our laboratory examined the effect of oral corticosteroids on esophageal acid contact times in a prospective, placebo-controlled, crossover trial in 20 stable, moderate-persistent asthmatics. Oral prednisone, 60 mg per day for 7 days, resulted in significant increases in esophageal acid contact times at the proximal and distal esophageal pH probes [30]. These factors may contribute to the increased GER prevalence in asthmatics.

Potential mechanisms of gastroesophageal reflux–triggered asthma

There are many mechanisms whereby the esophagus and lung can interact and result in esophageal acid–induced bronchoconstriction. Neurogenic inflammation plays a role in many of these mechanisms. Mechanisms include a vagally mediated reflex (whereby acid in the esophagus triggers airway responses), a direct axonal reflex (whereby the central nervous system [CNS] is not required to complete a reflex arc), heightened bronchial reactivity, and microaspiration [26]. Esophageal acid also causes increases in minute ventilation without altering pulmonary function [31].

Vagal reflex

The tracheobronchial tree and the esophagus share common embryonic foregut origins and autonomic innervation through the vagus nerve. In a dog model, Mansfield et al [32] noted that esophageal acid causes an increase in respiratory resistance that was abolished with vagotomy. We reproduced this finding in a human model noting that esophageal acid reduces PEF rates and increases specific airway resistance without evidence of microaspiration [33]. Wright et al [34] measured spirometry before and after esophageal acid infusions and reported that esophageal acid caused decreases in heart rate, FEV_1, and oxygen saturation, which did not occur with atropine pretreatment. These data show that a vagal mechanism is active.

Local axonal reflex

Fischer et al [35] noted, with morphologic studies, that there is a direct neuronal connection between the esophagus and the lung via nitric oxide–containing neurons. In a guinea pig model, when nociceptive afferent nerves are stimulated in the esophagus without CNS intervention, there is the release of tachykinins in the lung, including substance P and neurokinin-A, as the result of a local axonal reflex [36].

Heightened bronchial reactivity

Vincent et al [37] showed a correlation between the amount of methacholine required to reduce the FEV_1 by 20% and the number GER episodes on esophageal pH testing ($R = 0.56$, $P = 0.05$). This relationship was even stronger in asthmatics with documented GER by esophageal pH tests ($R = 0.98$, $P = 0.001$). Heightened bronchial reactivity with GER was noted during sleep by Cuttitta et al [38], who monitored esophageal pH and respiratory resistance in seven asthmatics with GER. Esophageal acid was associated with an increase in lower respiratory resistance. There was also a correlation between GER episode duration and increase in lower airway resistance. These studies illustrate that esophageal acid primes the respiratory system so that when asthmatics are exposed to another asthma trigger, such as cat dander, they have a heightened response.

Microaspiration

Microaspiration causes significant airway responses in animal models and in humans. In a cat model, Tuchman et al [39] noted that 50 μL of tracheal acid caused a 5-fold increase in total lung resistance compared with a 1.5-fold increase with 10 mL of esophageal acid. The vagus nerve also plays a role in the microaspiration model because vagotomy ablated the tracheal acidification response. In humans, Jack et al [40] monitored tracheal and esophageal pH and reported that GER episodes associated with tracheal and esophageal acidification decreased PEF rates by 84 L/min compared with 8 L/min when esophageal acid alone was present.

Neurogenic inflammation

All of these mechanisms can result in neurogenic inflammation. In a guinea pig model, Hamamato et al [41] noted that esophageal acid resulted in airway edema and the release of substance P. This airway edema was inhibited by a substance P receptor antagonist. Vagal and local axonal reflexes were responsible for these alterations. An acidic environment in the upper airway may also alter the inflammatory milieu [42]. Airway protective mechanisms may not be able to neutralize the acid load to the airway epithelium, thus exposing it to injury [43]. Esophageal contents may damage the airway epithelium, resulting in the release of cytokines and adhesion molecules, leading to neurogenic inflammation and the initiation of other inflammatory pathways [44].

Increased minute ventilation

Field et al [31] examined airway responses and respiratory mechanics in nonasthmatics during esophageal acid infusions. Minute ventilation increased with esophageal acid and decreased with esophageal acid clearance. Other respiratory parameters, including pulmonary function, did not change.

Asthma outcomes with anti-reflux therapy

Medical therapy

If GER is a potential asthma trigger, then aggressive GER therapy should improve asthma outcomes. Multiple studies have evaluated asthma outcomes, and most show an improvement in asthma symptoms. In reviewing the combined results of 12 studies examining medical therapy in 326 treated asthmatics with GER, asthma symptoms improved in 69%, medication use was reduced in 62%, and evening PEF rates improved in 26% of patients; however, pulmonary function did not improve [45]. Most trials used H_2 receptor antagonists (H_2RAs) and not proton pump inhibitors (PPIs) [45]. More recently, the Cochrane Airways Group registry examined controlled trials, and 12 trials met their inclusion criteria. Although they noted no overall improvement in asthma after GER therapy, subgroups of patients may benefit. They point out the importance of examining predictors of asthma response [46]. Coughlan et al performed a power analysis on available data, noting that a study sample size of 506 subjects would be needed to detect a 20 L/min improvement in PEF [47].

We performed a prospective pretest/post-test evaluation of 30 asthmatics with GER using a 3-month trial of acid suppressive therapy using omeprazole (20–60 mg/d). Seventy-three percent of asthmatics with GER had at least a 20% increase in PEF rate and/or a 20% decrease in asthma symptoms. The asthma responders had improvement in pulmonary function including FEV_1 and PEF rates. Asthma symptoms required significant time to improve. After 1 month of acid suppressive therapy there was a 30% reduction in asthma symptoms compared with baseline, and by 3 months there was a 57% reduction. Twelve weeks of acid suppressive therapy was required for asthma symptom improvement. Approximately 30% of asthmatics did not have adequate acid suppression, documented by esophageal pH testing, on 20 mg/d of omeprazole [48].

More recently, eight placebo-controlled trials in adults using PPIs have been reported (Table 2). There are no reported double blind, placebo-controlled trials using PPIs in children. All of the studies contained small subject numbers and had inadequate power to address asthma outcomes as noted by the Cochrane Airways Group [47]. Five of the eight PPI trials defined asthma by using clinical and objective data, including airway reactivity (bronchodilatory response or

Table 2
Adult-controlled[a] PPI trials in asthmatics with gastroesophageal reflux

Author	n	Crossover design	Treatment	Asthma outcome
Ford et al [50]	10	Yes	Omp 20 mg × 4 wk	No change
Meier et al [80]	15	Yes	Omp 40 mg × 6 wk	29% ↑ FEV_1 by 20% if esophagitis healed
Teichtahl et al [81]	20	Yes	Omp 40 mg × 4 wk	Mild improvement in PM PEF
Levin et al [82]	9	Yes	Omp 20 mg × 8 wk	Improved symptoms, PEF, and QOL
Boeree et al [49]	36	No	Omp 40 mg BID × 12 wk	Includes COPD, improved PM symptoms
Kiljander et al [83]	52	Yes	Omp 40 mg × 8 wk	Improved PM symptoms
Harmanci et al [84]	5	Yes	Omp 40 mg × 4 wk	Improved PM symptoms
Jiang et al [85]	30	No	Omp 20 mg + domperidone 10 mg TID × 6 wk	Improved FEV_1, PEF

Abbreviations: COPD, chronic obstructive pulmonary disease; FEV_1, forced expiratory volume at 1 s; Omp, omeprazole; PEF, peak expiratory flow; PPI, proton pump inhibitor; QOL, quality of life.
   [a] No pediatric-controlled PPI trials reported to date.

methacholine challenge tests). Six of the eight PPI trials were crossover in design, so that order and carryover effects could have interfered with results. Also, the duration of PPI therapy may have been too brief to show a treatment response. Only the Boeree et al [49] trial was of adequate duration (≥ 12 wk). Most trials did not document adequate acid suppression on therapy (eg, the Ford et al [50] trial used omeprazole 20 mg/d). Furthermore, asthma outcome variables were not consistently measured. Another potential limitation is that GER may not have been an asthma trigger for the individual subjects in the studies. A better study design may be a placebo-controlled parallel design with separate groups of treated and control subjects, using subjects who have GER as an asthma trigger. Not all asthmatics with GER have GER as a trigger of their asthma because asthma is heterogeneous concerning triggers and resultant bronchospasm.

A recently published abstract by Littner et al [51] reports asthma outcomes from the first multicentered, double blind, placebo-controlled trial using high-dose PPI therapy. Two hundred seven moderate to severe-persistent asthmatics with GER symptoms participated in this 24-week trial. Subjects were treated with lansoprazole 30 mg twice daily or placebo. Quality of life variables improved in the treatment group. Treated asthmatics had fewer asthma exacerbations and did not require prednisone bursts as often as the control asthmatics. This trial is the largest trial to date examining this topic.

Another potential way to examine asthma outcomes is to look at difficult-to-control or therapy-resistant asthmatics. Irwin et al [8] examined contributing factors in difficult-to-control asthmatics (those requiring 10 mg of prednisone at least every other day) by using a systematic management protocol. Treatment of GER and the addition of inhaled corticosteroids were the most helpful interventions. Heaney et al [52] examined predictors of therapy-resistant asthma using a systematic evaluation protocol and found that GER was prevalent in this population (57%). Khoshoo et al [53] examined the role of GER in children 5 to 10.5 years of age with persistent asthma and found that 59% had GER. Children with GER then had medical or surgical anti-reflux therapy [53]. All children with abnormal esophageal pH tests had a significant reduction in their asthma medications over the 1-year study period. Anti-reflux therapy resulted in the reduction of the use of short- and long-acting bronchodilators and inhaled cortico-steroids. Another important finding from this study is that at least 6 months of anti-reflux therapy was required to see an appreciable response in asthma outcome in these children [53].

Surgical therapy

Surgical trials have also examined asthmatics with GER. Most trials were case series and had many design flaws, including the lack of a control group, poor documentation of adequate GER control postoperatively, and poor documenta-tion of asthma outcomes. Field et al [54] examined asthma outcomes with anti-reflux surgery and identified 24 trials with 417 asthmatics. Anti-reflux surgery

Table 3
Surgical therapy in asthmatics with gastroesophageal reflux (all case series)

Author	n	Duration	Asthma outcome
Kennedy et al [86]	15	Unknown	100% improved
Overholt et al [87]	28	76 months	82% improved
Urschel et al [88]	27	Unknown	89% improved
Lomasney et al [89]	129	Unknown	75% improved
Sontag et al [90]	13	>1 y	55% improved
Tardif et al [91]	10	1.75 y	50% improved
Perrin-Fayolle et al [61]	44	>5 y	84% improved
DeMeester et al [92]	17	>3 y	82% improved
Johnson et al [93]	14	3 y	Group improved
So et al [94]	16	>1 y	48% improved
Patti et al [95]	39	2.3 y (median)	64% improved
Spivak et al [96]	39	2.7 y (median)	Group improved

improved GER variables in 90%, asthma symptoms in 79%, and asthma medication use in 80% of subjects. Pulmonary function improvement occurred in 27% of surgically treated asthmatics. Table 3 reviews the surgical outcome trials.

Randomized trials of medical versus surgical therapy

Two groups compared medical versus surgical therapy in GER-related asthma; however, PPIs were not used. Larrain et al [55] examined the effect of cimetidine 300 mg four times a day versus surgery in nonallergic asthmatics. After 6 months, there were improvements in pulmonary function, including FEV_1 and PEF, in both treatment groups but not in the placebo group. Medication use improved in both treatment groups. Asthma was improved in 74% of medically treated subjects and in 77% of surgically treated subjects, compared with 36% of control subjects. Sontag et al [56] performed a placebo-controlled randomized study comparing ranitidine 150 mg, three times a day, with surgery in 73 subjects. In the surgery group, 75% had improvement in asthma symptoms, compared with 9% of the medically treated group and 4% of the control group at 5-year follow-up. More recently, Sontag et al [57] examined 62 patients randomized to ranitidine, surgery, or placebo. At the end of 2 years, mean asthma symptom scores in the surgically treated group improved 43%, compared with < 10% in the medically treated and control groups. Some patients had up to 19 years of clinical follow-up after randomization.

Potential predictors of gastroesophageal reflux–responsive asthma

Despite the numerous design flaws in many of the studies, some studies have identified potential predictors for asthma response either by the use of selected patient populations or by evaluation of predictive variables in the responders

---

Box 1. Potential predictors of asthma response

Asthma characteristics:
- Difficult-to-control asthma [8]
- Nonallergic intrinsic asthma [55]
- Nocturnal asthma [61]
- Obesity (BMI > 29.7 kg/m^2) [60]

GER characteristics:
- Reflux-associated respiratory symptoms [58]
- Regurgitation more than once weekly [48]
- Proximal acid on pH testing [48,59]
- Distal acid on pH testing [59,60]

(Box 1). These predictors need to be verified in independent patient populations. Irwin et al [8] noted that difficult-to-control asthma is a potential predictor, whereas Ekström et al [58] noted that a history of reflux-associated respiratory symptoms predicted asthma improvement. Our laboratory noted that the presence of regurgitation more than once a week or the presence of proximal reflux on pH esophageal testing predicted asthma response [48]. Schnatz et al [59] noted that more severe distal reflux predicted asthma response. Kiljander et al [60] noted that higher esophageal acid contact times and a higher BMI predicted asthma improvement. Larrain et al [55] noted that their nonallergic intrinsic asthmatics had asthma improvement with anti-reflux therapy. Perrin-Fayolle et al [61] noted that nocturnal asthma predicted asthma response. If validated, these predictors could help the clinician identify which asthmatics are most likely to respond to anti-reflux therapy.

Diagnosis and therapy of gastroesophageal reflux in asthmatics

Diagnosis

Making the diagnosis of GER in asthmatics is similar to making the diagnosis in people without asthma. GER symptoms may be intermittent, or continuous and progressive. Classic esophageal symptoms include heartburn, regurgitation, retrosternal and epigastric pain, dysphagia, cervical discomfort (globus), and belching [62]. GER symptoms may be temporally associated with chest tightness, wheezing or other asthma symptoms, and inhaler use [4,6]. GER may cause arousals from sleep. It may also be clinically silent in up to 62% of asthmatics without GER symptoms [9]. Esophageal pH testing is required to identify these asthmatics [9]. Many diagnostic tests are available for GER (Table 4).

Table 4
Diagnostic tests for gastroesophageal reflux accuracy in adults

	Sensitivity (%)	Specificity (%)
Empiric PPI trial [63]	70–80	85
Esophageal pH [65]	77–100	85–100
Endoscopy [68]	60 at best	90–95
Barium esophagram [63]	40	Depends
Bernstein test [63]	32–100	40–100
^{99}Technetium-sulfur colloid [63]	14–90	Up to 90

Abbreviation: PPI, proton pump inhibitor.

An empiric trial of acid suppression using a PPI is a simple and potentially definitive method for diagnosing and assessing GER as a potential asthma trigger in selected asthmatics. Response to PPI therapy can also assure a cause-and-effect relationship between GER and specific symptoms [63]. GER symptoms usually respond to PPI therapy within 7 to 14 days [63]. A minimum 3-month empiric trial of PPI should be used to assess asthma symptom improvement [48]. Fass et al [64] found that a 7-day trial of omeprazole 40 mg in the morning and 20 mg in the evening had a sensitivity of 78% and a specificity of 86% for diagnosing GER as the cause of noncardiac chest pain. An empiric trial has advantages, such as its availability, with preliminary evidence showing that it may be cost effective as well.

Ambulatory 24-hour esophageal pH testing is the gold standard for diagnosing GER and has a sensitivity and specificity that approaches 90% [65]. This test entails placing a pH probe intra-nasally and positioning it 5 cm above the LES (distal). Often, multi-channel pH probes are used to monitor pH at the distal and more proximal regions, including the pharynx. An event marker can be activated when GER or pulmonary symptoms occur. A reflux event is defined as a drop in pH below 4.0. The total percentage of time that the pH is < 4.0 is the most useful measurement, with 5.5% being the upper limit of normal. Esophageal pH testing can be used to assess whether there is adequate control of esophageal acid while the patient is on anti-reflux therapy. More recently, a wireless pH probe (Bravo pH Probe; Medtronics, Minneapolis, MN) has become available that overcomes the disadvantages of catheter-related pH probes [66]. The wireless probe is endoscopically placed approximately 6 cm above the Z line that separates the gastric mucosa from the esophageal mucosa. The capsule gathers pH data for approximately 2 days [66]. Another new experimental technique is multi-channel intraluminal esophageal impedance that can be combined with pH monitoring [67]. This device measures the electrical impedance of the esophagus in multiple sites up and down the catheter system so that the movement of gases, liquids, and solids can be quantitated. This technique, when combined with esophageal pH, is useful when assessing for acidic and nonacidic GER [67].

Upper endoscopy is useful for detecting esophageal mucosal injury, including esophagitis, strictures, webs, Barrett's esophagitis, and esophageal tumors [68].

Endoscopy has a poor sensitivity, which limits its usefulness as a diagnostic test for GER. The same is true for the barium esophagram, which has a sensitivity of approximately 40% [63]. Other tests, including radio-labeled ^{99}technetium-sulfur colloid scintiscanning and the Bernstein test, have low sensitivities and are not useful [63]. In conclusion, an empiric trial of acid suppression using a PPI and 24-hour esophageal pH testing seem to be the best methods for detecting GER in asthmatics.

In children, the North American Society for Pediatric Gastroenterology, Hepatology, and Nutrition developed guidelines concerning esophageal pH testing [7]. Children should be questioned about typical GER symptoms, and esophageal pH testing is recommended if persistent asthma is present. As in adults, most children with GER-triggered asthma do not have esophagitis, so endoscopy has a low sensitivity [12]. Empiric PPI trials can be considered in children, although no validation studies have been reported [7].

Therapy

Lifestyle changes are the cornerstone of GER therapy [68]. Lifestyle changes include weight loss (if the patient is obese), avoiding large meals, and avoiding meals within 3 hours of bedtime. Patients should avoid acidic foods, including carbonated drinks. Caffeine, chocolate and peppermint (which decrease LES pressure), and fatty foods (which delay gastric emptying) should be avoided. Antacids can be used for acute relief of GER symptoms. Raising the head of the bed with blocks or a wedge can reduce nocturnal GER. Assess whether theophylline is required because it can worsen GER.

Medical therapy includes gastric acid secretion inhibitors such as H$_2$RAs and PPIs. Prokinetic agents improve esophageal motility, increase LES pressure, and can be combined with other GER medications. First introduced in the 1970s, H$_2$RAs are safe and well tolerated, and all agents have approximately the same efficacy. Commonly used agents include cimetidine up to 800 mg twice daily or 400 mg four times daily, ranitidine 150 mg twice daily, nizatidine 150 mg twice daily, and famotidine 20 mg twice daily. These agents provide complete relief of heartburn in approximately 60% of patients [68]. PPIs achieve superior gastric acid suppression and directly inhibit the acid-secreting parietal cells, so PPIs should be given approximately 30 minutes to 1 hour before meals [68]. PPIs have an excellent safety profile. Patients have been on long-term omeprazole therapy for more than 16 years [69]. Currently available PPIs include omeprazole (Prilosec) 20 mg and 40 mg up to twice daily, lansoprazole (Prevacid) 30 mg once or twice daily, pantoprazole (Protonix) 40 mg once or twice daily, rabeprazole (Aciphex) 20 mg daily, and esomeprazole (Nexium) 40 mg up to twice daily. There are minimal clinically relevant differences among the PPIs [70]. Rabeprazole has a slightly faster onset on action than other PPIs; omeprazole has the highest potential for drug interactions with warfarin, diazepam, phenytoin, and theophylline; and pantoprazole has the lowest potential for drug interactions. None of the PPIs requires dosing adjustments for hepatic or renal insufficiency [70].

The only prokinetic agent available in the United States is metoclopramide. The usual dosing of metoclopramide is 10 mg four times daily. Metoclopramide causes CNS side effects, including drowsiness, irritability, and extrapyramidal effects, in approximately 20% to 50% of patients.

Anti-reflux surgery options include open and laparoscopic procedures. Fundoplication results in GER symptom resolution in approximately 80% to 90% of patients. However, surgery rarely replaces the need for anti-reflux medications [71]. Spechler et al [72] performed a prospective randomized trial of medical and surgical therapy in 160 patients with complicated GER, having a median follow-up of 10 years. Sixty-two percent of surgically treated patients continued to use anti-reflux medications regularly. Surgery also has risks. For instance, laparoscopic fundoplication is associated with a 12% risk of dysphagia. Surgery for treatment of GER-triggered asthma should be reserved for asthmatics who have marked improvement in their asthma with medical anti-reflux therapy.

There are endoscopic methods to treat GER, including endoscopic gastroplasty and the Stretta procedure, which delivers radio frequency energy below the mucosa at the gastroesophageal junction [73]. These endoscopic methods do not have outcomes data in asthmatics with GER-triggered asthma and should be considered experimental in this population.

Therapy in children

Therapy in children older than 2 years of age is similar to that of adults [74]. Lifestyle measures should be implemented. Metoclopramide is widely used, but CNS effects are common, affecting up to 20% of children treated. H_2 receptor antagonists, including cimetidine, are FDA approved in doses of 20 to 40 mg/kg/d divided into four doses. Ranitidine, 4 to 6 mg/kg/d, can be divided into two or three doses. PPIs are also effective [75]. Although not FDA approved for use in children, omeprazole is effective; however, it has a wide range of dosing requirements for adequate acid suppression (ranging from 0.7–3.5 mg/kg/d) [76]. Lansoprazole is FDA approved for use in children at a dose of 15 or 30 mg/d, dependent on the child's weight [77]. Surgical fundoplication can be performed in children; however, careful evaluation of esophageal and pulmonary parameters should be performed before considering surgical therapy.

Potential management strategy of gastroesophageal reflux–triggered asthma

Because anti-reflux therapy has the potential to improve asthma outcome in selected patients, all asthmatics should be assessed for GER. If GER symptoms are present, then an empiric trial of acid suppressive therapy should be considered. A PPI should be used because of its superior effectiveness and should be given at high doses, twice daily, for at least 3 months. Asthma symptoms, PEF rates, and asthma medication use should be monitored before and during the empiric trial [78]. Also, an empiric trial should be considered in asthmatics with moderate or severe persistent asthma, especially in those requiring oral corticosteroids, even in the absence of GER symptoms. If asthma outcomes are improved at the end of the 3-month empiric trial, then GER therapy should be continued. Maintenance GER therapy could begin with tapering the PPI dose to once daily. Surgery could be considered in selected patients, especially in those with normal esophageal motility. If asthma outcomes are not improved at the end of the 3-month empiric trial, then GER is most likely not a trigger of the individual's asthma if GER is adequately controlled.

O'Connor et al [79] designed a disease model to examine the cost-effectiveness of strategies for diagnosing GER-triggered asthma and reported that an empiric omeprazole trial for 3 months, followed by 24-hour esophageal pH testing in the nonresponders, was the most cost-effective way to include or exclude GER as a trigger in individual asthmatics. There are no published trials examining the cost-effectiveness of medical versus surgical therapy in asthmatics with GER-triggered asthma.

Summary

GER is a potential asthma trigger. Further research is needed to elucidate the role of esophageal acid in perpetuating airway inflammation and for validating potential predictors for asthma response with anti-reflux therapy.

Acknowledgments

I thank Arren Graf for editorial assistance in the preparation of this manuscript.

References

[1] Locke III GR, Talley NJ, Fett SL, et al. Prevalence and clinical spectrum of gastroesophageal reflux: a population-based study in Olmsted County, Minnesota. Gastroenterology 1997;112: 1148–56.

[2] Osler WB. The principles and practice of medicine. 8th edition. New York: D Appleton; 1912.

[3] Harding SM. Gastroesophageal reflux and asthma: insight into the association. J Allergy Clin Immunol 1999;104:251–9.

[4] Field SK, Underwood M, Brant R, et al. Prevalence of gastroesophageal reflux symptoms in asthma. Chest 1996;109:316–22.

[5] Perrin-Fayolle M, Bel A, Kofman J, et al. Asthma and gastroesophageal reflux: results of a survey of over 150 cases. Poumon Coeur 1980;36:225–30.

[6] Harding SM, Guzzo MR, Richter JE. 24-hour esophageal pH testing in asthmatics: respiratory symptom correlation with esophageal acid events. Chest 1999;115:654–9.

[7] Rudolph CD, Mazur LJ, Liptak GS, et al. North American Society for Pediatric Gastro-enterology, Hepatology, and Nutrition. Guidelines for evaluation and treatment of gastro-esophageal reflux in infants and children: recommendations of the North American Society for

Pediatric Gastroenterology, Hepatology, and Nutrition. J Pediatr Gastroenterol Nutr 2001; 32(Suppl 2):S1–31.

[8] Irwin RS, Curley FJ, French CL. Difficult-to-control asthma: contributing factors and outcome of a systematic management protocol. Chest 1993;103:1662–9.

[9] Harding SM, Guzzo MR, Richter JE. The prevalence of gastroesophageal reflux in asthma patients without reflux symptoms. Am J Respir Crit Care Med 2000;162:34–9.

[10] Thomas EJ, Kumar R, Dasan JB, et al. Gastroesophageal reflux in asthmatic children not responding to asthma medication: a scintigraphic study in 126 patients with correlation between scintigraphic and clinical findings of reflux. Clin Imaging 2003;27:333–6.

[11] Sontag SJ, Schnell TG, Miller TQ, et al. Prevalence of oesophagitis in asthmatics. Gut 1992; 33:872–6.

[12] Cinquetti M, Micelli S, Voltolina C, et al. The pattern of gastroesophageal reflux in asthmatic children. J Asthma 2002;39:135–42.

[13] Sontag SJ, O'Connell S, Khandelwal S, et al. Most asthmatics have gastroesophageal reflux with or without bronchodilator therapy. Gastroenterology 1991;101:876–7.

[14] Tucci F, Resti M, Fontana R, et al. Gastroesophageal reflux and bronchial asthma: prevalence and effect of cisapride therapy. J Pediatr Gastroenterol Nutr 1994;17:265–70.

[15] el-Serag HB, Sonnenberg A. Comorbid occurrence of laryngeal or pulmonary disease with esophagitis in United States military veterans. Gastroenterology 1997;11:755–60.

[16] Gislason T, Janson C, Vermeire P, et al. Respiratory symptoms and nocturnal gastroesophageal reflux: a population-based study of young adults in three European countries. Chest 2002;121: 158–63.

[17] Diette GB, Krishnan JA, Dominici F, et al. Asthma in older patients. Arch Intern Med 2002; 162:1123–32.

[18] Shireman TI, Heaton PC, Gay WE, et al. Relationship between asthma drug therapy patterns and healthcare utilization. Ann Pharmacother 2002;36:557–64.

[19] el-Serag HB, Gilger M, Kuebeler M, et al. Extraesophageal associations of gastroesophageal reflux disease in children without neurologic defects. Gastroenterology 2001;121:1294–9.

[20] Mittal RK, Balaban DH. The esophagogastric junction. N Engl J Med 1997;336:924–32.

[21] Mittal RK, Holloway R, Dent J. Effect of atropine on the frequency of reflux and transient lower esophageal sphincter relaxation in normal subjects. Gastroenterology 1995;109:1547–54.

[22] Lodi U, Harding SM, Coghlan HC, et al. Autonomic regulation in asthmatics with gastro-esophageal reflux. Chest 1997;111:65–70.

[23] Roussos C, Macklem PT. The respiratory muscles. N Engl J Med 1982;307:786–97.

[24] Mays EE. Intrinsic asthma in adults: association with gastroesophageal reflux. JAMA 1976; 236:2626–8.

[25] Locke GR, Talley NJ, Fett SL, et al. Risk factors associated with symptoms of gastroesophageal reflux. Am J Med 1999;106:642–9.

[26] Harding SM. GERD, airway disease, and the mechanisms of interaction. In: Stein MR, editor. Lung biology in health and disease, vol. 129: gastroesophageal disease and airway disease. New York: Marcel Dekker; 1999. p. 139–78.

[27] Ekström T, Tibbling L. Influence of theophylline on gastro-oesophageal reflux and asthma. Eur J Clin Pharmacol 1988;35:353–6.

[28] Hubert D, Gaudric M, Guerre J, et al. Effect of theophylline on gastroesophageal reflux in patients with asthma. J Allergy Clin Immunol 1988;81:1168–74.

[29] Crowell MD, Zayat EN, Lacy BE, et al. The effects of an inhaled beta(2)-adrenergic agonist on lower esophageal function: a dose-response study. Chest 2001;120:1184–7.

[30] Lazenby JP, Guzzo MR, Harding SM, et al. Oral corticosteroids increase esophageal acid contact times in patients with stable asthma. Chest 2002;121:625–34.

[31] Field SK, Evans JA, Price LM. The effects of acid perfusion of the esophagus on ventilation and respiratory sensation. Am J Respir Crit Care Med 1998;157:1059–62.

[32] Mansfield LE, Hameister HH, Spaulding HS, et al. The role of the vagus nerve in airway narrowing caused by intraesophageal hydrochloric acid provocation and esophageal distention. Ann Allergy 1981;47:431–4.

[33] Harding SM, Schan CA, Guzzo MR, et al. Gastroesophageal reflux-induced bronchoconstriction: is microaspiration a factor? Chest 1995;108:1220–7.

[34] Wright RA, Miller SA, Corsello BF. Acid-induced esophagobronchial-cardiac reflexes in humans. Gastroenterology 1990;99:71–3.

[35] Fischer A, Canning BJ, Undem BJ, et al. Evidence for an esophageal origin of VIP-IR and NO synthase-IR nerves innervating the guinea pig trachealis: a retrograde neuronal tracing and immunohistochemical analysis. Comp Neurology 1998;394:326–34.

[36] Canning BJ. Inflammation in asthma: the roles of nerves and the potential influence of gastro-esophageal reflux disease. In: Stein MR, editor. Lung biology in health and disease, vol. 129: gastroesophageal disease and airway disease. New York: Marcel Dekker; 1999. p. 19–54.

[37] Vincent D, Cohen-Jonathan AM, Leport J, et al. Gastro-oesophageal reflux prevalence and relationship with bronchial reactivity in asthma. Eur Respir J 1997;10:2255–9.

[38] Cuttitta G, Cibella F, Visconti A, et al. Spontaneous gastroesophageal reflux and airway patency during the night in adult asthmatics. Am J Respir Crit Care Med 2000;161:177–81.

[39] Tuchman DN, Boyle JT, Pack AI, et al. Comparison of airway responses following tracheal or esophageal acidification in the cat. Gastroenterology 1984;87:872–81.

[40] Jack CIA, Calverley PMA, Donnelly RJ, et al. Simultaneous tracheal and oesophageal pH measurements in asthmatic patients with gastro-oesophageal reflux. Thorax 1995;50:201–4.

[41] Hamamato J, Kohrogi H, Kawano O, et al. Esophageal stimulation by hydrochloric acid causes neurogenic inflammation in the airways of guinea pigs. J Appl Physiol 1997;82:738–45.

[42] Hunt JF, Erwin E, Palmer L, et al. Expression and activity of pH-regulatory glutaminase in the human airway epithelium. Am J Respir Crit Care Med 2002;165:101–7.

[43] Ricciardolo FLM, Gaston B, Hunt J. Acid stress in the pathology of asthma. J Allergy Clin Immunol 2004;113:610–9.

[44] Stein MR. Advances in the approach to gastroesophageal reflux (GER) and asthma. J Asthma 1999;36:309–14.

[45] Field SK, Sutherland LR. Does medical anti-reflux therapy improve asthma in asthmatics with gastroesophageal reflux? A critical review of the literature. Chest 1998;114:274–83.

[46] Gibson PG, Henry HL, Coughlan JL. Gastro-oesophageal reflux treatment for asthma in adults and children. Syst Rev 2003 (2):CDOO1496.

[47] Coughlan JL, Gibson PG, Henry RC. Medical treatment for reflux oesophagitis does not consistently improve asthma control: a systematic review. Thorax 2001;56:198–204.

[48] Harding SM, Richter JE, Guzzo MR, et al. Asthma and gastroesophageal reflux: acid suppressive therapy improves asthma outcome. Am J Med 1996;100:395–405.

[49] Boeree MJ, Peters FTM, Postma DS, et al. No effects of high-dose omeprazole in patients with severe airway hyperresponsiveness and (a)symptomatic gastro-oesophageal reflux. Eur Respir J 1998;11:1070–4.

[50] Ford GA, Oliver PS, Prior JS, et al. Omeprazole in the treatment of asthmatics with nocturnal symptoms and gastro-oesophageal reflux: a placebo-controlled cross-over study. Postgrad Med J 1994;70:350–5.

[51] Littner MR, Ballard III D, Huang B, et al. Twenty-four weeks of lansoprazole reduces asthma exacerbation and improves asthma quality of life in subjects with symptoms of acid reflux [abstract]. Eur Respir J 2002;20(Suppl 38):428.

[52] Heaney LG, Conway E, Kelly C, et al. Predictors of therapy resistant asthma: outcomes of a systematic evaluation protocol. Thorax 2003;58:561–6.

[53] Khoshoo V, Le T, Haydel Jr RM, et al. Role of gastroesophageal reflux in older children with persistent asthma. Chest 2003;123:1008–13.

[54] Field SK, Gelfand GAJ, McFadden SD. The effects of anti-reflux surgery on asthmatics with gastroesophageal reflux. Chest 1999;116:766–74.

[55] Larrain A, Carrasco E, Galleguillos F, et al. Medical and surgical treatment of nonallergic asthma associated with gastroesophageal reflux. Chest 1991;99:1330–5.

[56] Sontag S, O'Connell S, Khandelwal S. Anti-reflux surgery in asthmatics with reflux (GER) improves pulmonary symptoms and function. Gastroenterology 1990;98:A128.

[57] Sontag SJ, O'Connell S, Khandelwal S, et al. Asthmatics with gastroesophageal reflux: long term results of a randomized trial of medical and surgical anti-reflux therapies. Am J Gastroenterol 2003;98:987–99.

[58] Ekström T, Lindgren BR, Tibbling L. Effects on ranitidine treatment on patients with asthma and a history of gastroesophageal reflux: a double blind crossover study. Thorax 1989;44: 19–23.

[59] Schnatz PF, Castell JA, Castell DO. Pulmonary symptoms associated with gastroesophageal reflux: use of ambulatory pH monitoring to diagnose and to direct therapy. Am J Gastroenterol 1996;91:1715–8.

[60] Kiljander TO, Salomaa ER, Hietanen EK. Asthma and gastro-oesophageal reflux: can the response to anti-reflux therapy by predicted? Respir Med 2001;95:387–92.

[61] Perrin-Fayolle M, Gormand F, Braillon G, et al. Long-term results of surgical treatment for gastroesophageal reflux in asthmatic patients. Chest 1989;96:40–5.

[62] Cioffi U, Rosso L, De Simone M. Gastroesophageal reflux disease. Minerva Gastroenterol Dietol 1999;45:43–9.

[63] Richter JE. Diagnostic tests for gastroesophageal reflux disease. Am J Med Sci 2003;326:300–8.

[64] Fass R, Ofman JJ, Gralnek IM, et al. Clinical and economic assessment of the omeprazole test in patients with symptoms suggestive of gastroesophageal reflux disease. Arch Intern Med 1999;159:2161–8.

[65] Kahrilas PJ, Quigley EM. Clinical esophageal pH recording: a technical review for practice guideline development. Gastroenterology 1996;110:1982–96.

[66] Pandolfino JE, Richter JE, Ours T, et al. Ambulatory esophageal pH monitoring using a wireless system. Am J Gastroenterol 2003;98:740–9.

[67] Shay S, Tutuian R, Sifrim D, et al. Twenty-four hour ambulatory simultaneous impedance and pH monitoring: a multicenter report of normal values from 60 healthy volunteers. Am J Gastroenterol 2004;99:1037–43.

[68] DeVault KR, Castell DO. Updated guideline for the diagnosis and treatment of gastroesophageal reflux disease. The Practice Parameters Committee of the American College of Gastroenterology. Am J Gastroenterol 1999;94:1434–42.

[69] Klinkenberg-Knol EC, Nelis F, Dent J, et al. Long-term omeprazole treatment in resistant gastroesophageal reflux disease: efficacy, safety, and influence on gastric mucosa. Gastroenterology 2000;118:795–8.

[70] Wolfe MM, Welage LS, Sachs G. Proton pump inhibitors and gastric acid secretion. Am J Gastroenterol 2001;96:3467–8.

[71] Kahrilas PJ. Management of GERD: medical versus surgical. Semin Gastrointest Dis 2001;12: 3–15.

[72] Spechler SJ, Lee E, Ahnen D, et al. Long-term outcome of medical and surgical therapies for gastroesophageal reflux disease: follow-up of a randomized control trial. JAMA 2001;285: 2331–8.

[73] Triadafilopoulos G. Changes in GERD symptoms scores correlate with improvement in esophageal acid exposure after the Stretta procedure. Surg Endosc 2004;18:1038–44.

[74] Cezard JP. Managing gastro-oesophageal reflux disease in children. Digestion 2004;69(Suppl 1): 3–8.

[75] Marchetti F, Gerarduzzi T, Ventura A. Proton pump inhibitors in children: a review. Dig Liver Dis 2003;35:738–46.

[76] Hassall E, Israel D, Shepherd R, et al. Omeprazole for treatment of chronic erosive esophagitis in children: a multicenter study of efficacy, safety, tolerability and dose requirements. International Pediatric Omeprazole Study Group. J Pediatr 2000;137:800–7.

[77] Scott LJ. Lansoprazole: in the management of gastroesophageal reflux disease in children. Paediatr Drugs 2003;5:56–62.

[78] Harding SM, Sontag SJ. Asthma and gastroesophageal reflux. Am J Gastroenterol 2000; 95(Suppl):S23–32.

[79] O'Connor JFB, Singer ME, Richter JE. The cost-effectiveness of strategies to assess gastroesophageal reflux as an exacerbating factor in asthma. Am J Gastroenterol 1999;94:1472–80.

[80] Meier JH, McNally PR, Punja M, et al. Does omeprazole (Prilosec) improve respiratory function in asthmatics with gastroesophageal reflux? A double-blind, placebo-controlled crossover study. Dig Dis Sci 1994;39:2127–33.

[81] Teichtahl H, Kronborg IJ, Yeomans ND, et al. Adult asthma and gastroesophageal reflux: the effects of omeprazole therapy on asthma. Aust N Z J Med 1996;26:671–6.

[82] Levin TR, Sperling RM, McQuaid KR. Omeprazole improves peak expiratory flow rate and quality of life in asthmatics with gastroesophageal reflux. Am J Gastroenterol 1998;93:1060–3.

[83] Kiljander TO, Salomaa ER, Hietanen EK, et al. Gastroesophageal reflux in asthmatics: a double-blind, placebo-controlled crossover study with omeprazole. Chest 1999;116:1257–64.

[84] Harmanci E, Entok E, Metintas M, et al. Gastroesophageal reflux in the patients with asthma. Allergol Immunopathol (Madr) 2001;29:123–8.

[85] Jiang SP, Liang RY, Zeng ZY, et al. Effects of anti-reflux treatment on bronchial hyper-responsiveness and lung function in asthmatic patients with gastroesophageal reflux disease. World J Gastroenterol 2003;9:1123–5.

[86] Kennedy JH. "Silent" gastroesophageal reflux. Dis Chest 1962;42:42–5.

[87] Overholt RH, Ashraf MM. Esophageal reflux as a trigger in asthma. N Y State J Med 1966; 66:3030–2.

[88] Urschel HC, Paulson DL. Gastroesophageal reflux and hiatal hernia; complications and therapy. J Thorac Cardiovasc Surg 1967;53:21–32.

[89] Lomasney TL. Hiatus hernia and the respiratory tract. Ann Thorac Surg 1977;24:448–50.

[90] Sontag S, O'Connell S, Greenlee H, et al. Is gastroesophageal reflux a factor in some asthmatics? Am J Gastroenterol 1984;82:119–26.

[91] Tardif C, Nouvet G, Denis P, et al. Surgical treatment of gastroesophageal reflux in 10 patients with severe asthma. Respiration 1989;56:110–5.

[92] DeMeester TR, Bonavina L, Iascone C, et al. Chronic respiratory symptoms and occult gastroesophageal reflux: a prospective clinical study and results of surgical therapy. Ann Surg 1900; 211:337–45.

[93] Johnson WE, Hagen JA, DeMeester TR, et al. Outcome of respiratory symptoms after anti-reflux surgery on patients with gastroesophageal reflux disease. Arch Surg 1996;131:489–92.

[94] So JBY, Zeitel SM, Rattner DW. Outcome of atypical symptoms attributed to gastroesophageal reflux treated by laparoscopic fundoplication. Surgery 1998;124:28–32.

[95] Patti MG, Arcerito M, Tamburini A, et al. Effect of laparoscopic fundoplication on gastroesophageal reflux disease-induced respiratory symptoms. J Gastrointest Surg 2000;4:143–9.

[96] Spivak H, Smith CD, Phichith A, et al. Asthma and gastroesophageal reflux: fundoplication decreases need for systemic corticosteroids. Gastrointest Surg 1999;3:477–82.

ELSEVIER
SAUNDERS

Immunol Allergy Clin N Am
25 (2005) 149–167

IMMUNOLOGY
AND ALLERGY
CLINICS
OF NORTH AMERICA

Food allergy and additives: triggers in asthma

Jonathan M. Spergel, MD, PhD*, Joel Fiedler, MD

Department of Pediatrics, Division of Allergy and Immunology,
The Children's Hospital of Philadelphia, University of Pennsylvania School of Medicine,
34th Sreet and Civic Center Blvd, Philadelphia, PA 19104, USA

Food allergies are increasing in occurrence in Westernized societies. Approximately 8% of children less than 3 years of age endure food allergies, and about 2% of adults are affected [1,2]. Cow's milk, egg, peanut, soy, wheat, fish, shellfish, and tree nuts are responsible for the majority of allergic reactions to foods in the United States. Adverse food reactions or food allergies can be broadly divided into immunologic and nonimmunologic responses. Nonimmunologic food reactions are subdivided into metabolic, pharmacologic, toxic, and infectious etiologies. Immunologic reactions occur after a food is absorbed, processed, and presented to an active immune system that reacts to the food. Food antigens can cause three types of immune responses: (1) IgE-mediated reactions, (2) non-IgE–mediated reaction, and (3) tolerance (ie, no reaction). IgE-mediated are the most common food allergies.

The most frequently observed clinical manifestations of IgE-mediated food allergies are cutaneous and gastrointestinal (GI) symptoms [3,4]. Foods can induce respiratory reactions with various consequences: (1) food-induced anaphylaxis, (2) food-induced rhinitis, (3) oral allergy syndrome, (4) food-induced asthma, (5) food-induced exercise-dependent anaphylaxis, (6) food-additive reactions, (7) occupational asthma due to foods, and (8) inhalation of food vapor particle (Box 1). This article discusses these scenarios and food allergy as a risk factor for precipitating an asthmatic response or episode.

Food allergy as risk factor for asthma

Longitudinal studies of patients with atopic dermatitis and food allergies have found that a history of food allergy increases the risk of asthma. Investigators

* Corresponding author.
E-mail address: Spergel@email.chop.edu (J.M. Spergel).

0889-8561/05/$ – see front matter © 2005 Elsevier Inc. All rights reserved.
doi:10.1016/j.iac.2004.09.012

Box 1. Respiratory-induced food reactions

Respiratory symptoms: 25% of food challenges
Isolated respiratory symptoms: 2% to 5% of food challenges
Isolated rhinitis symptoms: <1% of food challenges
Respiratory reactions to food additives: <0.5% of population
Occupational asthma: Up to 25% of grain workers

---

from the Isle of Wight reported in their 4-year follow-up of a birth cohort of 1218 children that 29 (2.4%) children developed egg allergy [5]. Rhinitis and asthma were associated with egg allergy, with an odds ratio (OR) of 5.0 compared with the population in general. Similarly, Gustafusson [6] found, in 94 children with atopic dermatitis, that a history of egg allergy increased the risk for the development of asthma. Kotaniemi-Syrjanen [7] identified 80 children with wheezing in the first 2 years of life and followed the subjects to school age; 40% (32 patients) developed persistent asthma. Persistent asthma was significantly associated with elevated specific IgE to egg and wheat, duplicating earlier observations. In the study with the longest follow-up (22 years), 100 atopic children were enrolled, and 63 were followed until 22 years of age. In those 63 adults, egg or milk allergy in the first year of life was a major risk for adult asthma [8]. These studies confirm that food allergy, and egg allergy in particular, in early infancy increases the risk for developing asthma later in life.

Food allergy as risk factor for severe asthma

Food allergy can be a risk factor for life-threatening asthma. A case-control study by Roberts et al [9] found that patients with asthma and food allergy had an OR of 8.58 for life-threatening asthma compared with allergic diseases (4.42) or frequent admissions (14.2). This study indicates that food allergy is a risk factor for life-threatening asthma but is not as significant a risk as multiple hospitalization or previous severe reactions.

Food-induced anaphylaxis

Foods can induce a wide spectrum of allergic response from mild isolated urticaria to life-threatening anaphylaxis with severe respiratory compromise. Egg, milk, peanut, soy, fish, shellfish, and tree nuts are the most common food allergens confirmed in well-controlled, blinded food challenges [4,10]. Food-elicited reactions with respiratory symptoms include difficulty breathing, wheezing, throat tightness, and nasal congestion, and these symptoms are significantly more likely in patients with underlying asthma. These respiratory reactions are typically more severe than GI or cutaneous reactions. This finding is consistent with the observation that patients with respiratory symptoms are more likely to have a fatal or near-fatal reaction after accidental ingestion of food to which they are allergic [11,12]. In a survey of six fatal and seven near-fatal anaphylactic reactions after food ingestion, all patients experienced asthma and respiratory symptoms as manifestations of their clinical presentation [11]. Furthermore, patients with asthma are at greater risk for severe and fatal anaphylaxis compared with patients with no history of asthma, allergic rhinitis, or atopic dermatitis. One study reported that in 31 of 32 cases of food-related fatalities, the patients had asthma in a physician-reported registry in the United States [13]. This finding was confirmed in a UK study, where eight out of eight patients with fatal anaphylaxis had a history of asthma [14].

The foods responsible for these serious reactions were peanut, tree nuts, egg, and cow's milk in the United States [11]. The causative food varies by region; for example, in Asia, the Chinese delicacy bird's nest soup (double-boiled edible nest of swift, *Collocalia* spp.), crustacean seafood, egg, and cow's milk are the most common reported foods to cause anaphylaxis [15]. In summary, patients with asthma are at greater risk for a life-threatening allergic reaction to foods, and experiencing respiratory symptoms as part of a food reaction increases the risk for severe reaction.

Food-induced rhinitis

Nasal symptoms are on occasion attributed to food ingestion, and roughly 20% of the children who underwent double-blind, placebo-controlled food challenges experienced nasal symptoms [16]. Rhinitis typically occurs in association with other clinical symptoms and rarely occurs in isolation [16].

Many patients associate the ingestion of cow milk and other dairy products with an increase in the production and thickness of nasal secretions or mucus. This association, although often anecdotally reported, cannot be ascribed to a specific allergic type reaction. Pinnock et al [17] investigated the relationship between milk intake and mucus production in adults. They found that milk and dairy product intake was not associated with an increase in upper or lower respiratory tract symptoms of congestion or increased amount nasal secretions whether patients were asymptomatic or symptomatic with rhinovirus infection. The amount of nasal secretions in tissue was not significantly related to overall milk consumption.

Oral allergy syndrome

Oral allergy syndrome represents a cross-reaction of plant proteins with airborne environmental allergens. The designation of the syndrome is derived from the fact that symptoms occur primarily, if not exclusively, in the oropharynx and do not involve other organ systems. The term "pollen food allergy" has also been proposed to reflect the clinical scenario of oral symptoms provoked by a food sensitivity as a response to previous exposure to a respiratory allergen with sensitization to a pollen [18]. Local IgE-mediated mast cell activation provokes sudden onset of pruritus affecting the oropharyngeal cavity. The symptoms often affect the lips, tongue, palate, and throat, with occasional reports of throat tightness. The symptoms are generally of short duration and respond well to antihistamines or can self-dissipate without medications.

The oral allergy syndrome can be elicited by a variety of plant proteins and occurs with the ingestion of various fresh fruits and fresh vegetables. The reactions do not occur when the fruit or vegetable is cooked or the antigenic form is altered. Often, removing the skin or peel of the fruit or vegetable can eliminate or reduce the tendency for the reaction.

The environmental allergens that have been most commonly reported to cross-react with the plant proteins often referred to as pathogenesis-related proteins are birch tree, ragweed, mugwort, and grasses [19]. Cross-reactivity occurs when two or more allergens share common epitopes and bind to the same IgE antibody. Sensitivity to pollens usually occurs before sensitivity to provoking foods. Oral allergy syndrome can begin as early as in the young school-age child.

The most common reported cross-reactivities include melons and banana with ragweed; apple, hazelnut, carrot, potato, kiwi, cherry, and pear with birch pollen; and celery and carrot with mugwort. The major apple allergen, Mal d 1, has 63% homology with the major birch pollen, Bet v 1 [20]. The birch pollen profilin, Bet v 2, cross-reacts with profilin found in pear, celery, and potato [19]. Because of cross-reactivity, patients with oral allergy syndrome with melons and ragweed allergy may experience more pronounced symptoms during the ragweed season due to the rise in ragweed-specific IgE.

The diagnosis of oral allergy syndrome is based on suggestive history in a patient with significant allergic rhinitis. The skin test with commercially prepared extracts can be negative because the responsible food allergen is often altered in the manufacturing process [21]. Use of the pure fresh fruit or vegetable for skin testing via a prick test often elicits a positive response when testing to the commercial extract is negative. Three studies [22–24] suggest that treatment of pollen-induced allergic rhinitis with immunotherapy can abate the oral allergy syndrome, but the natural history of this entity has not been well studied or characterized. However, Moller [25] was not able to demonstrate a change in oral allergy symptoms in patients undergoing desensitization to birch pollen.

There is no consensus among allergists regarding recommendations for these patients. A recent survey of board-certified allergists revealed that 50% recommended complete avoidance of the offending fruit or vegetable and that 9% never recommended avoidance [18]. The survey showed that 3% of allergists always prescribed an Epi-pen (Epinephrine, Dey Pharmaceutical), kit and 30% never prescribed one. The difficulty lies in defining the patient who may be at risk for a more severe type of reaction. Although oral allergy syndrome is not a typical food allergy, it should be considered a food-related allergic reaction. As with other food allergies, the treatment remains avoidance of the offending fruit or vegetable, especially during "cross-reacting" pollen season.

Food-allergy–induced asthma

Food sensitivities causing isolated asthma or lower airway symptoms are rare. Studies of food challenges suggest overall rates between 2% and 5%. Onorato et al [101] examined 300 asthmatic patients from a pulmonary clinic. Only 12% had a history of food allergy suggested by clinical symptoms and positive skin testing. Food-induced wheezing was confirmed in only 2% of cases, compared with 25% suggested by history alone. This substantially lower rate on direct challenge compared with history and a positive skin test is a common finding; positive skin testing is only about 50% predictive for food reactions. In a larger study of almost 600 pulmonary patients at the National Jewish Research and Medical Center in Denver, Colorado, 68% had a clinical history of food-induced allergic reactions. Subsequent food challenges were positive in 60% of the patients, with 25% of the patients experiencing wheezing on challenge but only 2% with isolated wheezing. Similar to our studies and others, wheezing occurs in about 25% of challenges in combination with cutaneous or GI symptoms [10,26]. These studies cite wheezing occurring often in combination with other systemic symptoms. Isolated asthma symptoms from food allergic reactions are rare, occurring in 2% of the patients.

Several studies have examined children with undefined food allergies. These children underwent food challenges to determine if they were clinically sensitive to the food. The rate for isolated lower airway symptoms in these studies ranged from 1% to 13% [27,28]. The highest rate occurred in patients with milk allergy [28]. In our study of over 1000 open food challenges in pediatric patients in a tertiary care center with food allergies, we documented isolated respiratory symptoms in less than 5% of our patients [10].

In a subset of food-allergic children, the chronic ingestion of an allergic food may result in increased airway hyper-responsiveness in the absence of acute symptoms on ingestion. In one study, 26 children with asthma and food allergy were evaluated for changes in their airway hyper-responsiveness [29] during methacholine inhalation challenges before blinded food challenges and 4 hours after the food challenge. Twelve out of 22 positive food challenges involved lower airway symptoms, including cough or wheezing. Significant increases in airway hyper-responsiveness occurred in 7 of the 12 patients who experienced chest symptoms during positive food challenges. Decreases in FEV_1 were not generally observed in these seven patients during the food challenges. These data indicate that food-induced allergic reactions may increase airway hyper-responsiveness, as demonstrated by increasing responsiveness to methacholine in a subset of patients with moderate to severe persistent asthma after ingestion of specific foods.

One small pilot study of milk and egg avoidance for 8 weeks found an improvement in asthmatic children with avoidance measures. The 13 children in the avoidance group had improvement in peak flow rate compared with nine children in the control group who did not show improvement in peak flow reading [30]. In contrast, Wood et al [31] investigated a high-risk population of 20 adults to assess whether milk consumption had an effect on asthma control and flares. They used a randomized, crossover, double-blind, placebo-controlled trial to examine the effects of dairy products in patients who perceived that their asthma worsened with the ingestion of milk products. Subjects complied with a dairy-free diet throughout the study. The active challenge was a single-dose drink equivalent to 300 mL of cow's milk. They found no difference in symptoms or in lung function after a milk challenge. Nguyen et al [32] found similar results with no effect of milk ingestion on FEV_1 and FVC 20 minutes after a milk challenge in 25 asthmatic adults. The latter two studies were done in more rigorous scientific manner compared with the pilot study of Yusoff [30] on milk and egg avoidance. Pinnock et al [33] examined 60 adult volunteers who were challenged with rhinovirus and had nasal mucus production measured over a 10-day period and assessed milk and total diary consumption. Pinnock found no evidence of increased mucus production with milk consumption. Therefore, dairy products are unlikely to cause isolated rhinitis or bronchoconstriction in patients with asthma.

A study in adults with asthma concluded that food allergy is an unlikely cause of increased airway hyper-responsiveness [34]. In eleven adults with asthma, a clinical history of food-induced wheezing and positive prick skin tests to the suspected foods were evaluated. Results demonstrated that an equal percentage of patients had increased airway hyper-responsiveness, which was determined by methacholine inhalation challenges, after blinded food challenges to food allergen or placebo. Therefore, it is unlikely that food allergy causes isolated increased airway hyper-responsiveness in a significant number of patients.

Food-dependent, exercise-induced anaphylaxis

Food-dependent, exercise-induced anaphylaxis (FDEIA) is a subset of exercise-induced anaphylaxis that is characterized by urticaria, airway obstruction, and hypotension after physical exercise. In some cases of FDEIA, the food ingestion can be any nonspecific meal, and in other cases the FDEIA occurs with exercise after ingestion of specific inciting foods [35,36]. In specific FDEIA, an IgE-mediated mechanism is likely because patients have positive testing for the causative foods [36].

FDEIA was first described in 1979 by Maulitz [37]. Numerous foods (eg, shrimp; shellfish; chicken; wheat; nuts; fruits such as apples, peaches and grapes; and vegetables such as celery, tomatoes, fennel, lettuce, and potatoes) have been implicated in this clinical entity [38,39]. Wheat is the most commonly identified allergen in many studies from Europe and Japan; in particular, the α- and γ-gladin–like peptides have been postulated to be the causative allergen [40].

In the United States, FDEIA is more common in females than males by 3 to 1 ratio, with shellfish as the most common specific food [41].

The mechanism of FDEIA has not been elucidated, but it has been hypothesized that exercise triggers allergic reactions in patients who have low-grade type I allergies specific for certain foods. Because serum histamine and tryptase levels are increased during symptomatic attacks, this finding supports a mechanism that indicates degranulation of mast cells in a probable IgE-mediated fashion [42]. Many other factors may play a role, including autonomic nervous system dysfunction, medication use, weather, humidity, stress, family tendency, and menstruation cycle in females [35,36]. It is hypothesized that rigorous exercise increases food allergen absorption by changes in splanchnic blood flow. FDEIA is rare but is a known cause of food-related wheezing and anaphylaxis.

Food-additive–induced asthma

Food additives have been thought by many people, including physicians, to be a precipitating cause of exacerbations of asthma and a cause of acute allergic-type reactions. Despite this common perception, there is a relative paucity of well-controlled, double-blinded studies to support this view.

There are more than 2500 substances that the FDA lists as food additives in the United States [43]. There are relatively few additives that have been linked to provoking bronchoconstriction in asthmatic patients, and in this article the most common additives that have been purported to trigger asthma are discussed.

The incidence of reactions to food additives is unknown but is generally overestimated by the public. European studies have extrapolated the prevalence as <0.5% of the total population and only as high as 2% in an atopic population [44]. A large British survey of more than 15,000 patients with self-reporting of challenges listed prevalence of adverse reactions as 0.01% to 0.23% [45].

The prevalence of allergic reactions to foods (2% to 8% in pediatric populations) [1,2] is much higher than the incidence of reactions to any of the food additives. Asthmatic responses to a variety of additives are not as prevalent as once suspected. Diets restricted in food additives have not been shown to be of benefit in asthmatic patients and should not be routinely recommended.

The most well known of the additives for which evidence exists to support an association of sensitivity and asthmatic responses are sulfating agents. The sulfating agents include sulfur dioxide, sodium sulfite, sodium and potassium bisulfite, and metabisulfites. These agents have long been used in food processing and have been used as preservatives and antioxidants [46]. Sodium metabisulfite is the most commonly used chemical preservative, and it has been estimated that 1 to 3 mg of sulfites are consumed per person per day, with an additional amount in those that consume beer and wine [47]. Sulfites have also been used as preservatives for inhalation and parenteral medications (including Epi-pen kit). Their main function is to delay the oxidation of foods and medications by being preferentially oxidized before the food or the medication. In 1986, the FDA moved to regulate the use of sulfites in fresh fruits and vegetables, and the previously common practice of using these agents in salad bars is no longer in practice. In addition, the FDA regulation requires specific labeling on products that exceed 10 parts per million. Foods that are highest in sulfite content include dried fruits, wine, molasses, sauerkraut, and white grape juice. Other foods that are relatively high in sulfite content include dried potatoes, gravies, fresh shrimp, pectin, corn syrup, pickles, and relishes.

The prevalence of adverse reactions to sulfating agents is not known, and few studies have been conducted in children. The reactions to sulfites have been reported primarily in patients with underlying asthma. The mechanism of action has not been clearly defined, but a number of hypotheses have been advanced, including IgE-mediated processes (skin testing by prick and intradermal methods have identified some individuals with positive skin test results and positive challenges) [48]. Another possible mechanism is SO_2-induced bronchospasm. SO_2 is a by-product of metabisulfite in an acidic environment and can produce bronchospasm in patients with asthma in concentrations as low as 1 ppm. A third possible mechanism of action is deficiency of the enzyme sulfite oxidase. Evidence for this mechanism is limited [49].

The diagnosis of sulfite sensitivity requires a specific challenge because history alone usually cannot establish the diagnosis. Patients may be challenged with various forms of the additive, such as capsules, neutral solutions, or acidic solutions of a sulfite preparation. Toxicity studies in normal individuals have shown that ingestion of up to 400 mg per day can be tolerated [50]. The role of sulfating agents in the production of nonasthmatic adverse reactions is controversial. Simon [51] conducted a challenge using potassium metabisulfite on 61 adult asthmatic patients and demonstrated a 25% decrease in FEV_1 in 5 of the 61 patients (8.2%). The largest study reported is that of Bush [52], in which 203 adult asthmatics (not preselected for sulfite sensitivity) were challenged with capsules and neutral solutions of sulfite; 3.9% had a 20% drop in FEV_1. The positive response rate was 8.4% in the group that was being treated with steroids (oral or inhaled) but was only 0.8% in the group that did not require steroids for the control of asthma. This observation suggests that the risk of reacting to sulfites may be much higher in the subgroup of patients with more severe asthma.

Observations have been made that the prevalence of sulfite sensitivity may increase with age in children with severe asthma. Towns and Mellis [53] performed challenges on 29 children with moderate to severe asthma (age range 5–14 years). Although two thirds of the children showed a fall in FEV_1 on challenge, none of the asthma symptoms improved on elimination and avoidance of sulfites. Other studies in children have shown reaction rates of 3.5% in asthmatic children challenged with sulfiting capsules or oral metabisulfite [54]. Differences in challenge procedures, such as capsule versus acidic beverage, may account for the discrepancies in reports of prevalence of reactions. The inhalation of metabisulfite may reflect a heightened bronchial sensitivity to inhaled SO_2 and may not indicate a concomitant risk of asthma episode from the ingestion of food containing a sulfiting agent [55].

The role of other food additives as precipitating agent for asthma is less clear. This is particularly true for tartrazine. The cause and effect of tartrazine sensitivity in triggering asthma has not been established. In an early textbook on childhood asthma, it was postulated that tartrazine precipitated asthma in some children [56]. Stevenson [57], in his review of tartrazine sensitivity, concluded that tartrazine does not induce asthma even among the group that was aspirin sensitive. Interpretation of many of the studies on the role of tartrazine sensitivity and asthma is difficult due to flaws in the study designs, such as withholding asthma medications during challenges. The most extensive study was performed by Stevenson [57]. In 240 patients, of whom 190 patients were aspirin intolerant, there was no asthmatic response in any of the patients who were challenged with tartrazine up to doses of 50 mg [57]. There is no compelling evidence that tartrazine induces asthmatic responses.

Tartrazine is also known as yellow dye #5, and other food colorants, including yellow dye #6 (sunset yellow), amaranth (red dye #2), and erythrosine (red dye #3), have been linked in sporadic case reports to triggering asthmatic responses, but conclusive evidence is lacking. Many natural colorants, such as annatto, carmine, carotene, and tumeric, have been added to foods and have been linked to an asthmatic response. IgE-mediated reactions, including asthma, have been reported in patients upon ingestion of carmine-containing foods and beverages [58]. Carmine has a red color and is a protein derived from an insect that lives as a parasite on the pear cactus.

Monosodium L-glutamate (MSG) is a popular flavor enhancer, and there are a few anecdotal reports of MSG sensitivity linked to asthma [59,60]. Woessner [61] found, in a study of 100 asthmatic patients (30 with a clinical history of asthma flare after MSG ingestion), that none of the 100 patients had a drop in FEV_1 after MSG challenges up to 2.5 mg. Thus, even in history-positive patients, the existence of MSG-induced asthma has not been reproducible. There is a report of delayed fall in pulmonary function beginning 6 hours after ingestion of MSG and not associated with Chinese restaurant syndrome [59,60]. This may be a separate entity. In most of the anecdotal reports, the quantity of MSG required to elicit a positive response was in the range of 2.5 to 3 mg, also in the absence of other foods eaten concurrently. This quantity is much higher than that usually ingested in typical Chinese restaurant syndrome. Studies examining the Chinese restaurant syndrome did not find consistent results in patients reacting to MSG, also suggesting that Chinese restaurant syndrome is not a clinically relevant syndrome for precipitating asthmatic responses [62].

Food additives are typically minor ingredients or components of the food. A few additives are allowed to be listed collectively, such as natural flavors, but a recent bill (The Food Allergen Labeling and Consumer Protection Act, S. 741) was approved by the House Energy and Commerce Committee, and the Senate will require stricter labeling guidelines [63].

Suspected food additive sensitivities are best studied by performing oral challenges (skin testing is not helpful). Challenges in asthmatic patients need to be done while patients are on their routine medications to avoid false-positive tests (a flaw in many studies). Challenges are also best performed in a double blind manner.

Protective roles of food in asthma (omega-3-fatty acids)

Foods that are rich in omega-3-polyunsaturated fatty acids may be protective of asthmatic response by virtue of their anti-inflammatory effects. High dietary levels of foods rich in omega fatty acids have been associated with a lower incidence of inflammatory diseases. However, only limited effects have been demonstrated in asthma, and few clinical studies have been done. Most of the evidence derives from in vitro work. A Japanese study was performed in a long-term hospital setting in which subjects received fish oil capsules containing eicosapentaenoic acid or control capsules with olive oil [64]. Asthma symptom scores and methacholine response decreased in the fish oil group but not in the olive oil control group. The results suggest that dietary supplementation with fish oil rich in omega fatty acids may be beneficial for children with asthma in a strictly controlled environment. The children in this 10-month study had minimal exposure to environmental inhaled allergens.

In the ongoing Childhood Asthma Prevention study, dust mite avoidance and dietary supplement of omega-3-fatty acids had a beneficial effect on childhood asthma. In the preliminary results of 700 mothers and their offspring, children in the dietary intervention group at 18 months of age had fewer wheezing episodes [65]. There was also a recent report from Salam in which asthmatic mothers who ate fish high in omega-3-fatty acids during pregnancy had offspring who were 70% less likely to develop asthma before age 5 than the mothers who never ate fish high in omega-3-fatty acids while pregnant [66]. These findings suggest that the omega-3-fatty acid consumption by pregnant asthmatic mothers may decrease the tendency for asthma in offspring who are predisposed to develop asthma. These results suggest that dietary intervention may play a role in preventing airway disease.

It has been suggested that anti-oxidants, especially vitamin C, may have a protective function for lung parameters [67]. In patients with asthma, diets high in antioxidants may decrease bronchial reactivity and may thereby have an affect in the prevention and treatment of asthma [68]. This is based on observations of lower levels of vitamin C in asthmatics than nonasthmatics because oxidant stress is thought to contribute to the pathogenesis of airway obstruction. Despite studies that have shown that ascorbic acid supplementation is associated with improved lung function [69], studies have not documented that the use of vitamin C has a beneficial effect on wheezing or asthma control [70]. Pretreatment with vitamin C has not been effective in preventing histamine- or allergen-induced bronchocon-striction [71,72], and no definitive study has documented the usefulness of vitamin C in the treatment of asthma. However, a recent report from Mexico City that looked at children with a genetic deficiency of glutathione transferase showed a decrease of asthma symptoms with supplementation with antioxidants vitamin C and E in a clinical trial [73]. This was in a group of children with high ambient ozone exposure, and it was hypothesized that asthmatic children genetically lacking in the glutathione enzyme have a greater susceptibility to deterioration of lung function with ozone exposure and greater benefit from antioxidant supplementation. Glutathione peroxidase, which is a component of the body antioxidant system, has been found to be reduced in asthmatic children compared with a control group. These children were given a supplement of 250 mg/d of vitamin C and 50 mg/d of vitamin E. It cannot be claimed that the routine use of antioxidant vitamin C or vitamin E is helpful in controlling asthma symptoms or asthma exacerbations. Although the concept that antioxidants can prevent free radical inflammatory damage to lung tissue is intriguing, clinical evidence to support the routine use of antioxidants is lacking.

Occupational asthma

Occupational asthma as a response to many low- and high-molecular-weight antigens has been well described. Airway hyper-reactivity can develop due to exposure to an occupational agent via inhalation in patients without pre-existing asthma. Numerous chemicals have been shown to cause occupational asthma on an IgE and a non-IgE basis. The list of agents includes a number of food products, with baker's asthma being one of the more commonly identified causes. This entity can be caused and mediated by specific IgE sensitization to a number of flours, including wheat, rye, barley, buckwheat, and soy. Significant cross-reactivity has been demonstrated among those grains because exposed workers often develop IgE antibodies to a number of different cereal proteins [74]. In addition to common food antigens, sensitivity has been noted to enzymes contained in the flour [75]. There is a family of alpha amylase inhibitor compounds (these compounds inhibit insect and mammalian alpha amylase and have a role in defending plants against parasitic infection) that have been shown to be sensitizers, and a recent report on limiting exposure to amylase has shown an overall decrease in symptomatic sensitization in bread workers over a 10-year period in a UK food company [76]. In addition to alpha amylase, other additives can be sensitizers that include hemicellulose, cellulase, and glucoamylase, all of which are enzymes derived from aspergillus mold. Bakers can also become sensitized to a number of contaminants, such as storage mites, fungi, and insect debris, which can be contained in the flour [77].

Wheat consists of four major protein fractions: albumin, gliadin, globulin, and gluten. Sensitivity can develop to a single fraction or a combination of proteins. Wheat allergens can also become antigenic after alteration during the processing of wheat. Studies on patterns of crossed immunoelectrophoresis show that 40 different wheat antigens have been identified when water-soluble extract was analyzed [78]. In most cases, baker's asthma is caused by IgE-mediated responses to a specific allergen.

Asthma and rhinitis have been described in bakers dating as far back as 1713 in a narrative by Ramazzini reporting that grain handlers were almost always short of breath [79]. A typical history for baker's asthma would begin as rhinitis followed by asthma occurring after exposure in the workplace. Flour allergy has been reported as high as 30% in bakers [76,80]. In a review by Popp [80], a combination of positive skin test and RAST to a cereal antigen and elevated IgE was predictive of developing baker's asthma; the diagnosis was confirmed with bronchial provocation. A recent report from Spain documented four bakery workers whose work-related allergic respiratory symptoms were induced upon exposure to egg aerosols [81]. Elucidating the specific antigen as cause for each case of baker's asthma remains difficult because a significant number of antigens have been reported to induce asthma.

Grain dust exposure has been linked to the development of asthmatic symptoms. A survey of farmers in England who engaged in harvesting grains showed that 25% complained of respiratory symptoms including cough, wheeze, and dyspnea after working on combine harvesters [82]. A 40-year-old Canadian study examined particle size of airborne dust collected during oat and wheat loading and found dust particles to be in the respirable range [83]. Another risk factor is a history of atopic disease for the development of baker's asthma [84].

A number of workers in various food industries have been described who have developed asthma in response to inhalation of specific food antigens. Occupational asthma has been described in garlic workers on the basis of developing specific IgE to inhalation of garlic dust [85]. All of the 12 patients in that report had allergy to pollens, and in all cases the asthma was preceded by rhinitis. It was postulated that atopic status increased the susceptibility of these patients to garlic dust sensitization.

Allergic sensitization has been reported in workers who process seafood. The prevalence of occupational asthma is higher in workers exposed to crustaceans than those exposed to mollusks and bony fish. One longitudinal study of crab-processing workers demonstrated that 25% of exposed workers developed new onset of asthma-like symptoms [86].

A careful and thorough history is of paramount importance in the evaluation of any patient thought to be manifesting occupational asthma. Symptom pattern may not always be obvious when there is delay in onset of symptoms or when exposure is intermittent. Variables may include duration and type of exposure and the patient's underlying atopic status. Skin testing and RAST testing may be helpful when a suitable agent is available. Specific inhalation challenges must be performed in specialized laboratory facilities and may not be readily available.

Once occupational asthma has been diagnosed, the ideal treatment is to remove the patient from that exposure, but this can be difficult. Specific levels of airborne exposure to some allergens that can cause asthma symptoms have been defined, and industrial hygiene measures can often help to minimize exposure [87]. However, once hypersensitivity to an agent develops, asthmatic responses may occur at low levels of exposure that are unavoidable in the workplace. The treatment is the same as for other types of asthma. Follow-up studies of patients with occupational asthma have suggested that a significant percentage of these individuals have ongoing symptoms [88]. The factors that affect long-term prognosis probably include duration of symptoms and disease severity.

The ideal treatment remains prevention. In many industries, prospective employees may undergo skin testing (eg, in the seafood industry) before beginning work. Compliance with protective devices to prevent aerosolized inhalation is often low due to the cumbersome nature of the masks. Occupational asthma remains a major concern and cost burden to the health care system and an economic and emotional burden for the patient who may be in a situation in which he may be forced to change occupation.

Inhalation of food particles triggering asthma

Exposure to airborne food particles can cause respiratory symptoms in a susceptible individual with known IgE-mediated symptoms to the food. These reactions have been reported most commonly with fish and shellfish. Patients with known fish allergy can develop wheezing or rhinitis when exposed to food particles during cooking or manipulation of the food [89]. Similar reactions have been reported to rice [90], legumes [91,92], and milk [93].

The best controlled study examining this problem was done by Roberts et al [94], who identified 12 children with reported reaction on inhalation of a food. Nine children and families agreed to be challenged to the causative food by inhalation in a double-blind placebo challenge. Five children had positive challenges with acute symptoms of asthma; two children had late-phase reactions with a decrease in lung function. The foods that the patients reacted to were fish, chickpea, and buckwheat. However, in a study of 30 children with peanut allergy, no reactions were noted on just smelling peanut butter or casual contact with peanut butter [95]. These studies indicate that only if a food protein can be aerosolized can a patient with known sensitivity to that particular food react if the food particles are inhaled.

Food testing

Prick skin tests to food extracts are a useful screening method as initial assessment. They are the quickest, most reliable, least costly, and best-studied screening method. Controls used include the glycerinated saline diluent (to rule out nonspecific or dermatographic reactions) and histamine (to screen for the presence of residual antihistamines in the tissues).

A positive prick skin test with appropriate controls strongly supports the diagnosis of immediate hypersensitivity to a food in patients with a compatible clinical history. Positive skin tests are defined as wheal 3 mm greater than a negative control. A patient with a positive skin test but a questionable clinical history should undergo a formal food challenge to clarify the diagnosis because the positive predictive accuracy of an isolated prick skin test is < 50% [96]. A negative prick skin test excludes an IgE-mediated food reaction, with a negative predictive accuracy of > 90% expected for all allergy syndrome. False-negative skin tests are possible but rare. When a false-negative test is suspected, testing should be repeated with fresh food, particularly for fruit and vegetables. When testing to fresh foods is performed, a control subject is helpful to rule out nonspecific irritant reactions.

In vitro tests such as CAP-RAST FEIA (Pharmacia) measure absolute values of food-specific IgE and are less sensitive than prick skin tests. RAST tests are useful in the following circumstances when skin tests cannot be performed: (1) patients who cannot discontinue antihistamines because of severe ongoing allergic symptoms, (2) patients who have significant dermatographism, and (3) patients with severe atopic dermatitis with little available surface area for appropriate skin testing. A major limitation of RAST testing is that interpretation can be difficult because sensitivity and specificity vary by each food. CAP-RAST tests are an improved in vitro measurement of specific IgE with less nonspecific IgE binding that can occur with standard RAST. However, similar to other RAST tests and skin tests, there are limitations in interpretation because sensitivity and specificity are not 100%. Knowledge of particular test characteristics (and the illness being evaluated) is required for appropriate application and interpretation of each method.

Various studies of the CAP-RAST FEIA (Pharmacia) in children have established 90% positive predictive values milk, egg, peanut, and fish [97–100]. These values varied by population studied and the age of the patient. A 90% predictive value could not be established for soy or wheat.

Summary

Exposure to food allergens can cause a varied pattern of respiratory symptoms as allergic responses (Table 1). Food allergy in a patient presenting with asthma

Table 1
Foods causing respiratory reactions

Food implicated	Reactions
Fish and shellfish	Occcupational asthma
	Inhalation of food particles triggering asthma
Wheat and other grains	Baker's asthma
Melons, banana, apple, hazelnut, carrot, potato, kiwi, cherry, pear, celery, and carrot	Oral allergy syndrome
Shrimp, chicken, wheat, nuts, apples, peaches, grapes, celery, tomatoes, fennel, lettuce, and potatoes	Food-dependent exercise-induced anaphylaxis
Peanut, tree nuts, and many others (including many of the foods above)	Food-induced anaphlyaxis

tends to indicate a more severe disease constellation. Patients with underlying asthma may experience more severe and life-threatening allergic food reactions. When a food reaction involves respiratory symptoms, it is almost always a more severe reaction compared with reactions that do not involve the respiratory tract. Susceptible patients may react to a causative food on inhalation without ingestion. Patients can react to food particles in work environments (eg, baker's asthma). However, isolated asthma or rhinitis symptoms without concomitant cutaneous or GI symptoms are rare events. Additionally, reactions to food additives can involve respiratory symptoms but are more unusual than reactions to foods.

References

[1] Young E, Stoneham MD, Petruckevitch A, et al. A population study of food intolerance. Lancet 1994;343:1127–30.

[2] Sloan A, Powers M. A perspective on popular perceptions of adverse reactions to foods. J Allergy Clin Immunol 1986;78:127–83.

[3] Sampson HA. Food allergy. Part 1: immunopathogenesis and clinical disorders. J Allergy Clin Immunol 1999;103:717–28.

[4] Bock SA, Atkins FM. Patterns of food hypersensitivity during sixteen years of double-blind, placebo-controlled food challenges. J Pediatr 1990;117:561–7.

[5] Tariq SM, Matthews SM, Hakim EA, et al. Egg allergy in infancy predicts respiratory allergic disease by 4 years of age. Pediatr Allergy Immunol 2000;11:162–7.

[6] Gustafsson D, Sjoberg O, Foucard T. Sensitization to food and airborne allergens in children with atopic dermatitis followed up to 7 years of age. Pediatr Allergy Immunol 2003;14:448–52.

[7] Kotaniemi-Syrjanen A, Reijonen T, Romppanen J, et al. Allergen-specific immunoglobulin E antibodies in wheezing infants: the risk for asthma in later childhood. Pediatrics 2003;111: e255–61.

[8] Rhodes H, Sporik R, Thomas P, et al. Early life risk factors for adult asthma: a birth cohort study of subjects at risk. J Allergy Clin Immun 2001;108:720–5.

[9] Roberts G, Patel N, Levi-Schaffer F, et al. Food allergy as a risk factor for life-threatening asthma in childhood: a case-controlled study. J Allergy Clin Immunol 2003;112:168–74.

[10] Spergel JM, Beausoleil JL, Fiedler JM, et al. Correlation of initial food reactions to observed reactions on challenges. Ann Allergy Asthma Immunol 2004;92:217–24.

[11] Sampson HA, Mendelson L, Rosen JP. Fatal and near-fatal anaphylactic reactions to food in children and adolescents. N Engl J Med 1992;327:380–4.

[12] Yunginger JW, Sweeney KG, Sturner WQ, et al. Fatal food-induced anaphylaxis. JAMA 1988;260:1450–2.

[13] Bock SA, Munoz-Furlong A, Sampson HA. Fatalities due to anaphylactic reactions to foods. J Allergy Clin Immunol 2001;107:191–3.

[14] Macdougall CF, Cant AJ, Colver AF. How dangerous is food allergy in childhood? The incidence of severe and fatal allergic reactions across the UK and Ireland. Arch Dis Child 2002; 86:236–9.

[15] Goh D, Lau Y, Chew F, et al. Pattern of food-induced anaphylaxis in children of an Asian community. Allergy 1999;57:78–92.

[16] James JM, Bernhisel-Broadbent J, Sampson HA. Respiratory reactions provoked by double-blind food challenges in children. Am J Respir Crit Care Med 1994;149:59–64.

[17] Pinnock C, Graham N, Mylvaganam A, et al. Relationship between milk intake and mucus production in adult volunteers challenged with rhinovirus-2. Am Rev Respir Dis 1990;141: 352–60.

[18] Ma S, Sicherer SH, Nowak-Wegrzyn A. A survey on the management of pollen-food allergy syndrome in allergy practices. J Allergy Clin Immunol 2003;112:784–8.

[19] Ebner C, Hoffmann-Sommergruber K, Breiteneder H. Plant food allergens homologous to pathogenesis-related proteins. Allergy 2001;56(Suppl 67):43–4.

[20] Fritsch R, Bohle B, Vollmann U, et al. Bet v 1, the major birch pollen allergen, and Mal d 1, the major apple allergen, cross-react at the level of allergen-specific T helper cells. J Allergy Clin Immunol 1998;102:679–86.

[21] Ortolani C, Ispano M, Pastorello EA, et al. Comparison of results of skin prick tests (with fresh foods and commercial food extracts) and RAST in 100 patients with oral allergy syndrome. J Allergy Clin Immunol 1989;83:683–90.

[22] Enberg RN, Leickly FE, McCullough J, et al. Watermelon and ragweed share allergens. J Allergy Clin Immunol 1987;79:867–75.

[23] Asero R. How long does the effect of birch pollen injection SIT on apple allergy last? Allergy 2003;58:435–8.

[24] Kelso JM, Jones RT, Tellez R, et al. Oral allergy syndrome successfully treated with pollen immunotherapy. Ann Allergy Asthma Immunol 1995;74:391–6.

[25] Moller C. Effect of pollen immunotherapy on food hypersensitivity in children with birch pollinosis. Ann Allergy 1989;62:343–5.

[26] Hill DJ, Firer MA, Shelton MJ, et al. Manifestations of milk allergy in infancy: clinical and immunologic findings. J Pediatr 1986;109:270–6.

[27] Novembre E, de Martino M, Vierucci A. Foods and respiratory allergy. J Allergy Clin Immunol 1988;81:1059–65.

[28] Businco L, Falconieri P, Giampietro P, et al. Food allergy and asthma. Pediatr Pulmonol Suppl 1995;11:59–60.

[29] James JM, Eigenmann PA, Eggleston PA, et al. Airway reactivity changes in asthmatic patients undergoing blinded food challenges. Am J Respir Crit Care Med 1996;153:597–603.

[30] Yusoff NA, Hampton SM, Dickerson JW, et al. The effects of exclusion of dietary egg and milk in the management of asthmatic children: a pilot study. J R Soc Health 2004;124:74–80.

[31] Woods RK, Weiner JM, Abramson M, et al. Do dairy products induce bronchoconstriction in adults with asthma? J Allergy Clin Immunol 1998;101:45–50.

[32] Nguyen MT. Effect of cow milk on pulmonary function in atopic asthmatic patients. Ann Allergy Asthma Immunol 1997;79:62–4.

[33] Pinnock CB, Arney WK. The milk-mucus belief: sensory analysis comparing cow's milk and a soy placebo. Appetite 1993;20:61–70.

[34] Zwetchkenbaum JF, Skufca R, Nelson HS. An examination of food hypersensitivity as a cause of increased bronchial responsiveness to inhaled methacholine. J Allergy Clin Immunol 1991;88:360–4.

[35] Castells MC, Horan RF, Sheffer AL. Exercise-induced anaphylaxis. Curr Allergy Asthma Rep 2003;3:15–21.

[36] Romano A, Di Fonso M, Giuffreda F, et al. Food-dependent exercise-induced anaphylaxis: clinical and laboratory findings in 54 subjects. Int Arch Allergy Immunol 2001;125:264–72.

[37] Maulitz R, Pratt D, Schocket A. Exercise-induced anaphylactic reaction to shellfish. J Allergy Clin Immunol 1979;63:433–4.

[38] Morita E, Matsuo H, Mihara S, et al. Fast omega-gliadin is a major allergen in wheat-dependent exercise-induced anaphylaxis. J Dermatol Sci 2003;33:99–104.

[39] Perez-Calderon R, Gonzalo-Garijo MA, Fernandez de Soria R. Exercise-induced anaphylaxis to onion. Allergy 2002;57:752–3.

[40] Palosuo K, Alenius H, Varjonen E, et al. A novel wheat gliadin as a cause of exercise-induced anaphylaxis. J Allergy Clin Immun 1999;103:912–7.

[41] Shadick NA, Liang MH, Partridge AJ, et al. The natural history of exercise-induced anaphylaxis: survey results from a 10-year follow-up study. J Allergy Clin Immunol 1999;104:123–7.

[42] Schwartz H. Elevated serum tryptase in exercise-induced anaphylaxis. J Allergy Clin Immun 1995;95:917–9.

[43] US Food and Drug Administration. EAFUS: a food additive database. Available at: http://vm.cfsan.fda.gov/~dms/eafus.html. Accessed October 21, 2004.

[44] Fuglsang G, Madsen C, Saval P, et al. Prevalence of intolerance to food additives among Danish school children. Pediatr Allergy Immunol 1993;4:123–9.

[45] Young E, Patel S, Stoneham M, et al. The prevalence of reaction to food additives in a survey population. J R Coll Physicians Lond 1987;21:241–7.

[46] Twarog F. Metabisulfite sensitivity in asthma: a review. N Engl Soc Allergy Proc 1983;4: 100–21.

[47] Salam MT, Li YF, Langholz B, Gilliland FD. Early-life environmental risk factors for asthma: findings from the Children's Health Study. Environ Health Perspect 2004;112:760–5.

[48] Boxer MB, Bush RK, Harris KE, et al. The laboratory evaluation of IgE antibody to metabisulfites in patients skin test positive to metabisulfites. J Allergy Clin Immunol 1988;82: 622–6.

[49] Simon RA. Sulfite sensitivity. Ann Allergy 1987;59:100–5.

[50] Hotzel D, Muskat E, Bitsch I, et al. [Thiamine deficiency and harmlessness of sulfite for man. I: problem arrangement, experiment planning, clinical studies]. Int Z Vitaminforsch 1969;39: 372–83.

[51] Stevenson DD, Simon RA. Sensitivity to ingested metabisulfites in asthmatic subjects. J Allergy Clin Immunol 1981;68:26–32.

[52] Bush RK, Taylor SL, Holden K, et al. Prevalence of sensitivity to sulfiting agents in asthmatic patients. Am J Med 1986;81:816–20.

[53] Towns SJ, Mellis CM. Role of acetyl salicylic acid and sodium metabisulfite in chronic childhood asthma. Pediatrics 1984;73:631–7.

[54] Boner AL, Guarise A, Vallone G, et al. Metabisulfite oral challenge: incidence of adverse responses in chronic childhood asthma and its relationship with bronchial hyperreactivity. J Allergy Clin Immunol 1990;85:479–83.

[55] Boushey HA. Bronchial hyperreactivity to sulfur dioxide: physiologic and political implications. J Allergy Clin Immunol 1982;69:335–8.

[56] Speer K. The management of childhood asthma. Springfield (IL): Charles C. Thomas; 1958.

[57] Stevenson DD, Simon RA, Lumry WR, et al. Adverse reactions to tartrazine. J Allergy Clin Immunol 1986;78:182–91.

[58] Burge PS, O'Brien IM, Harries MG, et al. Occupational asthma due to inhaled carmine. Clin Allergy 1979;9:185–9.

[59] Moneret-Vautrin DA. Monosodium glutamate-induced asthma: study of the potential risk of 30 asthmatics and review of the literature. Allerg Immunol (Paris) 1987;19:29–35.

[60] Allen DH, Delohery J, Baker G. Monosodium L-glutamate-induced asthma. J Allergy Clin Immunol 1987;80:530–7.

[61] Woessner KM, Simon RA, Stevenson DD. Monosodium glutamate sensitivity in asthma. J Allergy Clin Immunol 1999;104:305–10.

[62] Geha RS, Beiser A, Ren C, et al. Multicenter, double-blind, placebo-controlled, multiple-challenge evaluation of reported reactions to monosodium glutamate. J Allergy Clin Immunol 2000;106:973–80.

[63] Food-Allergy-Network. Food labeling. Available at: www.foodallergy.org/Advocacy/labeling.html. Accessed September 5, 2004.

[64] Nagakura T, Matsuda S, Shichijyo K, et al. Dietary supplementation with fish oil rich in omega-3 polyunsaturated fatty acids in children with bronchial asthma. Eur Respir J 2000;16:861–5.

[65] Mihrshahi S, Peat JK, Marks GB, et al. Eighteen-month outcomes of house dust mite avoidance and dietary fatty acid modification in the Childhood Asthma Prevention Study (CAPS). J Allergy Clin Immunol 2003;111:162–8.

[66] Salam M, Langholz B, Gilliland FD. Maternal fish comsumption during pregnancy and risk of childhood asthma [abstract]. Am J Respir Crit Care Med 2004;169:A722.

[67] Britton JR, Pavord ID, Richards KA, et al. Dietary antioxidant vitamin intake and lung function in the general population. Am J Respir Crit Care Med 1995;151:1383–7.

[68] Cook DG, Carey IM, Whincup PH, et al. Effect of fresh fruit consumption on lung function and wheeze in children. Thorax 1997;52:628–33.

[69] Grievink L, Smit HA, Ocke MC, et al. Dietary intake of antioxidant (pro)-vitamins, respiratory symptoms and pulmonary function: the MORGEN study. Thorax 1998;53:166–71.

[70] Mainous III AG, Hueston WJ, Connor MK. Serum vitamin C levels and use of health care resources for wheezing episodes. Arch Fam Med 2000;9:241–5.

[71] Cockcroft DW, Killian DN, Mellon JJ, et al. Protective effect of drugs on histamine-induced asthma. Thorax 1977;32:429–37.

[72] Kordansky DW, Rosenthal RR, Norman PS. The effect of vitamin C on antigen-induced bronchospasm. J Allergy Clin Immunol 1979;63:61–4.

[73] Romieu I, Sienra-Monge JJ, Ramirez-Aguilar M, et al. Genetic polymorphism of GSTM1 and antioxidant supplementation influence lung function in relation to ozone exposure in asthmatic children in Mexico City. Thorax 2004;59:8–10.

[74] Sandiford CP, Tee RD, Newman-Taylor AJ. Identification of crossreacting wheat, rye, barley and soya flour allergens using sera from individuals with wheat-induced asthma. Clin Exp Allergy 1995;25:340–9.

[75] Hendrick DJ, Davies RJ, Pepys J. Bakers' asthma. Clin Allergy 1976;6:241–50.

[76] Smith TA. Preventing baker's asthma: an alternative strategy. Occup Med (Lond) 2004;54:21–7.

[77] Baldo BA, Krilis S, Wrigley CW. Hypersensitivity to inhaled flour allergens: comparison between cereals. Allergy 1980;35:45–56.

[78] Blands J, Diamant B, Kallos P, et al. Flour allergy in bakers. I: identification of allergenic fractions in flour and comparison of diagnostic methods. Int Arch Allergy Appl Immunol 1976; 52:392–406.

[79] Mapp C. Agents, old and new, causing occupational asthma. Occup Environ Med 2001; 58–60:354–60.

[80] Popp W, Zwick H, Rauscher H. Short-term sensitizing antibodies in bakers' asthma. Int Arch Allergy Appl Immunol 1988;86:215–9.

[81] Escudero C, Quirce S, Fernandez-Nieto M, Miguel J, et al. Egg white proteins as inhalant allergens associated with baker's asthma. Allergy 2003;58:616–20.

[82] Darke CS, Knowelden J, Lacey J, et al. Respiratory disease of workers harvesting grain. Thorax 1976;31:294–302.

[83] Williams N, Skoulas A, Merriman JE. Exposure to Grain Dust. I: a survey of the effects. J Gnathol 1964;69:319–29.

[84] Herxheimer H. Skin sensitivity to flour in bakers' apprentices. Lancet 1967;1:83–4.

[85] Anibarro B, Fontela JL, De La Hoz F. Occupational asthma induced by garlic dust. J Allergy Clin Immunol 1997;100:734–8.

[86] Desjardins A, Malo JL, L'Archeveque J, et al. Occupational IgE-mediated sensitization and asthma caused by clam and shrimp. J Allergy Clin Immunol 1995;96:608–17.

[87] Baur X, Chen Z, Liebers V. Exposure-response relationships of occupational inhalative allergens. Clin Exp Allergy 1998;28:537–44.

[88] Chan-Yeung M. Evaluation of impairment/disability in patients with occupational asthma. Am Rev Respir Dis 1987;135:950–1.

[89] Pascual CY, Crespo JF, Dominguez Noche C, et al. IgE-binding proteins in fish and fish steam. Monogr Allergy 1996;32:174–80.

[90] Gonzalez-Mendiola R, Martin-Garcia C, Carnes J, et al. Asthma induced by the inhalation of vapours during the process of boiling rice. Allergy 2003;58:1202–3.

[91] Anto JM, Sunyer J, Reed CE, et al. Preventing asthma epidemics due to soybeans by dust-control measures. N Engl J Med 1993;329:1760–3.

[92] Martin JA, Compaired JA, de la Hoz B, et al. Bronchial asthma induced by chick pea and lentil. Allergy 1992;47:185–7.

[93] Nowak-Wegrzyn A, Shapiro GG, Beyer K, et al. Contamination of dry powder inhalers for asthma with milk proteins containing lactose. J Allergy Clin Immunol 2004;113:558–60.

[94] Roberts G, Golder N, Lack G. Bronchial challenges with aerosolized food in asthmatic, food-allergic children. Allergy 2002;57:713–7.

[95] Simonte SJ, Ma S, Mofidi S, Sicherer SH. Relevance of casual contact with peanut butter in children with peanut allergy. J Allergy Clin Immunol 2003;112:180–2.

[96] Eigenmann PA, Sampson HA. Interpreting skin prick tests in the evaluation of food allergy in children. Pediatr Allergy Immunol 1998;9:186–91.

[97] Garcia Ara MC, Boyano Martinez T, Diaz Pena JM, et al. Specific IgE levels in the diagnosis of immediate hypersensitivity to cows' milk protien in the infant. J Allergy Clin Immunol 2001; 107:185–90.

[98] Sampson HA. Utility of food-specific IgE concentrations in predicting symptomatic food allergy. J Allergy Clin Immunol 2001;107:891–6.

[99] Boyano Martinez T, Garcia-Ara C, Diaz-Pena JM, et al. Validity of specific IgE antibodies in children with egg allergy. Clin Exp Allergy 2001;31:1464–9.

[100] Rance F, Abbal M, Lauwers-Cances V. Improved screening for peanut allergy by the combined use of skin prick tests and specific IgE assays. J Allergy Clin Immunol 2002;109:1027–33.

[101] Onorato J, Merland N, Terral C, et al. Placebo-controlled double-blind food challenge in asthma. J Allergy Clin Immunol 1986;78:1139–146.

ELSEVIER
SAUNDERS

Immunol Allergy Clin N Am
25 (2005) 169–190

IMMUNOLOGY
AND ALLERGY
CLINICS
OF NORTH AMERICA

Medications as asthma triggers

Ronina A. Covar, MD*, Beth A. Macomber, MD,
Stanley J. Szefler, MD

*Department of Pediatrics, Division of Allergy-Clinical Immunology,
National Jewish Medical and Research Center, 1400 Jackson Street A303, Denver, CO 80206, USA*

Of all the identifiable asthma triggers, drugs or medications probably comprise a minority, yet they can occur with grave consequences [1]. Aspirin (acetylsalicylic acid, ASA) and other nonsteroidal anti-inflammatory drugs (NSAIDs) are responsible for a vast majority, and other agents, such as β-blockers, angiotensin-converting enzyme (ACE) inhibitors, cholinergic agonists, cholinomimetic alkaloids, chemotherapeutic agents, diuretics, corticosteroids, antibiotics, radiocontrast, neuromuscular, and anesthetic agents have been reported to cause bronchospasm or mimic asthma [1]. Most of the agents inducing respiratory reactions also cause multisystemic manifestations. There are a number of pharmacologic stimuli directly or indirectly causing bronchial responsiveness, such as acetylcholine, methacholine, carbachol, histamine, prostaglandin (PG)D_2, leukotriene (LT)C_4/D_4/E_4, adenosine, tachykinins, bradykinin, metabisulfite/SO_2, and propranolol [2]. This article focuses on the common medications intended to provide "beneficial pharmacologic and medical effect" that have the potential to cause a distinct respiratory reaction in mostly susceptible individuals due to various mechanisms versus drugs that cause multisystemic adverse reactions. The three main groups are ASA/NSAIDs, β-blockers, and ACE inhibitors.

Aspirin and nonsteroidal anti-inflammatory drugs

Although willow bark had been used for centuries for its curative properties such as antipyresis, salicin as its active ingredient was first isolated in its pure form in the eighteenth century. Chemical manipulations to prepare acetylsalicylic

---

* Corresponding author.
E-mail address: covarr@njc.org (R.A. Covar).

0889-8561/05/$ – see front matter © 2005 Elsevier Inc. All rights reserved.
doi:10.1016/j.iac.2004.09.009

acid (ASA) followed for many years before it was formally introduced as "aspirin" in the medical literature in 1899 [3]. Although there had been anecdotal reports of angioedema, urticaria, and bronchospastic reactions associated with ASA almost a hundred years after salicin was first isolated and only 3 years after the drug was first synthesized, the first description of a clinically distinct syndrome of ASA sensitivity, asthma, and nasal polyposis was published in 1922 [4,5]. It had taken many more years before the triad became a popular clinical entity recognized by Samter and Beers in 1968 [5]. Cellular, molecular, and genetic mechanisms have been elucidated in the last two decades.

NSAIDs, including ASA, are commonly used for relief of inflammation, fever, and pain. The chronic use of ASA has gained popularity because of evidence of its protective effect for cardiovascular disease and colorectal adenomas and carcinomas. Most individuals are able to use NSAIDs/ASA without developing adverse reactions, but a substantial minority develop a specific clinical syndrome characterized by a persistent inflammatory disease of the airways preceding manifestations of ASA sensitivity, labeled as ASA-exacerbated respiratory disease (AERD), more popularly recognized as ASA-induced or ASA-intolerant asthma (AIA) or ASA triad. Complete avoidance of this class of medications does not necessarily alter the progression of the underlying disease process, suggesting that the relationship is not directly causal.

The relationship between ASA sensitivity and airway disease seems to be complex. Although there is a direct temporal development of upper and lower airway symptomatology within minutes to hours of drug exposure, there has been evidence of its association with a chronic asthma course or severity, for reasons still unclear. In a study of 1000 adult patients with asthma seen at a university hospital in Poland, ASA intolerance confirmed by inhalation challenge was found in 9%. Almost a third of cases with severe asthma had ASA intolerance, and this was found to be a significant factor for the development of severe asthma (odds ratio [OR] 5.44, 95% confidence interval [CI] 2.47–8.41; $P < 0.001$), confirmed further by multiple logistic regression analysis [6]. In a cross-sectional study of asthmatics from Western Australia, using a detailed questionnaire that addressed food, chemical, and drug sensitivities, ASA intolerance was associated with more severe asthma (OR 2.96, 95% CI 1.18–4.86; $P = 0.023$) [7]. Patients with AIA seemed to have a more severe and unstable disease course based on number of asthma attacks, doctor's visits, and self-rated asthma severity. In some European studies, 14% to 24% of asthmatics requiring mechanical ventilation were found to have a history of NSAID/ASA sensitivity [8,9]. These studies support the association between asthma severity and ASA sensitivity.

Prevalence

A comprehensive review [10] published recently of the prevalence of AIA substantiates the discrepancy in prevalence rates reported in many studies, likely reflecting differences in diagnostic methods used in the evaluation of ASA intolerance (eg, questionnaire versus provocation challenges) or differences in populations studied. In this meta-analysis in which the primary outcome was to determine whether ASA ingestion triggered an asthmatic response, participants were grouped according to the following to account for selection bias: (1) All patients with asthma with or without a history of AIA, (2) subjects preselected based on a reliable history of AIA or markers of an increased risk of the syndrome, or (3) patients with no evidence of AIA. The pooled prevalence rates of AIA based on oral provocation testing for the unselected asthma population, preselected population with history of AIA, and preselected population with no history of sensitivity were 21.1% (95% CI 13.6–28.6), 29.5% (95% CI 18.2–40.8), and 9% (95% CI 3.7–14.3), respectively. Much lower rates for ASA sensitivity for the unselected asthma population and preselected population with history of AIA (2.7% [95% CI 1.6–3.8] and 12.2% [95% CI 8.0–16.4], respectively) were found from verbal report alone. Lower prevalence found from questionnaire-based studies or verbal history may be attributed to intentional precautionary avoidance of NSAIDs by asthmatics due to general awareness of potential risk of adverse reactions or to a lack of perception of mild drug-induced reactions because of their relatively delayed onset of reaction.

Mechanisms

Precipitation of an asthmatic attack by ASA/NSAIDs is not based on an antigen–antibody reaction; cross-reactivity to structurally different NSAIDs is well established. In a similar manner, after ASA desensitization, tolerance to other NSAIDs that inhibit cyclooxygenase (COX) is observed [11]. The primary mechanism of the pharmacologic action of and intolerance to ASA/NSAIDs is thought to involve the inhibition of the COX enzyme and PG synthesis and activation of the LT pathways in the respiratory tract (Fig. 1). COX enzymes exist in at least two isoforms, COX1 (constitutive) and COX2 (inducible), which are encoded by distinct genes [12]. COX1 is found in most mammalian cells, including respiratory epithelial and endothelial cells, airway smooth muscle, fibroblasts, mast cells, and alveolar macrophages. COX2 is induced during inflammation and synthesizes inflammatory prostanoids, which participate in some inflammatory diseases, such as arthritis.

The cysteinyl-LT pathway has been well characterized. Its three primary enzymes are 5-lipoxygenase, 5-lipoxygenase activating protein (FLAP or ALOX5), and LTC_4 synthase. Cysteinyl-LTs are potent proinflammatory mediators known to cause bronchospasm, mucus hypersecretion, vascular permeability, airway edema, and eosinophil recruitment to the airways. Although speculative, ASA/NSAIDs, as COX inhibitors, preferentially shunt arachidonic acid metabolism into the 5-lipoxygenase pathway by depleting PGE_2 [13], a known inhibitor of LT synthesis that has anti-inflammatory and smooth muscle relaxant properties [14].

That enhanced production of cysteinyl-LTs is present in patients with clinically stable AIA compared with ATA subjects has been found in many

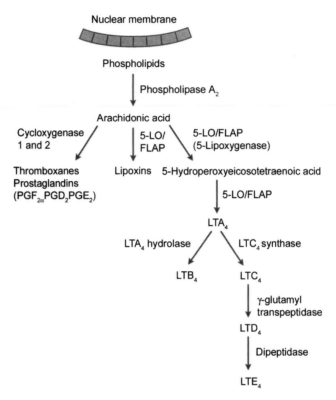

Fig. 1. Arachidonic acid cascade through the cyclooxygenase and the 5-lipoxygenase (5-LO) pathways. FLAP, 5-lipoxygenase activating protein (or ALOX5); LT, leukotriene; PG, prostaglandin. (*From* Stevenson DD, Simon RA, Zuraw BL. Sensitivity to aspirin and nonsteroidal antiinflammatory drugs. In: Middleton E, Reed C, Ellis E, et al. Allergy principles & practice. St. Louis (MO): Mosby, Inc.; 2001. p. 1701; with permission.)

studies showing elevated LTE_4 levels in the urine [15–17]. Furthermore, urinary LTE_4 levels increased after oral or inhaled ASA provocation challenges. Whether COX inhibition (measured by a fall in urinary thromboxane $[TX]A_2$ metabolite, 11-dehydro-TXB_2) is associated with enhanced cysteinyl-LT production in AIA who underwent an inhaled ASA and methacholine challenges was explored by Sladek and Szczeklik [18]. In this study, although both provocation challenges elicited a significant drop in lung function, only after the ASA challenge was there an evidence of eicosanoid alteration, demonstrated by a fall in urinary 11-dehydro-TXB_2 and a sevenfold increase in urinary LTE_4 excretion. An extension of these findings focusing on changes in arachidonic acid metabolites in the airway has been evaluated [19]. After provocation challenge with inhaled L-lysine-ASA, patients with AIA had decreases in PGE_2, $PGF_2\alpha$, TXB_2, and PGD_2 and an increase in LTE_4 levels. These findings suggest that small amounts of inhaled ASA can incite bronchospasm accompanied by diminished PG formation and enhanced 5-lipoxygenase activity leading to an elevation in LTE_4 in the airway of patients with AIA. No alterations in 12- and 15-hydroxyeicosate-traenoic production in bronchoalveolar lavage fluid (BALF) were found. Although it was possible that not enough L-lysine ASA was used to provoke this specific change, it could also be surmised that ASA-induced COX inhibition does not activate the 15-lipoxygenase pathway.

A study by Szczeklik et al [20] demonstrated that the ASA-precipitated increase in cysteinyl-LT in the respiratory tract is specific for the clinical syndrome of AIA. Bronchoscopy performed 15 minutes after a bronchial instillation of L-lysine ASA revealed an elevation in LTC_4, LTD_4, and LTE_4 levels and IL-5 only in AIA, with a concomitant reduction in PGE_2 and TXB_2 in AIA and ATA subjects. In ATA, ASA caused a reduction in PGD_2, $PGF_2\alpha$, 9α, 11β-PGF_2 levels, wheras no such change in these COX metabolites in AIA subjects was found, which further predisposes for airway obstruction, given that PGE_2 is already reduced. In addition, the AIA group had a significant increase in eosinophil count in the BALF. There was also evidence of mast cell activation based on the elevation in histamine levels after the bronchial challenge with highly significant correlations between levels of histamine and LTs, although no increase in tryptase levels in the airway was detected.

Another arachidonic acid metabolite that is upregulated with ASA-induced COX inhibition and may offer another mechanism in AIA is mast cell activation causing increased PGD_2 synthesis or release. PGD_2 is a major COX metabolite in mast cells (which can infiltrate an airway smooth muscle cell) and alveolar macrophages. Unlike PGE_2, it is known to cause bronchospasm. AIA subjects were found to have elevated baseline plasma PGD_2 metabolite (9α,11β-PGF_2), serum tryptase, and urinary LTE_4 levels compared with ATA and healthy nonatopic control subjects. These findings indicate that there could be an ongoing process of mast cell or macrophage activation even in clinically stable AIA. However, the findings of elevated products of mast cell activation have not been consistently found in other studies [20,21].

The genetic mechanisms involved in why this condition exists only in a subgroup of asthmatics have been of significant interest given numerous reports published recently. Only differences in LTC_4 synthase expression distinguish patients with AIA from ATA. LTC_4 synthase is a membrane-bound glutathione transferase expressed in eosinophils, basophils, and monocyte-macrophages and is a key enzyme in the synthesis of cysteinyl-LTs, converting LTA_4 to LTC_4. In a study by Cowburn et al [22], there was a fivefold over-representation of cells expressing LTC_4 synthase in bronchial biopsies from AIA subjects compared with ATA. In addition, no difference in immunostaining of bronchial biopsy specimens for COX1, COX2, 5-lipoxygenase, ALOX5, and LTA_4 hydrolase between ASA and ATA patients was found. Only the LTC_4 synthase cell counts in the submucosa, and none of the other eicosanoid pathway enzymes, correlated with basal cysteinyl-LT levels in the BALF and bronchial responsiveness to L-lysine-ASA. Furthermore, the expression of LTC_4 synthase mRNA in AIA biopsies was found mostly in EG2+ eosinophils, with only a small proportion from activated mast cells and macrophages. The gene coding LTC_4 synthase is located on the long arm of chromosome 5 (5q35) in a region implicated in asthma by linkage analysis and adjacent to a region (5q31–33) that includes a number of candidate asthma genes [23,24].

Sanak et al [23] described an adenine (A) to cytosine (C) transversion 444 base pairs (bp) upstream (−444) of the translation start site of the LTC_4 synthase gene during screening of the 5′ region of the gene and reported that the polymorphic C_{-444} allele occurred more commonly in patients with AIA (relative risk 2.62–3.89). In a population of asthmatic patients in Poland, the allele C frequency was 39% in patients with AIA and 26% and 25% in ATA subjects and healthy controls, respectively. Although LTC_4 synthase has been identified as a likely candidate gene for the AIA phenotype, the polymorphic C_{-444} allele has been found to be associated with AIA in a Polish population but not in American, Japanese, and Australian populations [25–27].

In conclusion, increased production of cysteinyl-LT at baseline and after ASA provocation suggests that these mediators contribute significantly to the pathogenesis of AIA. AIA subjects have an over-expression of the LTC_4 synthase in their airways. Although the LTC_4 synthase genotype is the likely component that could characterize AIA because the association of the C_{-444} allele in the promoter region of the LTC_4 synthase gene and AIA has been established, it has not been shown in several populations.

Approach to diagnosis and treatment

Clinical features and natural history

ASA/NSAID sensitivity is strongly suggested by a history of distinct clinical reactions (such as bronchospasm or rhinitis or urticaria/angioedema or anaphylaxis) that occur in proximity of ingestion of the medication, much like an allergic reaction, although the mechanisms are entirely different and are thought to be primarily mediated by COX inhibition. Some manifestations may be drug specific and are likely immune mediated and may have a delayed onset (eg, aseptic meningitis, hypersensitivity pneumonitis, hepatitis, erythema multiforme, anemia, interstitial nephritis, toxic epidermal necrolysis, and Steven Johnson syndrome) [28].

From a large survey ($n = 500$) in 10 countries participating in the European Network on Aspirin-Induced Asthma, the natural history and clinical characteristics of AIA were studied [29]. The diagnosis of AIA was based on a typical history, with 91% of the patients being able to perform ASA inhalation challenges. The inhaled provocation challenges were not done in the 9% of patients with an unequivocal history due to clinical instability or lack of consent. AIA developed according to a characteristic pattern: Perennial rhinitis first appeared at a mean age of 29.7 ± 12.5 years (in half it was thought to be related to a flu-like/viral illness) followed by asthma and ASA intolerance occurring about 4 years later; eventually nasal polyp formation develops. Females outnumbered males by

2.3:1, having rhinitis and ASA intolerance manifestations occurring earlier and with more progressive and severe courses than males. Although a third of patients could not identify any precipitating factors that led to the first attack of asthma, upper respiratory infection, NSAID/ASA ingestion, and allergen or industrial exposure were identified in 45%, 14%, and 11% of subjects. Symptoms of ASA reaction included dyspnea, nasal discharge and obstruction, skin reactions, conjunctival irritation, angioedema, and shock (hypotension and loss of consciousness in 6%). Inhaled corticosteroids were used by 80% of patients, and 51% of patients were oral corticosteroid dependent (mean dose of 8 mg prednisone per day). Fifteen percent of subjects with nasal polyps or sinus disease did not report a known ASA reaction but had a positive bronchial challenge. In 2 of the 16 centers, skin prick tests and measurements of serum IgE were performed. At least a third of patients were atopic and had an earlier onset of rhinitis and asthma, although they did not seem to have a different age at which ASA intolerance or nasal polyposis was detected.

A study of the natural history of AERD in patients admitted to the Scripps Clinic in California was published recently [30]. Three hundred fifty-two consecutive patients with a presumptive diagnosis of AERD were evaluated, and 85% experienced a respiratory reaction during single-blind, oral ASA challenges. The types of respiratory responses were more encompassing in the United States study, in which they included upper and lower respiratory reactions. In those with a confirmed AERD, similar to the European study, the average age at onset of AERD was 34 years, and the majority (57%) were female. In contrast to the European study in which female patients seemed to acquire a more severe disease, there were no significant gender differences in regard to the clinical characteristics in the United States study. The patients had averaged 2.3 hospitalizations and five emergency room visits for asthma. Thirty percent were on a chronic oral corticosteroid medication. There was no ethnic or familial distribution of AERD. The patients had experienced five sinus infections per year and had undergone an average of three sinus surgeries. Only 6% had not had any sinus operation. Over two thirds of patients had at least two prior reactions to NSAIDs including ASA. Although two thirds of patients were atopic, only 1% reported a family history of AERD.

Although the two studies may have used subjects who may have different features in terms of disease severity, they demonstrate that AERD is a distinct clinical syndrome in which a characteristic pattern emerges (eg, respiratory tract manifestations frequently preceding ASA/NSAID-induced reactions), which seems to be influenced by gender and atopic status, and in whom a majority develop a severe protracted course.

Diagnosis

There are no clinically available in vitro or cutaneous tests to diagnose AERD or ASA/NSAID sensitivity. The history is not always accurate because many subjects are unaware of their intolerance to ASA. The gold standard is a provocation challenge testing by oral, inhaled L-lysine ASA, nasal, or intravenous (only done in Japan) ASA [31]. The primary indication for the challenge is an ill-defined history of ASA tolerance or a suspected intolerance for desensitization or research purposes. Provocation tests should be performed by specialists in settings with adequate facilities for resuscitation.

Oral challenges are most commonly performed because this route resembles real-life exposure; hence, multisystemic symptoms, such as bronchial, upper airway, ocular, cutaneous, gastrointestinal, etc., can be elicited. In some centers, measurement of urinary LTE_4 is obtained for research purposes. The test is conclusive if a 20% drop in FEV_1 is documented, if significant symptoms arise, or if the maximum dose is attained (500–650 mg). The oral challenge protocol to detect respiratory reactions induced by ASA that was developed at the Scripps Clinic is depicted in Table 1 [11].

Inhaled ASA challenges are less risky (the reaction is easily reversed with an inhaled beta-agonist) and shorter (the elapsed time to bronchospasm is less than 30 minutes, and the entire test can be completed in less than 5 hours) to perform than the oral test, and, although both are reported to have similar specificity, an oral challenge can be more sensitive especially in drawing out extrabronchial symptoms [32]. The nasal challenge is performed by instillation of L-lysine ASA into the inferior nasal conchae. Anterior rhinomanometry is used to evaluate for changes in nasal patency and flow. However, the challenge cannot be performed in patients with severe nasal obstruction or who have large fluctuations in nasal flow at baseline. It is an option for patients in whom bronchial or provocation tests cannot be performed due to significant bronchial reactivity [31,33].

Treatment of aspirin-exacerbated respiratory disease

Available clinical practice guidelines for asthma treatment are applicable for the treatment of AIA. Corticosteroid therapy remains a mainstay in the treatment

Table 1
Oral challenge protocol to detect respiratory reactions by acetylsalicylic acid

| Time | ASA doses (mg)[a] | | |
	Day 1	Day 2	Day 3
7 AM	Placebo	30	100–150
10 AM	Placebo	45–60	150–325
1 PM	Placebo	60–100	650

Start challenges, if baseline FEV_1 is 70% or greater than predicted, without bronchodilator. Alternatively, if the absolute FEV_1 is greater than 1.5 liters and represents the best prior FEV_1 value, proceed with oral challenge. On the placebo day, FEV_1 values should vary by <10% from baseline, and starting FEV_1 value on day 2 should be within 10% of the starting value on day 1.

[a] ASA doses should be individualized: Start with 30 mg of ASA in everyone but increase to 45 mg for the second dose if the historic reaction was severe or to 60 mg if the historic reaction was milder.
From Stevenson DD, Simon R, Zuraw B. Sensitivity to aspirin and NSAID drugs. In: Adkinson NF, John Yunginger J, Busse W, Bochner B, Holgate S, Middleton E, editors. Middleton's allergy: principles and practice. 6th edition, vol 2. St Louis: Mosby; 2003. p. 1698; with permission.

of persistent asthma, even for AIA individuals, who often require aggressive anti-inflammatory coverage such as oral corticosteroids. Given the convincing evidence that cysteinyl-LT production is upregulated presumed to be secondary to a diversion of the arachidonate metabolism from COX inhibition, it would seem reasonable that LT-modifying agents would play a prominent role in alleviating ASA/NSAID-induced reactions. LT modifiers (5-lipoxygenase inhibitors and LT antagonists) have been found to be effective in the chronic therapy of patients with AIA and rhinitis in addition to those provided by inhaled corticosteroid therapy [34,35].

Rhinosinusitis and nasal polyposis greatly affect the morbidity and quality of life of AIA patients. Due to a high recurrence rate of at least 30%, polypectomy alone is not recommended, and other medications or desensitization are almost always necessary [36]. Topical corticosteroids are the treatment of choice. LT receptor antagonists are also reported effective in alleviating symptoms of nasal polyposis in these patients.

Education for the patient that includes discussion of adverse effects and cross-reactivity between ASA and other COX1-inhibiting drugs is crucial. For the physician, flagging medical records and appropriate communication with the patient and other members of the medical or surgical team is important.

Cross-reactivity and therapeutic implications

Individuals with AIA should be provided with a list of contraindicated drugs that are nonselective COX inhibitors and safe alternative medications (Box 1). The potency of these agents in causing bronchospasm seems to be in proportion to their relative potency or specificity in inhibiting COX, so that weak COX1 inhibitors tend to be tolerated at usual doses [37]. Common anti-inflammatory agents thought to be safe for use in asthmatic patients in usual doses include sodium salicylate, choline salicylate, salicylamide, dextropropoxyphene, benzydamine, and chloroquine [33,38]. Salsalate (Disalcid), nimesulide, and meloxicam (preferential inhibitors of COX2 but also inhibit COX1) induce bronchospasm at higher doses [39–41].

Acetaminophen, which preferentially blocks COX3 and is a known weak COX1 inhibitor, has been shown at doses of 150 to 600 mg to induce bronchospasm in only 6% of AIA patients [38]. From the Scripps Clinic, in AIA patients who underwent a single-blind acetaminophen challenge procedure, 24% and 32% developed bronchospasm at 1000- and 1500-mg doses, respectively [43]. There were no positive acetaminophen challenge results in patients with negative ASA challenge. Hence, the general recommendation on the use of acetaminophen in AIA stable patients include avoidance of acetaminophen at doses of 1000 mg or greater, especially in exquisitely ASA-sensitive patients.

The safety of recently developed highly selective COX2 inhibitors (eg, celecoxib and rofecoxib) has been demonstrated in numerous studies, and these can be recommended as alternative medications in AIA due to their analgesic,

Box 1. Drugs or chemicals that inhibit COX1 and cross-react or only partially inhibit COX1 and drugs that are selective COX2 inhibitors

NSAIDs that inhibit COX1

- Ibuprofen (Motrin, Rufen, Advil)
- Indomethacin (Indocin)
- Sulindac (Clinoril)
- Tolmetin (Tolectin)
- Naproxen sodium (Anaprox)
- Fenoprofen (Nalfon)
- Naproxen (Naprosyn)
- Meclofenamine (Meclomen)
- Ketorolac tromethamine (Toradol)
- Etodolac (Lodine)
- Oxaprozin (Daypro)
- Diclofenac (Voltaren)
- Ketoprofen (Orudis, Oruvail)
- Flurbiprofen (Ansaid)
- Piroxicam (Feldene)
- Nabumatone (Relafen)
- Mefenamic acid (Ponstel)

Low incidence of cross-reactivity: analgesics that are poor inhibitors of COX1 enzymes and only with high concentrations of the drug

- Acetaminophen (Paracetamol)
- Disalicylic acid (Disalcid)
- Meloxicam [40]

Selective COX2 inhibitors

- Nimesulide [41]
- Rofecoxib [45,46]
- Celecoxib [42,44]

Data from Stevenson DD. Approach to the patient with a history of adverse reactions to aspirin or NSAIDs: diagnosis and treatment. Allergy Asthma Proc 2000;21:25–31.

antipyretic, and anti-inflammatory properties [29,44–46]. None of the AIA patients developed bronchospasm to celecoxib or rofecoxib. Even with almost complete tolerance to COX2 inhibitors by AIA patients, the use of these medications in NSAID-intolerant subjects may not be generalizable, especially for patients who manifest with NSAID-induced urticaria/angioedema or anaphylaxis in whom cutaneous or anaphylactoid reactions can still develop [47,48]. Hence, careful use of COX2 inhibitors or performing a supervised provocation challenge may be recommended for these patients.

Acetylsalicylic acid desensitization

ASA desensitization refers to the process of inducing refractoriness to ASA or NSAIDs by administration of incremental doses of oral or inhaled ASA until all reactions disappear. A protocol that was developed and refined at the Scripps Clinic by Stevenson et al uses increasing doses of ASA in 5 days until the maximum dose of 650 mg is tolerated [11,49]. Daily doses of ASA (325 to 650 mg twice daily) are administered, and improvement in the underlying chronic respiratory symptoms can be achieved during maintenance of the desensitized state. The refractory state lasts 2 to 5 days, with gradual return to sensitivity between 2 and 4 days when ASA is withheld [50]. Cross-desensitization is also attained for other NSAIDs; hence, these can be used as substitutes for ongoing ASA treatment. ASA desensitization should be considered for AIA patients with recalcitrant respiratory symptoms and polyp formation, despite optimal pharmacotheraphy including high doses of systemic corticosteroids and repeated sinus surgery, and in patients with concomitant medical conditions requiring the use of ASA/NSAIDs, such as arthritis and other rheumatologic or cardiac disease.

Several reports from the Scripps Clinic of their experience with ASA desensitization have consistently shown significant improvement in nasal/sinus and asthma symptoms [51–53]. In their latest publication, of 172 patients with AIA who underwent desensitization between 1995 and 2000, 67% responded favorably to ASA treatment in terms of significant improvement in nasal (including sense of smell) and asthma symptoms and reduction in sinus infections, hospitalizations/ER visits for asthma, and requirement for systemic corticosteroids, most of which were apparent by the first 6 months of treatment and persisted for 1 to 5 years [51]. Fourteen percent discontinued treatment because of adverse effects (of which gastritis is the most common), and in 19% ASA treatment was discontinued for different reasons such as those unrelated to side effects, lack of adherence, or lack of effects.

Although ASA desensitization can be successful for improvement of asthma and rhinosinusitis, the mechanisms are not clear. A possible conjecture is that continued inhibition of COX1 and phospholipase A_2 could lead to a decrease in LT synthesis and other proinflammatory prostanoids by downregulation of cysteinyl-LT receptors [54]. Chronic desensitization has been associated with a decline in LTB_4 synthesis [55] and reduction in urinary LTE_4 levels [54].

Although considerable strides have been made in the past two decades in understanding the pathogenesis of this syndrome, there are many unanswered questions that relate to what stimulates the initial inflammatory response in the upper and lower airway, why COX inhibition does not produce significant reactions in most asthmatics, and what the mechanism is behind the chronic severe asthma and rhinosinusitis in AIA despite avoidance of ASA/NSAIDs. In addition, it is not certain why distinct clinical reactions (respiratory versus cutaneous versus cardiovascular) are triggered and how the intolerance is acquired.

Beta-blockers

β-adrenergic blocking agents are indicated for common medical conditions such as stable angina, myocardial infarctions (MIs), hypertension, heart failure, coronary artery disease, and arrhythmias. In addition, these medications are used in the management of hyperthyroid disease, acute stress reactions, generalized anxiety, essential tremor, glaucoma, and prophylaxis for migraines. Due to the extensive medical conditions for which β-blockers are proven effective and for which they can have a major impact on survival and quality of life, there is a large population, including asthmatics, who could benefit from their use. For instance, in over 100,000 adult survivors of MI, 21% were found to have asthma or chronic obstructive pulmonary disease [56]. Historically, β-blockers have been contraindicated in asthma due to concern for exacerbating asthma symptoms. However, the availability of newer formulations and more information on the benefits of β-blockers are causing a re-examination of their role in the asthmatic population.

In almost all asthmatics, nonselective β-blockade causes bronchoconstriction and increases bronchial hyper-responsiveness to methacholine and histamine [57,58]. It is likely that multiple mechanisms underlie this effect. The involvement of parasympathetic nerves seems rational because they are the dominant bronchoconstrictor neural pathway in the airways [59]. In support of parasympathetic involvement, cholinergic receptor blockade by oxitropium bromide was shown to inhibit propranolol-induced bronchospasm (PIB) [60]. Atropine [57] and pilocarpine also inhibited PIB in asthmatics [61]. The degree of the protective effect of atropine on PIB varied between individual asthmatics, suggesting heterogeneity in the cause of PIB in asthma [57].

There is evidence of other mechanisms contributing to the bronchoconstriction caused by β-blockers in asthmatics. One such pathway may include the non-adrenergic noncholinergic (NANC) nerves. Vasoactive intestinal peptide is a neurotransmitter of NANC nerves in the airways, and it has been shown to attenuate PIB independent of cholinergic blockage [62]. Another pathway may involve endogenous epinephrine tonically inhibiting cholinergic neurotransmission. A β-blocker may remove this effect, causing an increase in acetylcholine release to airway smooth muscle cells, promoting bronchoconstriction. This would affect asthmatics who are hyper-responsive to acetylcholine but would not affect healthy individuals [59].

Cellular mechanisms may play a role because cromones attenuate PIB to varying degrees [63,64]. It was proposed that PIB may be due to blockade of β-receptors on the mast cell surface, causing the release of chemical mediators such as histamine, cysteinyl-LT, and TXA_2. However, neither a LT-receptor nor a TXA_2 receptor antagonist was effective at alleviating PIB in asthmatics [65], and histamine levels were not found to be elevated with PIB [66].

Description of relevant pharmacologic and pharmacokinetic properties

β-adrenergic receptors ($β_1$ and $β_2$) are part of a large family of hormone and neurotransmitter receptors that initiate their function by coupling to a guanine nucleotide-binding protein [67]. When β-blockers occupy the receptor site, they act as a competitive antagonist that binds to the β-adrenergic receptor without activation [68]. Although $β_1$ and $β_2$-adrenoreceptors are widely distributed in the cardiovascular [67] and the respiratory systems [69], $β_2$-receptors are found four times more frequently in the airways [70], whereas $β_1$-adrenoceptors predominate in the heart. The stimulation of $β_2$-adrenoceptors causes muscular relaxation [67], blood pressure reduction [71], and bronchoconstriction [72]; $β_1$ cardiac stimulation causes an increase in the rate and force of contraction [67]. Nonselective β-adrenoceptor blockers block $β_1$ and $β_2$ receptors. Lower doses of $β_1$ antagonists preferentially bind to $β_1$ receptors, but as the plasma concentration of the $β_1$ blocker increases, its binding becomes less selective and increasingly inhibits $β_2$ receptors [73,74].

Different β-blockers have inherent properties (Table 2) [75] that help determine which β-blocker is indicated for the patient, and some features might have a more prominent impact on an asthmatic patient. β-blockers can be divided into those with or without intrinsic sympathomimetic activity (ISA). For those with ISA, in the presence of high-background sympathomimetic activity the

Table 2
Pharmacologic characteristics of β-adrenergic antagonists

Medication	Receptors	Lipophilicity	ISA
Acebutolol	$β_1$	Moderate	Yes
Atenolol	$β_1$	Low	No
Metoprolol	$β_1$	Moderate	No
Pindolol	$β_1, β_2$	Moderate	Yes
Timolol	$β_1, β_2$	Moderate	No
Nadolol	$β_1, β_2$	Low	No
Propranolol	$β_1, β_2$	High	No

Abbreviation: ISA, intrinsic sympathomimetic activity.
Data from Hoffman BB. Catecholamines, sympathomimetic drugs, and adrenergic receptor antagonists. In: Hardman JG, Limbird LE, Gillman AG. Goodman & Gilman's the pharmacological basis of therapeutics. New York: McGraw-Hill; 2001. p. 215–53.

medication acts as an antagonist, and with low or absent background sympathetic activity it acts as an agonist [67].

Therapeutic implications

Nonselective β-blockers are contraindicated in asthma because they have been shown to significantly decrease pulmonary function and place the patient at risk for acute bronchospasm. Regular use of noncardioselective β-blockers was demonstrated to cause a 13.5% decrease in FEV_1 [76]. This reduction is significant for asthmatics with severe airflow obstruction. In addition, severe bronchoconstriction and fatal attacks have been reported even with a topical ophthalmic application of a β-blocker [77,78]. This is important in conditions for which nonselective β-blockers are indicated; hence, alternative medications should be used.

Although a few studies have demonstrated significant effects of cardioselective β-blockers on lung function [79], their use may be tolerated in some asthmatics [80]. A meta-analysis of randomized, blinded, placebo-controlled trials that studied the effects of cardioselective β-blockers on FEV_1, symptoms, and inhaled $β_2$-agonist use in patients with mild to moderate reactive airway disease was recently reported [76]. Administration of a single dose of a cardioselective β-blocker was associated with a 7.46% (95% CI 5.59–9.32) reduction in FEV_1 and a 4.63% (95% CI 2.47–6.78) bronchodilator reversibility in FEV_1 compared with placebo, with no concomitant increase in symptoms. Analysis of several trials lasting from 3 days to 4 weeks demonstrated no significant change in FEV_1 (−0.42%; 95% CI −3.74–2.91), symptoms, or inhaler use compared with placebo but maintained an 8.74% (95% CI 1.96–15.52) increase in β-agonist bronchodilator response. Hence, it seems that cardioselective β-blockers do not produce clinically significant adverse respiratory effects in patients with mild to moderate reactive airway disease and can therefore be used for these patients. However, this meta-analysis has significant limitations, which include variable and generally short medication courses, exclusion of severe asthmatics, and lack of information on the effects of cardioselective β-blockers on asthma exacerbations. Long-term studies are needed to fully define the safety profile of cardioselective β-blocker use in asthmatics [81].

There is evolving evidence that in specific circumstances the benefits of cardioselective β-blockers outweigh the risks for asthmatics. A study of 3800 asthmatics showed a protective effect of a β-blocker on mortality within 2 years after MI (12% versus 20% mortality rate in β-blocker–treated and untreated asthmatics, respectively, with a relative risk of 0.6) [82]. The guidelines established by the American College of Cardiology and the American Heart Association suggest that β-blocker therapy after MI is appropriate for many elderly patients with asthma as long as they are closely monitored for adverse events [83]. Ipratropium bromide is the treatment of choice for β-blocker–induced bronchospasm [80]. Other drugs, including $β_2$ agonists, atropine, aminophylline, isoproterenol, steroids, halothane, and glucagon, have also reversed the broncho-spastic effects of β-blocking agents [84].

Angiotensin-converting enzyme inhibitors

ACE inhibitors are considered to be an effective and, in some cases preferred, intervention for the treatment or prevention of hypertension, cardiovascular diseases and their complications, and diabetic nephropathy. ACE inhibitors are usually well tolerated, and in the general population the more common side effects include cough, hypotension, and hyperkalemia [85]. Angioedema has been reported in rare cases [86], and there is a risk of teratogenicity during the second and third semester of pregnancy [87].

The reported incidence of ACE inhibitor–associated cough is 10% to 20% [88–90]. Prior asthma or bronchospasm is not a risk factor for developing cough as an ACE inhibitor adverse effect [91]. The cough has been described as dry, nonproductive, persistent, or hacking; often starting as a tickling sensation in the back of the throat; sometimes worse at night or on lying down; and as being episodic [90]. It can occur 1 day to several months after starting the medication and normally persists while taking the medication. It usually disappears within several days but may persist for up to 4 weeks after discontinuing the medication [86]. In asthmatics, the cough does not cause a decrease in lung function [92] and should not be responsive to treatment with albuterol. In patients with congestive heart failure, it is important to consider cough as a possible ACE inhibitor side effect before attributing it to pulmonary congestion [86].

ACE inhibitors are generally safe in most asthmatics [93]. Studies in patients with chronic airflow obstruction showed no significant change in their FEV_1 over the treatment period [92,94,95]. In addition, bronchial reactivity has been shown to remain unchanged with ACE inhibitors [92,95,96].

There have been few reports of bronchoconstriction and bronchial reactivity associated with this class of medication [91,97,98]. In one case report, a 51-year-old man developed intermittent shortness of breath and wheezing within a month of starting captopril that resolved upon discontinuation of the medication [97]. In another case report, a known asthmatic developed immediate worsening of dyspnea and wheezing upon starting enalapril [98]. The New Zealand Adverse Reactions Center registered 596 adverse respiratory events to enalapril, capto-pril, and lisinopril, including cough in 86% and bronchospasm and dyspnea in 8%. Unspecified reactions in 6% were noted [91]. Based on these reports, significant respiratory compromise seems rare but is a possible adverse effect of an ACE inhibitor.

ACE inhibitors have varying pharmacologic and pharmacokinetic profiles in regard to their lipophilic properties and requirement for hepatic biotransformation [85,99]. Although these properties may affect the potency and duration of activity of ACE inhibitors and consequently create practical prescription preferences to allow for once-daily dosing, there may be other factors, such as race and gender, that can affect the efficacy and side-effect profile of these medications. Studies have shown that the adverse effect of cough occurs nearly three times more often in women [86,100,101], and African Americans and Asians have a three- to fourfold higher risk of angioedema [71].

Mechanisms of angiotensin-converting enzyme inhibitor–induced respiratory reactions

The mechanisms of ACE inhibitor–induced cough are not completely defined but may be mediated by bradykinin and substance P [102]. ACE is present in membrane-bound form in endothelial cells, epithelial cells, and in the brain; and in a soluble form in the blood and other body fluids [99]. It catalyzes the conversion of angiotensin I into angiotensin II [85], which acts directly on vascular smooth muscle, increasing the peripheral and central vascular tone. It also stimulates aldosterone secretion, leading to sodium and water retention [99].

ACE acts as a kininase enzyme that degrades inflammatory compounds such as bradykinin, substance P, and neurokinin A [2,103]. Bradykinin increases vascular permeability and promotes vasodilation through stimulating arachidonic acid metabolite production and nitric oxide production [99]. Substance P is a tachykinin present in neurons arising from the vagus nerve beneath the epithelium of the trachea and major bronchi. It may mediate the afferent vagal impulses to the medullary cough center, resulting in cough [90]. Therefore, ACE inhibitors have the potential to create an abundance of kinins (eg, bradykinin, substance P, and neurokinin A) by inhibition of the ACE kininase enzyme action.

A mechanism that invokes substance P involvement in the causation of cough as an adverse reaction to an ACE inhibitor in some patients may be an increased cough reflex sensitivity. This theory is supported by the fact that patients with ACE inhibitor cough, compared with those without, have an increased cough response to capsaicin [104]. Capsaicin acts by depolarizing sensory neurons, causing release of substance P [105], and has been used to quantify the sensitivity of the cough reflex [106]. The involvement of PGs in the mechanism causing cough is also evidenced by the fact that the COX inhibitor sulindac has been shown to relieve the ACE inhibitor–induced cough in some patients [107,108].

As in ACE inhibitor–induced cough, the mechanism involved in ACE inhibitor–induced bronchoconstriction is elusive. There are reports implicating a specific sensitivity to bradykinin. Inhalation of bradykinin has been shown to decrease FEV_1 and cause bronchoconstriction in asthmatics but not significantly in healthy control subjects [109,110]. How bradykinin induces bronchoconstriction is not clear but may be due to cholinergic vagal reflex mechanisms and selective stimulation of C-fiber afferent nerves [109]. Histamine and prostanoids may contribute a small component to the response [108,111].

Approach to management and therapeutic implications

When an ACE inhibitor–induced respiratory reaction is suspected, the most practical approach seems to be a trial off the ACE inhibitor before pursuing multiple tests because this may save the patient from undergoing an extensive work-up [86]. If a person experiences cough with one ACE inhibitor, they will likely have cough with another ACE inhibitor and therefore should try a different type of medication [86,90]. One possible alternative is an angiotensin II receptor blocker, which produces hemodynamic effects similar to those of ACE inhibitors but does not have the adverse side effect of cough [103]. The alternative medication chosen is dictated by each individual's clinical situation. In patients who have a cough side effect where it is deemed important that they remain on an ACE inhibitor, oral theophylline [112] or cromolyn sodium can help to treat the cough, causing it to remit in some patients [113]. Treatment with the COX inhibitor sulindac has been shown to help reduce ACE inhibitor cough, but more information is needed on the long-term effects of sulindac used in combination with an ACE inhibitor before it can be recommended [107].

Summary

The means by which certain medications can trigger asthma vary in terms of acuity of onset, severity, and mechanisms involved. Certain medications, such as nonselective β-blockers, are expected to cause bronchoconstriction in almost all asthmatics and therefore should be avoided. Although ASA/NSAIDs or β-blockers can induce immediate bronchoconstriction, ACE inhibitors can manifest with adverse respiratory reactions within a day to weeks of use. ASA-induced reactions tend to occur several years after the onset of rhinitis/asthma phenotype, suggesting that an underlying inflammatory process triggers the development of ASA sensitivity. The severity of reactions in AERD can range from mere naso-ocular to profound anaphylactoid presentation, attributed most likely to COX inhibition. The mechanisms involved in bronchospasm or increased responsiveness to β-blockers or ACE inhibitors also need further investigation.

The general and most practical approach is avoidance and cautious use of the drugs, especially if susceptibility is known for an asthmatic. However, these medications can exert a major role in the management of common diseases, some of which have serious and debilitating complications. Fortunately, controller therapy for asthma and equally efficacious alternatives (eg, angiotensin II receptor blockers) or more selective medications (eg, selective COX2 inhibitors and cardioselective β-blockers) for the treatment of these conditions are now available. In the case of ASA sensitivity, desensitization is another worthy option.

References

[1] Hunt LW, Rosenow III EC. Asthma-producing drugs. Ann Allergy 1992;68:453–62.
[2] Van Schoor J, Joos GF, Pauwels RA. Indirect bronchial hyperresponsiveness in asthma: mechanisms, pharmacology and implications for clinical research. Eur Respir J 2000;16:514–33.
[3] Roberts II LJ, Morrow JD. Analgesic-antipyretic and antiinflammatory agents and drugs

employed in the treatment of gout. In: Hardman JG, Limbird LE, Gilman AG, editors. Good-man & Gilman's the pharmacological basis of therapeutics. New York: McGraw-Hill; 2001. p. 687–8.

[4] Widal F, Abrami P, Lermoyez J. First complete description of the aspirin idiosyncrasy-asthma-nasal polyposis syndrome (plus urticaria). Presse Med 1922;18:189–92.

[5] Samter M, Beers RFJ. Intolerance to aspirin: clinical studies and consideration of its patho-genesis. Ann Intern Med 1968;68:975–83.

[6] Kupczyk M, Kuprys I, Gorski P, et al. Aspirin intolerance and allergy to house dust mites: important factors associated with development of severe asthma. Ann Allergy Asthma Immunol 2004;92:453–8.

[7] Vally H, Taylor ML, Thompson PJ. The prevalence of aspirin tolerant asthma (AIA) in Australian asthmatic patients. Thorax 2002;57:569–74.

[8] Picado C, Castillo JA, Montserrat JM, et al. Aspirin-intolerance as a precipitating factor of life-threatening attacks of asthma requiring mechanical ventilation. Eur Respir J 1989;2: 127–9.

[9] Marquette CH, Saulnier F, Leroy O, et al. Long-term prognosis of near-fatal asthma. Am Rev Respir Dis 1992;146:76–81.

[10] Jenkins C, Costello J, Hodge L. Systematic review of prevalence of aspirin-induced asthma and its implications for clinical practice. BMJ 2004;328:434–40.

[11] Namazy JA, Simon RA. Sensitivity to nonsteroidal anti-inflammatory drugs. Ann Allergy Asthma Immunol 2002;89:542–50.

[12] Pang L, Pitt A, Petkova D, et al. The COX-1/COX-2 balance in asthma. Clin Exp Allergy 1998; 28:1050–8.

[13] Vane JR. Inhibition of prostaglandin synthesis as a mechanism of action for aspirin-like drugs. Nature 1971;231:232–5.

[14] Pavord ID. Bronchoprotective role for endogenous prostaglandin E_2. Lancet 1994;345:436–8.

[15] Kumlin M, Dahlen B, Bjorck T, et al. Urinary excretion of leukotriene E_4 and 11-dehydro-thromboxane B_2 in response to bronchial provocations with allergen, aspirin, leukotriene D_4, and histamine in asthmatics. Am Rev Respir Dis 1992;146:96–103.

[16] Christie PE, Tagari P, Ford-Hutchinson AW, et al. Urinary leukotriene E_4 concentrations increase after aspirin challenge in aspirin-sensitive asthmatic subjects. Am Rev Respir Dis 1991;143:1025–9.

[17] Higashi N, Taniguchi M, Mita H, et al. Clinical features of asthmatic patients with increased urinary leukotriene E4 excretion (hyperleukotrienuria): involvement of chronic hyperplastic rhinosinusitis with nasal polyposis. J Allergy Clin Immunol 2004;113:277–83.

[18] Sladek K, Szczeklik A. Cysteinyl leukotrienes overproduction and mast cell activation in aspirin-provoked bronchospasm in asthma. Eur Respir J 1993;6:391–9.

[19] Sladek K, Dworski R, Soja J, et al. Eicosanoids in bronchoalveolar lavage fluid of aspirin-intolerant patients with asthma after aspirin challenge. Am J Respir Crit Care Med 1994; 149:940–6.

[20] Szczeklik A, Sladek K, Dworski R, et al. Bronchial aspirin challenge causes specific eicosanoid response in aspirin-sensitive asthmatics. Am J Respir Crit Care Med 1996;154:1608–14.

[21] Bosso JV, Schwartz LB, Stevenson DD. Tryptase and histamine release during aspirin-induced respiratory reactions. J Allergy Clin Immunol 1991;88:830–7.

[22] Cowburn AS, Sladek K, Soja J, et al. Overexpression of leukotriene C_4 synthase in bronchial biopsies from patients with aspirin-intolerant asthma. J Clin Invest 1998;101:834–46.

[23] Sanak M, Simon H-U, Szczeklik A. Leukotriene C_4 synthase promoter polymorphism and risk of aspirin-induced asthma. Lancet 1997;350:1599–600.

[24] Penrose JF, Spector J, Baldasaro M, et al. Molecular cloning of the gene for human leukotriene C4 synthase: organization, nucleotide sequence, and chromosomal localization to 5q35. J Biol Chem 1996;271:11356–61.

[25] Kedda M-A, Shi J, Duffy D, et al. Characterization of two polymorphisms in the leukotriene C_4 synthase gene in an Australian population of subjects with mild, moderate, and severe asthma. J Allergy Clin Immunol 2004;113:889–95.

[26] Kawagishi Y, Mita H, Taniguchi M, et al. Leukotriene C_4 synthase promoter polymorphism in Japanese patients with aspirin-induced asthma. J Allergy Clin Immunol 2002;109:936–42.

[27] Van Sambeck R, Stevenson DD, Baldasaro M, et al. 5′ flanking region polymorphism of the gene encoding leukotriene C_4 synthase does not correlate wth the aspirin-intolerant asthma phenotype in the United States. J Allergy Clin Immunol 2000;106:72–6.

[28] Stevenson DD, Sanchez-Borges M, Szczeklik A. Classification of allergic and pseudoallergic reactions to drugs that inhibit cyclooxygenase enzymes. Ann Allergy Asthma Immunol 2001; 87:177–80.

[29] Szczeklik A, Nizankowska E, Duplaga M. Natural history of aspirin-induced asthma. Eur Respir J 2000;16:432–6.

[30] Berges-Gimeno MP, Simon RA, Stevenson DD. The natural history and clinical characteristics of aspirin-exacerbated respiratory disease. Ann Allergy Asthma Immunol 2002;89:474–8.

[31] Melillo E, Balzano G, Bianco S, et al. Report of the INTERASMA Working Group on standardization of inhalation provocation tests in aspirin-induced asthma: oral and inhalation provocation tests for the diagnosis of aspirin-induced asthma. Allergy 2001;56:899–911.

[32] Nizankowska E, Bestynska-Krypel A, Cmiel A, et al. Oral and bronchial provocation tests with aspirin for diagnosis of aspirin-induced asthma. Eur Respir J 2000;15:863–9.

[33] Stevenson DD, Simon RA, Zuraw BL. Sensitivity to aspirin and nonsteroidal antiinflammatory drugs. In: Middleton E, Reed C, Ellis E, Adkinson NF, Yunginger JW, Busse WW, Bochner B, Simons FE, editors. Allergy principles & practice. St. Louis (MO): Mosby; 2001. p. 1695–710.

[34] Dahlen B, Nizankowska E, Szczeklik A, et al. Benefits from adding the 5-lipoxygenase inhibitor zileuton to conventional therapy in aspirin-intolerant asthmatics. Am J Respir Crit Care Med 1998;157:1187–94.

[35] Dahlen S-E, Malmstrom K, Nizankowska E, et al. Improvement of aspirin-intolerant asthma by montelukast, a leukotriene antagonist. Am J Respir Crit Care Med 2002;165:9–14.

[36] Hosemann W. Surgical treatment of nasal polyposis in patient with aspirin intolerance. Thorax 2000;55(Suppl 2):S87–90.

[37] Stevenson DD. Approach to the patient with a history of adverse reactions to aspirin or NSAIDs: diagnosis and treatment. Allergy Asthma Proc 2000;21:25–31.

[38] Szczeklik A, Gryglewski RJ, Czerniawska-Mysik G. Clinical patterns of hypersensitivity to nonsteroidal anti-inflammatory drugs and their pathogenesis. J Allergy Clin Immunol 1977; 60:276–84.

[39] Stevenson DD, Hougham A, Schrank P, et al. Salsalate cross-sensitivity in aspirin-sensitive patients with asthma. J Allergy Clin Immunol 1990;86:749–58.

[40] Kosnik M, Music E, Matjaz F, et al. Relative safety of meloxicam in NSAID-intolerant patients. Allergy 1998;53:1231–3.

[41] Andri L, Senna G, Betteli C, et al. Tolerability of nimesulide in aspirin-sensitive patients. Ann Allergy 1994;72:29–32.

[42] Dahlen B, Szczeklik A, Murray JJ. Celecoxib in patients with asthma and aspirin intolerance. N Engl J Med 2001;344:142.

[43] Settipane RA, Schrank P, Simon RA, et al. Prevalence of cross-sensitivity with acetaminophen in aspirin-sensitive asthmatic subjects. J Allergy Clin Immunol 1995;96:480–5.

[44] Gyllfors P, Bochenek G, Overholt J, et al. Biochemical and clinical evidence that aspirin-intolerant asthmatic subjects tolerate the cyclooxygenase 2-selective analgetic drug celecoxib. J Allergy Clin Immunol 2003;111:1116–21.

[45] Martin-Garcia C, Hinojosa M, Berges P, et al. Safety of a cyclooxygenase-2 inhibitor in patients with aspirin-sensitive asthma. Chest 2002;121:1812–7.

[46] Stevenson DD, Simon RA. Lack of cross-reactivity between rofecoxib and aspirin in aspirin-sensitive patients with asthma. J Allergy Clin Immunol 2001;108:47–51.

[47] Sanchez-Borges M, Capriles-Hulett A, Caballero-Fonsenca F, et al. Tolerability to new COX-2 inhibitors in NSAID-sensitive patients with cutaneous reactions. Ann Allergy Asthma Immunol 2001;87:201–4.

[48] Schellenberg RR, Isserow SH. Anaphylactoid reaction to a cyclooxygenase-2 inhibitor in a patient who had a reaction to a cyclooxygenase-1 inhibitor. N Engl J Med 2001;345:1856.

[49] Stevenson DD, Simon RA, Mathison DA. Aspirin-sensitive asthma: tolerance to aspirin after positive oral aspirin challenges. J Allergy Clin Immunol 1980;66:82–8.

[50] Pleskow WW, Stevenson DD, Mathison DA, et al. Aspirin desensitization in aspirin sensitive asthmatic patients: clinical manifestations and characterization of the refractory period. J Allergy Clin Immunol 1982;69:11–9.

[51] Berges-Gimeno MP, Simon RA, Stevenson DD. Long-term treatment with aspirin desensitization in asthmatic patients with aspirin-exacerbated respiratory disease. J Allergy Clin Immunol 2003;111:180–6.

[52] Sweet JM, Stevenson DD, Simon RA, et al. Long-term effects of aspirin desensitization: treatment for aspirin-sensitive rhinosinusitis-asthma. J Allergy Clin Immunol 1990;85:59–65.

[53] Stevenson DD, Hankammer MA, Mathison DA, et al. Aspirin desensitization treatment of aspirin-sensitive patients with rhinosinusitis-asthma: long-term outcomes. J Allergy Clin Immunol 1996;98:751–8.

[54] Nasser SM, Patel M, Bell GS, et al. The effect of aspirin desensitization on urinary leukotriene E4 concentrations in aspirin-sensitive asthma. Am J Respir Crit Care Med 1995;151:1326–30.

[55] Juergens UR, Christiansen SC, Stevenson DD, et al. Inhibition of monocyte leukotriene B4 production following aspirin desensitization. J Allergy Clin Immunol 1995;96:148–56.

[56] Krumholz HM, Radford MJ, Wang YMS, et al. National use and effectiveness of β-blockers for the treatment of elderly patients after acute myocardial infarction: National Cooperative Cardiovascular Project. JAMA 1998;280:623–9.

[57] Okayama M, Yafuso N, Nogami H, et al. A new method of inhalation challenge with propranolol: comparison with methacholine-induced bronchoconstriction and role of vagal nerve activity. J Allergy Clin Immunol 1987;80:291–9.

[58] Zaid G, Beall GN. Bronchial response to beta-adrenergic blockade. N Engl J Med 1966;275:580–4.

[59] Barnes PJ. Neural control of human airways in health and disease. Am Rev Respir Dis 1986;134:1289–314.

[60] Ind PW, Dixon CM, Fuller RW, et al. Anticholinergic blockade of beta-blocker-induced bronchoconstriction. Am Rev Respir Dis 1989;139:1390–4.

[61] Okayama M, Shen T, Midorikawa J, et al. Effect of Pilocarpine on propranolol-induced bronchoconstriction in asthma. Am J Respir Crit Care Med 1994;149:76–80.

[62] Crimi N, Palermo F, Oliveri R, et al. Effect of vasoactive intestinal peptide (VIP) on propranolol-induced bronchoconstriction. J Allergy Clin Immunol 1988;82:617–21.

[63] Koeter GH, Meurs H, De Monchy JG, et al. Protective effect of disodium cromoglycate on propranolol challenge. Allergy 1982;37:587–90.

[64] Foresi A, Chetta A, Pelucchi A, et al. Effect of inhaled disodium cromoglycate and nedocromil sodium on propranolol-induced bronchoconstriction. Ann Allergy 1993;70:159–63.

[65] Fujimura M, Abo M, Kamio Y, et al. Effect of leukotriene and thromboxane antagoinist on propranolol-induced bronchoconstriction. Am J Respir Crit Care Med 1999;160:2100–3.

[66] Ind PW, Barnes PJ, Brown MJ, et al. Plasma histamine concentration during propranolol induced bronchoconstriction. Thorax 1985;40:903–9.

[67] Emilien G, Maloteaux J-M. Current therapeutic uses and potential of β-adrenoceptor agonists and antagonists. Eur J Clin Pharmacol 1998;53:389–404.

[68] Boskabady MH, Snashall PD. Bronchial responsiveness to beta-adrenergic stimulation and enhanced beta-blockade in asthma. Respirology 2000;5:111–8.

[69] Carstairs JR, Nimmo AJ, Barnes PJ. Autoradiogaphic visualization of beta-adrenoceptor subtypes in human lung. Am Rev Respir Dis 1985;132:541–7.

[70] Spina D, Rigby PJ, Paterson JW, et al. Autoradiographic localization of beta-adrenoceptors in asthmatic human lung. Am Rev Respir Dis 1989;140:1410–5.

[71] Chobanian AV, Bakris GL, Black HR, et al. Seventh report of the Joint National Committee on Prevention, Detection, Evaluation, and Treatment of High Blood Pressure. Hypertension 2003;42:1206–52.

[72] Schoene RB, Martin TR, Charan NB, et al. Timolol-induced bronchospasm in asthmatic bronchitis. JAMA 1981;245:1460–1.

[73] Kendall MJ. Clinical relevance of pharmacokinetic differences between beta blockers. Am J Cardiol 1997;80:15J–9.

[74] Wood AJ. Pharmacologic differences between beta blockers. Am Heart J 1984;108:1070–7.

[75] Hoffman BB. Catecholamines, sympathomimetic drugs, and adrenergic receptor antagonists. In: Hardman JG, Limbird LE, Gilman AG, editors. Goodman & Gilman's the pharmacological basis of therapeutics. New York: McGraw-Hill; 2001. p. 215–53.

[76] Salpeter SR, Ormiston TM, Salpeter EE. Cardioselective β-blockers in patients with reactive airway disease: a meta-analysis. Ann Intern Med 2002;137:715–25.

[77] Dunn TL, Gerber MJ, Shen AS, et al. The effect of topical ophthalmic instillation of Timolol and Betaxolol on lung function in asthmatic subjects. Am Rev Respir Dis 1986;133:264–8.

[78] Fraunfelder FT, Barker AF. Respiratory effects of Timolol. N Engl J Med 1984;311:1441.

[79] Cazzola M, Noschese P, D'Amato G, et al. Comparison of the effects of single oral doses of nebivolol and celiprolol on airways in patients with mild asthma. Chest 2000;118:1322–6.

[80] National Asthma Education and Prevention Program. Expert Panel Report II. Guidelines for the diagnosis and management of asthma. Bethesda: National Heart, Lung, and Blood Institute/National Institute of Health; 1997.

[81] Shulan DJ, Katlan M. Use of β-blockers in patients with reactive airway disease. Ann Intern Med 2003;139:304.

[82] Gottlieb SS, McCarter RJ, Vogel RA. Effect of beta-blockade on mortality among high-risk and low-risk patients after myocardial infarction. N Engl J Med 1998;339:489–97.

[83] Ryan TJ, Antman EM, Brooks NH, et al. 1999 update: ACC/AHA guidelines for the management of patients with acute myocardial infarction: executive summary and recommendations. Circulation 1999;100:1016–30.

[84] Mohammad JT, Weinacker AB. Beta-adrenergic-blocking agents in bronchospastic diseases: a therapeutic dilemma. Pharmacotherapy 1999;19:974–8.

[85] Piepho RW. Role of angiotensin-converting-enzyme inhibition in contemporary cardiovascular therapy. Am J Health Syst Pharm 2000;57(Suppl 1):S2.

[86] Israili ZH, Hall WD. Cough and angioneurotic edema associated with angiotensin-converting enzyme inhibitor therapy. Ann Intern Med 1992;117:234–42.

[87] Schaefer BM, Caracciolo V, Frishman WH, et al. Gender, ethnicity, and genes in cardiovascular disease. Part 2: implications for pharmacotherapy. Heart Dis 2003;5:202–14.

[88] Simon SR, Black HR, Moser M, et al. Cough and ACE inhibitors. Arch Intern Med 1992;152:1698–700.

[89] Goldszer RC, Lilly LS, Solomon HS. Prevalence of cough during angiotensin-converting enzyme inhibitor therapy. Am J Med 1988;85:887.

[90] Just PM. The positive association of cough with angiotensin-converting enzyme inhibitors. Pharmacotherapy 1989;9:82–7.

[91] Wood R. Bronchospasm and cough as adverse reactions to the ACE inhibitors captopril, enalapril and lisinopril: a controlled retrospective cohort study. Br J Clin Pharmacol 1995;39:265–70.

[92] Kaufman J, Schmitt S, Barnard J, et al. Angiotensin-coverting enzyme inhibitors in patients with bronchial responsiveness and asthma. Chest 1992;101:922–5.

[93] Craig TJ. Drugs to be used with caution in patients with asthma. Am Fam Physician 1996;54:947–53.

[94] Peacock AJ, Matthews AW. The effect of captorpril on pulmonary haemodynamics and lung function in patients with chronic airflow obstruction. Thorax 1986;41:225.

[95] Dixon CM, Fuller RW, Barnes PJ. The effect of an angiotensin converting enzyme inhibitor, ramipril, on bronchial responses to inhaled histamine and bradykinin in asthmatic subjects. Br J Clin Pharmacol 1987;23:91–3.

[96] Boulet L-P, Milot J, Lampron N, et al. Pulmonary function and airway responsiveness during long-term therapy with captopril. JAMA 1989;261:413–6.

[97] Popa V. Captopril-related (and -induced?) asthma. Am Rev Respir Dis 1987;136:999–1000.

[98] Semple PF, Herd GW. Cough and wheeze caused by inhibitors of angiotensin-converting enzyme. N Engl J Med 1986;314:61.

[99] Brown NJ, Vaughan DE. Angiotensin-converting enzyme inhibitors. Circulation 1998;97: 1411–20.

[100] Os I, Bratland B, Dahlof B, et al. Female sex as an important determinant of lisinopril-induced cough. Lancet 1992;339:372.

[101] Gibson GR. Enalapril-induced cough. Arch Intern Med 1989;149:2701–3.

[102] Kawakami Y, Munakata M, Yamaguchi E, et al. Molecular studies of bronchial asthma, sarcoidosis and angiotensin converting enzyme inhibitor-induced cough. Respirology 1998; 3:45–9.

[103] Dart RA, Gollub S, Lazar J, et al. Treatment of systemic hypertension in patients with pulmonary disease. Chest 2003;123:222–43.

[104] Fuller RW, Choudry NB. Increased cough reflex associated with angiotensin converting enzyme inhibitor cough. BMJ 1987;295:1025–6.

[105] Buck SH, Burks TF. Capsaicin: hot new pharmacological tool. Trends Pharmacol Sci 1983; 4:84–7.

[106] McEwan JR, Fuller RW. Angiotensin converting enzyme inhibitors and cough. J Cardiovasc Pharmacol 1989;13(Suppl 3):S67–9.

[107] Nicholls MG, Gilchrist NL. Sulindac and cough induced by converting enzyme inhibitors. Lancet 1987;I:872.

[108] Fuller RW, McEwan JR, Choudry NB. The abnormal cough reflex: role of prostaglandins. Am Rev Respir Dis 1989;139:A586.

[109] Fuller RW, Dixon CM, Cuss FM, et al. Bradykinin-induced bronchoconstriction in humans. Am Rev Respir Dis 1987;135:176–80.

[110] Varonier HS, Panzani R. The effect of inhalations of bradykinin on healthy and atopic (asthmatic) children. Int Arch Allergy 1968;34:293–6.

[111] Polosa R, Phillips GD, Lai CK, et al. Contribution of histamine and prostanoids to bronchoconstriction provoked by inhaled bradykinin in atopic asthma. Allergy 1990;45:174–82.

[112] Cazzola M, Matera MG, Liccardi G, et al. Theophylline in the inhibition of angiotensin-converting enzyme inhibitor-induced cough. Respiration (Herrlisheim) 1993;60:212–5.

[113] Hargreaves M. Sodium cromoglycate: a remedy for ace inhibitor-induced cough. Br J Clin Pract 1993;47:319–20.

ELSEVIER
SAUNDERS

Immunol Allergy Clin N Am
25 (2005) 191–205

IMMUNOLOGY
AND ALLERGY
CLINICS
OF NORTH AMERICA

Occupational exposures as triggers of asthma

Paul G. Vigo, MD, Mitchell H. Grayson, MD*

*Department of Medicine, Division of Allergy and Immunology,
Washington University School of Medicine, Campus Box 8122, 660 South Euclid Avenue,
St. Louis, MO 63110, USA*

The influence of environment on laborers has been noted since ancient times. Hippocrates (460–370 BC) observed that workers handling agricultural grains and products seemed to have more frequent respiratory complaints than workers in other trades. In the early 1700s, Ramazzini, the father of occupational medicine, wrote a discourse about the maladies of grain handlers [1]. Whether these people had pneumoconiosis or asthma is hard to determine. Nonetheless, Hippocrates and Ramazzini showed an increased awareness of factors in the environment that have an impact on the health of laborers. Factories and manufacturing plants abound with fumes, particles, dusts, and gases that can trigger respiratory symptoms upon exposure.

Respiratory complaints rank second to dermatologic manifestations as the most prevalent work-related disorders worldwide, and occupational asthma (OA) is the most common nonacute occupational lung disease of this group [2]. By the mid-1990s, approximately 250 agents had been identified as possible causes of OA [3]. With the introduction of new organic and inorganic chemicals, the list continues to grow. The clinician has the responsibility to identify patients suffering from OA and better manage their disease to minimize morbidity.

OA is characterized by variable airflow limitation and airway hyperresponsiveness directly attributable to a particular work environment. This airflow obstruction is brought about by inflammation of the respiratory tract and is frequently reversible. Although the presumed environmental agents may not be elucidated in all cases, the patient may be diagnosed with OA. Somewhat controversial is how to deal with evidence of pre-existing asthma in making the diagnosis of OA. The American College of Chest Physicians argues that asthma

---

* Corresponding author.
E-mail address: mgrayson@wustl.edu (M.H. Grayson).

0889-8561/05/$ – see front matter © 2005 Elsevier Inc. All rights reserved.
doi:10.1016/j.iac.2004.09.004

antedating the occupational exposure precludes the diagnosis of OA; however, Wagner and Wegman [4] have proposed a new definition of OA that includes pre-existing asthma exacerbated by occupational triggers.

Because more cases of OA are being identified, the economic, medico-legal, and social repercussions are difficult to ignore. Once a patient is diagnosed with OA, the employer should minimize and eliminate identified agents to pro-tect the diagnosed employee and survey the work environment to verify that there are no potential exposures remaining that might endanger other workers. The OA patient should undergo work rehabilitation and proper retraining for another job if continuing the current job is not possible. In Quebec, it is estimated that this surveying, verifying, and retraining costs somewhere around CAD $75,000 (approximately USD $60,000) [5]. This figure is roughly the equivalent of 2 years' salary, which is the usual amount of time for retraining and job hunting if the patient cannot stay in his or her current employment [5,6]. A survey of 134 OA workers 2 years after diagnosis showed that the unemployment rate can be as high as 8%. This financial burden does not include compensation for medical care, which is needed for an indefinite amount of time by as many as 75% of OA patients (see Prognosis section). Adding to the overall burden are the cost of lost productivity, "pain and suffering," diminished quality of life from continued symptoms, and social displacement if the patient needs to relocate for a different job. Thus, the true financial cost of OA cannot easily or reliably be determined but is likely quite high. In this article we discuss the prevalence, etiology (including presumed causative agents), diagnosis, and treatment of this high-burden disease.

Prevalence

The prevalence of occupational asthma is unknown because of several factors that hinder estimates. First, development of de novo asthma in adults is common; often in these cases, the role of the workplace is overlooked. Second, devel-opment of respiratory symptoms may result in patients leaving a work envi-ronment before a diagnosis of OA can be made. Third, no appropriate reporting system or registry exists in most countries to monitor the disease. Complicating our understanding about OA is the fact that much of the published literature is derived from anecdotal reports, small series, or retrospective data with no pro-spective long-term studies. Additionally, physicians may be hesitant to make the diagnosis of OA. Some of this hesitancy may be explained by living in a litigious society where the burden lies with the patient and physician to prove the respi-ratory condition is a direct consequence of employment.

Some data are available on OA prevalence. Reports place the prevalence of OA at 5% to 25% of exposed workers. The widely varying OA prevalence figures come from different industries, presumably indicating that prevalence is dependent upon the putative agents involved [7,8]. Workers that are regularly exposed to di-isocyanate compounds report a 10% prevalence rate [8], whereas one of the highest prevalence rates quoted involves the platinum refining industry, where one out of four chronically exposed workers are reported to develop OA [9]. From 5% to 15% of rubber industry and health care/lab workers have evidence of latex sensitization [10,11]. Up to 50% of these workers have some form of respiratory symptoms, the severity of which correlates with amount and duration of exposure. Health care workers who complain of rhinoconjunctival symptoms after inhalation exposure to powdered latex particles have a higher prevalence of OA. One estimate put the cumulative incidence of OA from latex exposure at 4.5% [12].

Despite the wide discrepancy in reported prevalence rates, it is believed that approximately 2% to 10% of asthma cases worldwide may have occupational triggers [13]. Of these, only 2% to 5% of cases likely developed asthma strictly from workplace exposures [14]. Therefore, the risk of OA is fairly low when examining all individuals in a society, but the risk rises substantially when the patient works in an environment where occupational triggers are abundant. In one study, 26% of all new cases of asthma in adults (15–55 years of age) were felt to be caused by exposures received at work [15].

Pathophysiology

Although certain occupations or industries have long been associated with increased prevalence of asthma among workers, the mechanism by which putative occupational "asthma triggers" induce disease remains unclear. Most patients do not report a family history of atopy or asthma. Similar to non-occupational asthma, other factors besides a history of atopy seem to play a significant role in the development of the disease.

Four mechanisms are postulated to explain the development of OA. The first two are broadly described as "occupational asthma with latency" because of the lag time between purported sensitization and appearance of symptoms. Both are immunologic in nature but can be differentiated by the ability of the putative agent to elicit an IgE response with exposure. The third mechanism attributes the symptoms to an irritant effect, and the fourth uses the pharmaco-physiologic action of the agent without participation of the immune system. The last two mechanisms (irritant and pharmaco-physiologic) can be thought of as "occupational asthma without latency" because symptoms appear nearly instantly after exposure to the offending agent. Table 1 highlights different clinical characteristics and proposed mechanisms for the four forms of occupational asthma.

The two "occupational asthma with latency" mechanisms can be divided by the purported role of IgE in the reaction. In the IgE-mediated explanation, high-molecular-weight (HMW) (ie, >5 kD) and low-molecular-weight (LMW) molecules are able to induce an IgE response on their own or after haptenation with a human protein, forming a functional antigen. This mechanism is also seen with inhalant allergens leading to typical allergic rhinitis or allergic asthma. The appearance of symptoms is usually preceded by a period of latency that may last months to years after first exposure or sensitization to the agent. During this time,

Table 1
Proposed mechanisms and clinical characteristics of occupational asthma

	Asthma with latency		Asthma without latency	
	IgE involved	No IgE involved	RADS	Pharmaco-physiologic
Agents implicated	HMW agents	LMW agents	Noxious chemicals	Organic or inorganic compounds
Atopic history	Commonly present	May or may not be present	May or may not be present	May or may not be present
Skin testing	Positive	Negative	Negative	Negative
Onset of symptoms after sensitization	Months to years, insidiously	Months to years, insidiously	Acutely after accidental exposure or insidiously with chronic exposure	Acutely after exposures
Pattern of inflammatory response	Biphasic (early and late)	Late or biphasic	Late or irregular	Late or irregular

Abbreviations: HMW, high molecular weight; LMW, low molecular weight; RADS, reactive airways dysfunction syndrome.

respiratory symptoms, if present, may not be as prominent as nasal or ocular ones. After specific IgE against the sensitizing agent has been produced, reintroduction of the occupational allergen leads to cross-linking of IgE antibodies on the surface of mast cells and basophils. This leads to degranulation of these cells with release of preformed and newly synthesized inflammatory mediators including histamine, cysteinyl leukotrienes, prostaglandins, cytokines, and other chemotactic factors. These substances initiate a cascade of events that manifest as an immediate or biphasic (immediate and late) inflammatory response.

The second immunologic mechanism does not seem to involve the formation of IgE antibodies. This mechanism is often invoked when LMW agents are the purported cause of OA. These agents generally induce a lone late or atypical inflammatory reaction [16,17]. There are studies showing a different mechanism separate from IgE-mediated that might be operative when these agents cause disease. For example, it is believed that isocyanates [18] and plicatic acid (a water-soluble, nonvolatile compound) from Western Red Cedar [19] may be able to elicit IgE and IgG antibody responses. In the case of Western Red Cedar asthma, only 20% of subjects were shown to have IgE against plicatic acid despite having symptoms [19]. Bronchial biopsies from these patients revealed activated lymphocytes in the bronchial mucosal wall. When incubated with plicatic acid, peripheral blood lymphocytes from these patients proliferate, suggesting that plicatic acid-specific T cell clones have been generated in affected individuals [20,21]. Whether the formation of specific IgE leads to disease or represents only a sign of exposure remains unknown. Even less well defined than the role of IgE is the role of antigen-specific IgG [22]. It is anticipated that further studies focusing on the role of the cellular immune response [20] to LMW agents may yield clues to the pathogenesis of OA.

The third mechanism (without latency) proposes a neurogenic reflex that may result from insult to the bronchial epithelium. This insult may be in the form of gases, fumes, particles, or vapor. The damage that ensues leads to epithelial denudation, mucus hypersecretion, increased bronchial smooth muscle tone, and inflammatory cell recruitment with subsequent fibrosis. The ability of the agent to cause harm depends on its physical and chemical properties rather than its ability to stimulate an immune response [23]. This is the mechanism of reactive airways dysfunction syndrome (RADS), an entity that was first described in 1981 by Brooks and Lockey [24]. Some of the more common agents believed to cause RADS include chlorine gas, phosgene, ozone, acids (sulfuric, phosphoric, and hydrochloric), dioxides (sulfur and nitrogen), anhydrous ammonia, and toluene diisocyanate (which can also cause asthma with latency) [23,25].

The fourth mechanism (without latency) involves the pharmaco-physiologic action of the agent causing symptoms during or immediately after exposure. A classic example of this type of reaction is exposure of the respiratory tract to organophosphates. These insecticides can cause mucus hypersecretion and interfere with the normal cholinergic control of airway caliber, leading to broncho-constriction. Byssinosis is the development of bronchoconstriction, coughing, wheezing, or shortness of breath after inhalation of cotton, hemp, or flax dust. The underlying mechanism of byssinosis is not known but may be related to non-IgE–mediated degranulation of mast cells with subsequent release of histamine; therefore, antihistamines have a role in treatment of this disease [26]. Chronic exposure to these types of agents is thought to cause inflammatory responses that may lead to permanent remodeling of the airway.

Although these mechanistic models are convenient and relatively simple to comprehend, the actual operative mechanisms are likely more complex and may involve a combination of each of these processes. Further research is needed to more fully comprehend the mechanisms by which OA develops. Until this occurs, it is unlikely that OA-specific therapeutics will be developed or will have a significant hope of making an impact in this disease.

Common agents and occupational exposures

There are more than 250 identified putative causes of OA, and, in general, these agents are organic macromolecules or inorganic chemicals found, used, or produced in the workplace [3]. These compounds can be divided into two groups based on their molecular weights. Some common HMW and LMW agents are described in Table 2.

Most HWM agents are plant or animal proteins and polysaccharides that are able to induce an antibody (IgE) response on their own without the need for haptenization. Natural rubber latex has become an important sensitizer in the rubber, health care, and laboratory industries [10,27]. Wheat and rye flour are important causative agents in many cases of so-called "baker's asthma." In

Table 2
Common sensitizers and exposures

Occupation/industry	HMW agents	LMW agents
Sawmill/woodworking/ carpentry	Wood dust (mahogany, oak, California redwood)	Plicatic acid (Western Red cedar)
Health care	Latex (powdered gloves)	Ethylene oxide (sterilizer) Glutaraldehyde (sterilizer)
Lab workers	Laboratory animals (dander, excreta, serum, feathers) Papain powder (tissue digestion)	Formalin (tissue fixing)
Pharmaceuticals	Psyllium Pancreatic enzymes	Ampicillin/penicillin Piperazine Tetracycline Salbutamol
Bird/pigeon fanciers poultry industry	Avian proteins (feathers, droppings)	Amprolium HCl (antiparasitic)
Beauticians	Henna extract (dye)	Monoethanolamine Hexamethylamine Ammonium thioglycolate Persulfate salts
Textile/dye industry	Cotton, wool, hemp Weevils	Paraphenylenediamine (fur dyers) Anthraquinone methyl blue (cloth dyers)
Paint/epoxy/chemicals		(Anhydrides) trimellitic, phthalic, hexamethylene
Polyurethane/plastics		Toluene diisocyanate
Platinum workers		Platinum salts (refinery)
Platers		Sodium bichromate Nickel sulphate
Solderers		Colophony (flux) Propylene glycol
Welders		Nickel
Cement workers		Potassium dichromate
Grains/baking/brewing	Wheat, buckwheat, rye flour Hops (brewery) Flour mites *Aspergillus* spp	
Nursery/greenhouse	Spider mite (*Tetranychus urticae*)	
Seafood processing	Crab/prawn proteins	
Printing/book binding	Acacia and arabic gum	
Detergent manufacturing	*Bacillus subtilis*	

Abbreviations: HMW, high molecular weight; LMW, low molecular weight.

addition to the flour, these workers are exposed to products of the mold genus *Aspergillus*, flour mites, insect debris, and other contaminants, all of which are potential HWM agents [28]. Proteins found in mammalian dander, saliva, serum, and excreta are associated with disease in veterinarians, laboratory workers, and animal handlers or fanciers. The reported prevalence rate of sensitization to rat or mouse urinary allergen is as high as 30%, with as many as a third of these individuals having symptoms of OA [29,30]. Nearly all avian species produce allergens found in their feathers and droppings. Even insect and arthropod handlers, such as entomologists and sericulturists, are exposed to allergens found in the wings and other body parts of moths, flies, grain weevils, and worms. Farmers, because of their contact with livestock and crops, are susceptible to sensitization to these mammalian-, avian-, and insect-derived allergens [31–33].

Other HWM agents that can induce asthma symptoms in the workplace include plant- and animal-derived enzymes. Pancreatic enzymes extracted from pig [34] include trypsin, lipase, and amylase, all of which are used in the pharmaceutical industry. Often enzymes of plant origin are used in food preparation, breweries, and pharmaceutical/research laboratories. Other enzymes that have been associated with the IgE-mediated mechanism of OA include papain [35,36] (a proteolytic enzyme from the papaya tree) and bromelain [37,38] (a pineapple-derived) enzyme.

LMW agents that may cause asthma symptoms include organic or small inorganic chemicals that are readily inhaled into the respiratory tract and are encountered in a variety of settings including workplaces in pharmaceutical manufacturing, automobile assembly, paint/plastics/adhesives manufacturing, electronics and welding, and chemical production. Among the LMW agents, diisocyanates and anhydrides are the most common [8]. Toluene diisocyanate (TDI) is a highly reactive compound that can denature biomolecules. Inhalation of TDI at high concentrations is irritating to the respiratory and nasal mucosa. Lower concentration contact is also dangerous: These exposures have been shown to cause sensitization and subsequent respiratory symptoms [39]. Anhydrides are also commonly encountered; they are used in plastics, epoxy resin, and paint manufacturing. Occupational exposure to high concentrations of trimellitic anhydrate (TMA) can lead to lacrimation, rhinorrhea, coughing, shortness of breath, and hemoptysis in previously unexposed workers. Furthermore, sensitization can develop because TMA-protein, conjugate-specific IgE antibodies have been documented in patients having asthmatic symptoms [40]. Other commonly encountered LWM agents include metals and metal products handled by platers, solderers, welders, and workers in refineries, electronic, and chemical plants.

Symptomatology, history, and physical examination

Obtaining a detailed medical and occupational history is critical in evaluating a patient presenting with respiratory symptoms suggestive of OA. The history should be used to recreate a timeline of symptom onset and circumstances in and out of the workplace that surrounded the onset of symptoms. Ocular, skin, and nasal symptoms may be more prominent and may precede lower respiratory complaints, especially in OA with an extended latency period [12,41,42]. It is important to determine any aggravation or improvement of symptoms that is temporally related to the work schedule. OA complaints tend to worsen during (or for several hours after) work [17]. Because symptoms occur after work hours, many employees (and providers) do not attribute the symptoms to work. Examples of this include patients with byssinosis frequently waking at night with coughing fits or patients who are sensitized to plicatic acid having significant nocturnal asthmatic attacks. Improvement of symptoms on weekends, vacations, or days off strengthens the hypothesis that the symptoms are due to a workplace exposure [14]. However, in some cases this pattern may not be evident, especially if there has been significant chronic inflammation between exposure episodes leading to the development of constant symptoms. The appearance of constitutional symptoms should also be noted because their presence widens the differential to include infections, tumors, hypersensitivity pneumonitis, or other inflammatory pneumonitides.

Personal and family history of atopy must be determined. Studies have shown that patients with atopy have a higher sensitization rate than those who do not have an atopic background [43]. This is most important when HMW antigens or other organic compounds are suspected as the causative agents. Atopic detergent workers or atopic workers who have been exposed to latex or laboratory animals show higher incidences of occupational asthma when compared with nonatopic workers in the same field [10,12,30,41]. Patients with aeroallergen allergies may have baseline bronchial hyper-responsiveness that may be aggravated further by additional or repeated exposure to agents encountered in the workplace.

In addition to pertinent medical questions, inquiries should be made about current and previous work situations, possible exposures, accidental spills, and adherence to Occupational Safety and Health Administration regulations. Questions as to whether colleagues are having similar symptoms and whether they work in the same area as the patient should be asked. The typical occupational health history contains questions such as What kind of work do you do? What does that involve? Are there any health hazards that you are aware of or concerned about?

It is advisable for the clinician to obtain materials safety data sheets from the employer to be able to learn of the properties and idiosyncrasies of chemicals and agents to which the worker was exposed. The duration and intensity of exposure should be determined. This allows for a better attempt at elucidating the extent of disease and possibly even the mechanism behind the symptoms. For example, a massive but short exposure to a particular agent instantly provoking ocular, nasal, and respiratory symptoms suggests RADS, not OA with latency, as the operative mechanism behind the symptoms [23].

During the evaluation, use of illicit drugs and cigarette smoking should be determined because these agents have irritant effects on the respiratory mucosa. Chronic smokers may have chronic obstructive pulmonary disease (COPD) that may be misdiagnosed as OA. Some evidence exists suggesting that cigarette smokers have a four to six times higher risk of OA upon exposure to platinum salts, laboratory animals, or acid anhydrides [44–46].

The physical examination should be thorough and complete. In addition to pulmonary findings, special attention should be directed to skin, ocular, oropharyngeal, and nasal examinations because these may hold clues to the cause and mechanism involved. It is not surprising that in some cases the physical examination is normal, especially when the office visit occurs during the worker's vacation or days off when no recent exposure to the sensitizers has occurred.

Diagnosis

Although the history and physical examination may suggest OA, objective testing is needed to confirm the diagnosis. It is important to recognize that there is no gold standard test for OA; diagnosis is based on interpretation of subjective and objective data in the context of the clinical picture. A brief overview of the diagnostic approach and treatment of occupational asthma is given in Box 1.

After taking a thorough history, it is important to confirm the presence of an atopic state, preferably by performing skin tests to common aeroallergens. Significant positive skin tests may suggest an allergic component to the symptoms. The patient may have subclinical asthma that has been unmasked by sensitizers or nonspecific irritants in the workplace. Skin testing for HWM agents encountered in the workplace may be of value in establishing a causal relationship between exposure and symptoms. To skin test to HWM agents, clinicians may have to resort to titration skin prick testing on non-exposed, nonatopic individuals to determine the minimum irritating concentration for a particular agent. One note of caution involves the unknown positive predictive value of a skin test to HWM agents: A positive skin test may not indicate IgE sensitization to the agent and may represent an irritant or nonspecific response.

Although skin testing may seem manageable for HMW agents, it is impractical or even impossible for most LMW agents. This is because for these agents to form functional antigenic determinants, they must become haptenated with a

---

Box 1. Diagnosis and management of occupational asthma

1. Clearly document and understand progression of symptoms.
2. Obtain a good medical and occupational history.
3. Establish presence of atopy.
4. Document level of bronchial hyper-responsiveness.
5. Exclude all other possible causes of lung disease.
6. Minimize further exposure for patient and coworkers in the offending work environment (may involve change of duties or job).
7. Control bronchial hyper-responsiveness and symptoms.
8. Monitor pulmonary status over time.

serum protein. It is possible that the act of haptenization changes the tertiary structure of the antigen-hapten complex that leads to the formation of conformational epitopes, which elicit production of specific IgE. Testing with the pure LMW agent alone, without haptenization, may prove useless because may be unable to elicit a wheal and flare reaction, which indicates presence of specific IgE.

Serum-specific IgE antibodies to HWM and some LWM agents are available by radioallergosorbent testing or enzyme-linked immunoassay and may be used to confirm atopy as well. However, the presence of such antibodies does not necessarily indicate that IgE sensitivity causes the patient's symptoms. As in allergic rhinitis and asymptomatic bronchial hyper-responsiveness, positive test results can occur in asymptomatic patients with subclinical sensitization.

The next step in the diagnosis of OA is to document airway hyper-reactivity by pulmonary function tests (PFTs). Assessing forced expiratory volume in 1 second (FEV_1) and the response to a bronchodilator before, during, and after work is often useful in establishing the diagnosis. However, the logistics of this— a technician and equipment to administer pulmonary function testing at home and at work—often makes this a difficult task to undertake. A more viable option is to have the patient record peak expiratory flow using a handheld peak flow meter before, during, and after work, together with measuring response to bronchodilator treatment [44]. Improper technique by the patient, falsification of results, or the presence of nonspecific bronchial irritants in the workplace and at home may limit the usefulness of the recorded data. If bronchial hyper-responsiveness cannot be determined by any of these methods, a methacholine challenge must be performed. A negative methacholine challenge rules out OA because the patient must have some evidence of bronchial hyper-responsiveness for the diagnosis to be made. Parameters for a positive bronchodilator response, PEFR variability, and methacholine provocation are the same for diagnosing OA as those used in diagnosing non-occupational asthma.

Specific challenge testing to simulate the work environment is done at a few centers. Although this may be considered the gold standard by some clinicians, it is impractical and potentially fraught with false-positive or false-negative results. This is because the correct concentration, combination, and duration of exposure may not be duplicated or otherwise match that which would be encountered in the workplace. Furthermore, the choice of agent and its physical form (dust, vapor, gas, fumes, etc.) may affect the outcome of testing [47]. Finally, this kind of testing may be harmful to the patient, especially if it is done in a facility that does not regularly perform these tests and therefore has had little experience with these issues.

Newer diagnostic techniques are being investigated to evaluate their usefulness in diagnosing OA. Some of these tests include measurement of exhaled nitric oxide, sputum eosinophil counts, and exhaled breath pH. Rather than "ruling-in" OA, there are diagnostic tests that may be useful to "rule out" other causes for respiratory symptoms. A chest x-ray is a good screening test to look for signs of COPD, pneumonia, foreign bodies, and pneumonitides. A limited sinus CT is often useful to exclude chronic sinus disease if the patient has a significant history and symptoms. Esophogastric pH monitoring or a therapeutic trial of an H2 receptor blocker or proton pump inhibitor may be necessary to rule out any contribution of gastro-esophageal reflux disease to the symptoms. Tests that have not proven useful in the workup of OA and should be avoided include lymphocyte proliferation assays and quantification of total IgG or IgM [48].

Differential diagnosis

During the sensitization phase, the most prominent presenting symptoms may be cough and nasal catarrh. Because wheezing may not manifest until later in the course of disease, many patients are misdiagnosed early as having recurrent respiratory infections. Shortness of breath is not an early symptom of OA but may be present in RADS, especially if the agent is extremely noxious or the exposure significant. Symptoms of RADS usually occur immediately or within 24 hours and may persist for months without further exposure. This is in contrast to OA where symptoms occur hours, if not days, after exposure (this follows several weeks after the initial sensitizing exposure) and cease with avoidance of the offending agent.

Mimics of OA include non-occupational asthma and its masqueraders. With the current definition of OA, the patient cannot have a pre-existing or prior history of asthma. It is therefore critical to determine if the patient has asthma that was unmasked or aggravated by factors in the workplace rather than caused by those agents [43]. In addition to non-occupational asthma, the major diagnosis to consider in the differential is COPD. This is a common disorder in workers with a significant smoking history and a symptom complex that includes shortness of breath, wheezing, chest tightness, and cough. Vocal cord dysfunction (VCD), another asthma masquerader, should be considered as a cause of symptoms similar to that seen in OA. VCD is more common in young adult women, competitive athletes, or patients with significant psychologic factors affecting their life [49]. Although VCD is often mistaken for asthma, it may present as acute shortness of breath where the perceived blockage is in the "throat" area, and symptoms often develop when the patient is engaged in some form of physical activity or exertion. The physiologic cause of VCD is paradoxic adduction of the vocal cords during inspiration leading to a localized obstruction of airflow into the lungs. A clue to the diagnosis is a flattened or attenuated inspiratory loop in the flow-volume curve during pulmonary function testing.

Occupational lung diseases, such as farmer's lung, coal miner's pneumoconiosis, silo filler's disease, or chemical worker's lung, can be mimics of OA. Patients with these conditions also present with work-related coughing, wheezing, chest tightness, and shortness of breath. These are not IgE-mediated diseases and do not cause obstructive disease (as assessed by PFT monitoring). Unfortunately, it is only retrospectively, or when index of suspicion is high, that these patients are worked up appropriately for OA.

Treatment

The management of occupational asthma is two pronged. The main principle is avoidance of further exposure and minimization of morbidity. To achieve this, exposure to the offending agent should be eliminated, and future exposures should be prevented. The employer should find a substitute for the offending agent or change the work process (engineering change). Alternatively, the employee could be moved within the company to a location where there is no risk of exposure. If these strategies cannot be implemented, use of personal respiratory protective equipment should be considered. Adherence to this avoidance measure is critical, and this approach must be emphasized to the patient. If the use of protective gear is impractical or impossible, then a change in occupation or trade may be the only acceptable alternative. Because factors outside of the workplace may aggravate symptoms due to existing inflammation in the respiratory tract, cigarette smoke, strong odors, dusts, humidity, cold air, or heavy aeroallergen exposure should be avoided as much as possible.

The second direction of treatment is to control the underlying respiratory inflammation. This can be achieved using the same pharmacologic agents as are used to treat non-occupational asthma. Even though no formal guidelines for assessing and treating OA exist, the clinician can be guided by the stepwise approach of the National Asthma Education and Prevention Program/Global Initiative for Asthma guidelines (available at www.nhlbi.nih.gov/guidelines/asthma/asthgdln.htm). It may be necessary to use a burst of oral corticosteroids to abate an acute or a severe episode. Maintenance inhaled corticosteroids may be used as controller therapy to diminish persistent airway hyper-responsiveness. Inhaled short-acting beta-agonists may be used as rescue medication. Specific immunotherapy injections may not be useful unless sensitivity to animal dander is the known cause of OA. However, pharmacotherapy alone treats symptoms but does nothing to resolve the underlying cause of disease; this is why primary therapy must be avoidance of the offending agent. Avoidance lessens the severity of the patient's disease and allows for more effective pharmacologic treatment at lower doses with fewer potential side effects.

Prognosis

The prognosis of patients with OA depends on several factors. Duration and level of exposure [29,30,50], baseline lung function, degree of initial decline in FEV_1, and intrinsic factors relating to the sensitizing or irritating agents [51] seem to dictate the level of improvement the patient derives after prompt removal from the offending environment. In the case of western red cedar OA, about 50% of workers had resolution of their symptoms when removed from the workplace [52]. Other studies [40,53,54], however, have not shown such positive results—especially when avoidance is not stringently applied. In one series, most red cedar OA patients who continued to work in sawmills for more than 6.5 years continued to have symptoms, with a majority of patients deteriorating and fewer than 10% showing any improvement [55,56]. Prognostic factors are not well defined; however, patients whose bronchial hyper-responsiveness persisted continued to have symptoms for years even after switching employment [54,57]. Therefore, early removal from exposure is recommended to try and minimize morbidity. Identification of an index patient with OA should prompt an examination of the workplace for possible exposures, other workers that might be affected, and ways to prevent all workers, including asymptomatic ones, from additional exposures.

Summary

With diligent employers, inquisitive physicians, and compliant patients, the prevalence of OA and its impact on our society may decline in the near future. To achieve this requires that care providers routinely inquire about work and workplace exposures of all of their patients. Otherwise too many OA patients will go undiagnosed. Additional research on the mechanisms of OA and new treatments are needed so that we will be able to offer improved prognosis for those who do develop OA in the future.

Acknowledgments

We thank Deborah L. Grayson, RN, MSN, MPH, COHN-S, for helpful advice and critical review of this manuscript.

References

[1] Pepys J, Bernstein IL. Historical aspects of occupational asthma. In: Bernstein IL, Chan-Yeung M, Malo J-L, et al, editors. Asthma in the workplace. 2nd edition. New York: Marcel Dekker; 1999. p. 299–322.

[2] Centers for Disease Control and Prevention. National occupational research agenda. Washington, DC: National Institute for Occupational Safety and Health, US Department of Health and Human Services; 1996. Pub. No. 96-115.

[3] Chan-Yeung M, Malo JL. Occupational asthma. N Engl J Med 1995;333:107–12.

[4] Wagner GR, Wegman DH. Occupational asthma: prevention by definition. Am J Ind Med 1998; 33:427–9.

[5] Dewitte JD, Chan-Yeung M, Malo JL. Medicolegal and compensation aspects of occupational asthma. Eur Respir J 1994;7:969–80.

[6] Malo JL, Boulet LP, Dewitte JD, et al. Quality of life of subjects with occupational asthma. J Allergy Clin Immunol 1993;91:1121–7.

[7] Beckett WS. The epidemiology of occupational asthma. Eur Respir J 1994;7:161–4.

[8] Bernstein DI. Allergic reactions to workplace allergens. JAMA 1997;278:1907–13.

[9] Cromwell O, Pepys J, Parish WE, et al. Specific IgE antibodies to platinum salts in sensitized workers. Clin Allergy 1979;9:109–17.

[10] Fish JE. Occupational asthma and rhinoconjunctivitis induced by natural rubber latex exposure. J Allergy Clin Immunol 2002;110(Suppl):S75–81.

[11] Liss GM, Sussman GL. Latex sensitization: occupational versus general population prevalence rates. Am J Ind Med 1999;35:196–200.

[12] Archambault S, Malo JL, Infante-Rivard C, Ghezzo H, Gautrin D. Incidence of sensitization, symptoms, and probable occupational rhinoconjunctivitis and asthma in apprentices starting exposure to latex. J Allergy Clin Immunol 2001;107:921–3.

[13] Blanc PD, Eisner MD, Israel L, Yelin EH. The association between occupation and asthma in general medical practice. Chest 1999;115:1259–64.

[14] Tarlo SM, Leung K, Broder I, Silverman F, Holness DL. Asthmatic subjects symptomatically worse at work: prevalence and characterization among a general asthma clinic population. Chest 2000;118:1309–14.

[15] Milton D. Risk and incidence of asthma attributable to occupational exposure among HMO members. Am J Ind Med 1998;33:1–10.

[16] Chan-Yeung M, Lam S, Koener S. Clinical features and natural history of occupational asthma due to western red cedar (Thuja plicata). Am J Med 1982;72:411–5.

[17] Perrin B, Cartier A, Ghezzo H, et al. Reassessment of the temporal patterns of bronchial obstruction after exposure to occupational sensitizing agents. J Allergy Clin Immunol 1991;87:630–9.

[18] Cartier A, Grammer L, Malo JL, et al. Specific serum antibodies against isocyanates: association with occupational asthma. J Allergy Clin Immunol 1989;84:507–14.

[19] Chan-Yeung M. Mechanism of occupational asthma due to western red cedar (Thuja plicata). Am J Ind Med 1994;25:13–8.

[20] Frew AJ, Chan H, Lam S, Chan-Yeung M. Bronchial inflammation in occupational asthma due to western red cedar. Am J Respir Crit Care Med 1995;151:340–4.

[21] Frew A, Chan H, Dryden P, Salari H, Lam S, Chan-Yeung M. Immunologic studies of the mechanisms of occupational asthma caused by western red cedar. J Allergy Clin Immunol 1993;92:466–78.

[22] Grammer L, Shaughnessy M, Kenamore B. Utility of antibody in identifying individuals who have or will develop anhydride-induced respiratory disease. Chest 1998;114:1199–202.

[23] Brooks SM, Weiss MA, Bernstein IL. Reactive airways dysfunction syndrome (RADS): persistent asthma syndrome after high level irritant exposures. Chest 1985;88:376–84.

[24] Brooks SM, Lockey J. Reactive airways disease syndrome (RADS): a newly defined occupational disease [abstract]. Am Rev Respir Dis 1981;123(Suppl):A133.

[25] Alberts WM, Brooks SM. Reactive airways dysfunction syndrome. Curr Opin Pulm Med 1996;2:104–10.

[26] Montanaro A. Occupational asthma. Immunol Allergy Clin North Am 2001;21:489–501.

[27] Hunt LW, Fransway AF, Reed CE, et al. An epidemic of occupational allergy to latex involving health care workers. J Occup Environ Med 1995;37:1204–9.

[28] Quirce S, Polo F, Figueredo E, Gonzalez R, Sastre J. Occupational asthma caused by soybean flour in bakers: differences with soybean-induced epidemic asthma. Clin Exp Allergy 2000;30:839–46.

[29] Hollander A, Heederik D, Doekes G. Respiratory allergy to rats: exposure-response relationships in laboratory animal workers. Am J Respir Crit Care Med 1997;155:562–7.

[30] Venables KM. Low molecular weight chemicals, hypersensitivity, and direct toxicity: the acid anhydrides. Br J Ind Med 1989;46:222–32.

[31] Lutsky I, Teichtahl H, Bar-Sela S. Occupational asthma due to poultry mites. J Allergy Clin Immunol 1984;73:56–60.

[32] Kronqvist M, Johansson E, Pershagen G, Johansson SG, van Hage-Hamsten M. Increasing prevalence of asthma over 12 years among dairy farmers on Gotland, Sweden: storage mites remain dominant allergens. Clin Exp Allergy 1999;29:35–41.

[33] Kronqvist M, Johansson E, Pershagen G, Johansson SG, van Hage-Hamsten M. Risk factors associated with asthma and rhinoconjunctivitis among Swedish farmers. Allergy 1999;54:1142–9.

[34] Aiken TC, Ward R, Peel ET, Hendrick DJ. Occupational asthma due to porcine pancreatic amylase. Occup Environ Med 1997;54:762–4.

[35] Baur X, Konig G, Bencze K, Fruhmann G. Clinical symptoms and results of skin test, RAST and bronchial provocation test in thirty-three papain workers: evidence for strong immunogenic potency and clinically relevant 'proteolytic effects of airborne papain'. Clin Allergy 1982;12: 9–17.

[36] Milne J, Brand S. Occupational asthma after inhalation of dust of the proteolytic enzyme, papain. Br J Ind Med 1975;32:302–7.

[37] Galleguillos F, Rodriguez JC. Asthma caused by bromelin inhalation. Clin Allergy 1978;8:21–4.

[38] Gailhofer G, Wilders-Truschnig M, Smolle J, Ludvan M. Asthma caused by bromelain: an occupational allergy. Clin Allergy 1988;18:445–50.

[39] Raulf-Heimsoth M, Baur X. Pathomechanisms and pathophysiology of isocyanate-induced diseases: summary of present knowledge. Am J Ind Med 1998;34:137–43.

[40] Grammar L, Shaughnessy M, Henderson J, et al. A clinical and immunologic study of workers with trimellitic-anhydride-induced immunologic lung disease after transfer to low exposure jobs. Am Rev Respir Dis 1993;148:547.

[41] Gautrin D, Ghezzo H, Infante-Rivard C, Malo JL. Incidence and determinants of IgE-mediated sensitization in apprentices: a prospective study. Am J Respir Crit Care Med 2000;162:1222–8.

[42] Malo JL, Lemiere C, Desjardins A, Cartier A. Prevalence and intensity of rhinoconjunctivitis in subjects with occupational asthma. Eur Respir J 1997;10:1513–5.

[43] Tilles SA, Jerath-Tatum A. Differential diagnosis of occupational asthma. Immunol Allergy Clin North Am 2003;23:167–76.

[44] Moscato G, Dellabianca A, Maestrelli P, et al. Features and severity of occupational asthma upon diagnosis: an Italian multicentric case review. Allergy 2002;57:236–42.

[45] Venables KM, Upton JL, Hawkins ER, Tee RD, Longbottom JL, Newman Taylor AJ. Smoking, atopy, and laboratory animal allergy. Br J Ind Med 1988;45:667–71.

[46] Venables KM, Topping MD, Howe W, Luczynska CM, Hawkins R, Taylor AJ. Interaction of smoking and atopy in producing specific IgE antibody against a hapten protein conjugate. Br Med J (Clin Res Ed) 1985;290:201–4.

[47] Zacharisen MC. Occupational asthma. Med Clin North Am 2002;86:951–71.

[48] Franz T, McMurrain KD, Brooks S, Bernstein IL. Clinical, immunologic, and physiologic observations in factory workers exposed to B. subtilis enzyme dust. J Allergy 1971;47:170–80.

[49] Newman KB, Mason III UG, Schmaling KB. Clinical features of vocal cord dysfunction. Am J Respir Crit Care Med 1995;152:1382–6.

[50] Baur X, Chen Z, Liebers V. Exposure-response relationships of occupational inhalative allergens. Clin Exp Allergy 1998;28:537–44.

[51] Montanaro A. Prognosis of occupational asthma. Ann Allergy Asthma Immunol 1999;83: 593–6.

[52] Chan-Yeung M, Lam S, Koener S. Evaluation of impairment/disability in patients with occupational asthma. Am Rev Respir Dis 1987;135:9501.

[53] Banks DE, Rando RJ, Barkman Jr HW. Persistence of toluene diisocyanate-induced asthma despite negligible workplace exposures. Chest 1990;97:121–5.

[54] Hudson P, Cartier A, Pineau L, et al. Follow-up of occupational asthma caused by crab and various agents. J Allergy Clin Immunol 1985;76:682–8.

[55] Cote J, Kennedy S, Chan-Yeung M. Outcome of patients with cedar asthma with continuous exposure. Am Rev Respir Dis 1990;141:373–6.

[56] Chan-Yeung M, MacLean L, Paggiaro PL. Follow-up study of 232 patients with occupational asthma caused by western red cedar (Thuja plicata). J Allergy Clin Immunol 1987;79:792–6.

[57] Malo JL, Cartier A, Cote J, Milot J, Leblanc C, Paquette L. Influence of inhaled steroids on recovery from occupational asthma after cessation of exposure: an 18-month double-blind crossover study. Am J Respir Crit Care Med 1996;153:953–60.

ELSEVIER
SAUNDERS

Immunol Allergy Clin N Am
25 (2005) 207–214

IMMUNOLOGY
AND ALLERGY
CLINICS
OF NORTH AMERICA

Index

Note: Page numbers of article titles are in **boldface** type.

0889-8561/05/$ – see front matter © 2005 Elsevier Inc. All rights reserved.
doi:10.1016/S0889-8561(04)00133-X